Textbook of Histology
COLOUR ATLAS

Revised Fifth Edition

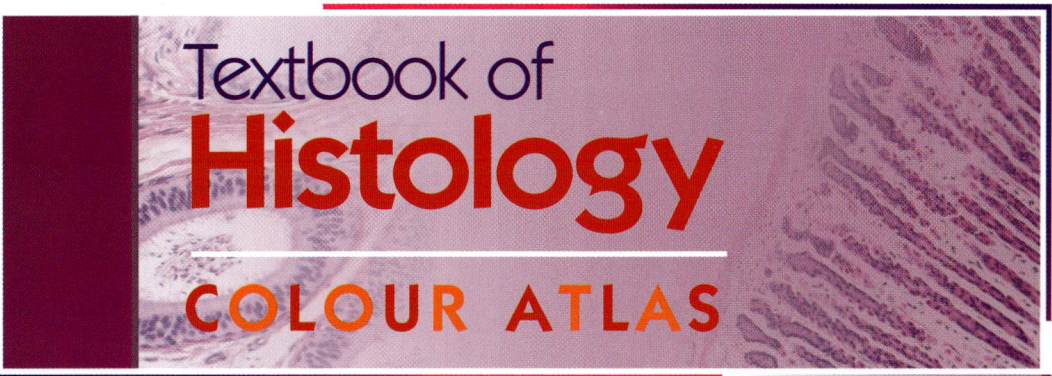

Textbook of Histology
COLOUR ATLAS
Revised Fifth Edition

Krishna Garg MS, PhD, FAMS, FIMSA, FIAMS
Ex-Professor and Head
Department of Anatomy
Lady Hardinge Medical College, New Delhi

Indira Bahl MS, FIMSA, FIAMS, ISA (Japan)
Ex-Professor and Head
Department of Anatomy
Maulana Azad Medical College, New Delhi

Mohini Kaul MS, MAMS
Ex-Professor and Head
Department of Anatomy
Maulana Azad Medical College, New Delhi

with contribution from
Sandip Mukherjee MSc, PhD
Assistant Professor, Serampore College, West Bengal

CBS Publishers & Distributors Pvt Ltd

New Delhi • Bengaluru • Chennai • Kochi • Kolkata • Mumbai
Bhopal • Bhubaneswar • Hyderabad • Jharkhand • Nagpur • Patna • Pune • Uttarakhand • Dhaka (Bangladesh)

Disclaimer

Science and technology are constantly changing fields. New research and experience broaden the scope of information and knowledge. The authors have tried their best in giving information available to them while preparing the material for this book. Although all efforts have been made to ensure optimum accuracy of the material, yet it is quite possible some errors might have been left uncorrected. The publisher, the printer, the authors, and the editors will not be held responsible for any inadvertent errors, omissions or inaccuracies.

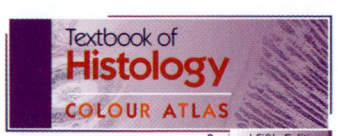

ISBN: 978-81-239-2464-9

Copyright © Authors and Publisher

Fifth Edition   2014
Reprint: 2016
Revised Reprint: 2017, 2019
First Edition   1982
Second Edition 1987
Third Edition   1999
Fourth Edition   2009

All rights reserved. No part of this book may be reproduced or transmitted in any form or by any means, electronic or mechanical, including photocopying, recording, or any information storage and retrieval system without permission, in writing, from the authors.

Published by Satish Kumar Jain and Produced by Varun Jain for
CBS Publishers & Distributors Pvt Ltd
4819/XI Prahlad Street, 24 Ansari Road, Daryaganj, New Delhi 110 002, India.

Ph: 23289259, 23266861, 23266867   Fax: 011-23243014   Website: www.cbspd.com
                                                                                              e-mail: delhi@cbspd.com; cbspubs@airtelmail.in.

Corporate Office: 204 FIE, Industrial Area, Patparganj, Delhi 110 092
Ph: 4934 4934   Fax: 4934 4935   e-mail: publishing@cbspd.com; publicity@cbspd.com

Branches

- **Bengaluru:** Seema House 2975, 17th Cross, K.R. Road,
  Banasankari 2nd Stage, Bengaluru 560 070, Karnataka
  Ph: +91-80-26771678/79   Fax: +91-80-26771680   e-mail: bangalore@cbspd.com
- **Chennai:** 7, Subbaraya Street, Shenoy Nagar, Chennai 600 030, Tamil Nadu
  Ph: +91-44-26680620, 26681266   Fax: +91-44-42032115   e-mail: chennai@cbspd.com
- **Kochi:** 42/1325, 1326, Power House Road, Opp KSEB Power House, Ernakulam 682 018, Kochi, Kerala
  Ph: +91-484-4059061-65   Fax: +91-484-4059065   e-mail: kochi@cbspd.com
- **Kolkata:** 6/B, Ground Floor, Rameswar Shaw Road, Kolkata-700 014, West Bengal
  Ph: +91-33-22891126, 22891127, 22891128   e-mail: kolkata@cbspd.com
- **Mumbai:** 83-C, Dr E Moses Road, Worli, Mumbai-400018, Maharashtra
  Ph: +91-22-24902340/41   Fax: +91-22-24902342   e-mail: mumbai@cbspd.com

Representatives

• **Bhopal**	0-8319310552	• **Bhubaneswar**	0-9911037372	• **Hyderabad**	0-9885175004
• **Jharkhand**	0-9811541605	• **Nagpur**	0-9021734563	• **Patna**	0-9334159340
• **Pune**	0-9623451994	• **Uttarakhand**	0-9716462459	• **Dhaka (Bangladesh)**	01912-003485

Printed at Magic International, Greater Noida, UP, India

Preface to Fifth Edition

The fourth edition of *Textbook of Histology: Colour Atlas* was received well, still there were comments about the small size of photomicrographs and figures. To overcome the problem, the fifth edition has been designed as our earlier first–third editions. Now the text is on one page and its figure on the facing page. Since figures are more important in providing visual impact, these along with the requisite photomicrographs and three points of identification as Facts to Remember are mostly given on the right hand pages of the book. The revision of these pages will help the students clear the professional examination with high scores.

The histology part of this book is "Must Know" only without any elaboration on the "Nice to Know" and "Good to Know" components as the time frame of First MBBS is rather short. Some figures have been supplemented by "Insets" and a few diagrammatic figures are given to provide the third-dimensional (3-D) view. The last chapter has been enlarged to give a bird's eye view of various fixatives and stains. This would help students studying their BSc and MSc courses. Multiple choice questions are given at the end of every chapter for revision.

This book is primarily meant for undergraduate students of medical, dental, homeopathic, physiotherapy and occupational therapy and allied health sciences courses.

Dr Sandip Mukherjee has gone through the whole text and figures and given necessary inputs.

Authors are grateful to Dr Mithlesh Chandra, an eminent pathologist, for providing us normal tissue photomicrographs. She is CEO of DIGISCAN, engaged in the production of virtual/digital slides in histology and pathology to facilitate teaching and learning in the classroom or during self-study.

Dr Medha Joshi MBBS, FCGP has been assisting us all the while. Her sincerity is admirable. We are indebted to her.

The excellent graphic work has been patiently and painstakingly done by Sanjay Chauhan and the formatting part of the book is done by Jyoti Kaur who is quick, correct and above board.

Mr SK Jain, Chairman and Managing Director; Mr Varun Jain, Director; Mr YN Arjuna, Senior Vice-President—Publishing, Editorial and Promotion, Mrs Ritu Chawla, Production Manager, and their team have been giving suggestions whenever required; without their continuous support, this edition would not have seen the light of the day.

Last but not the least, our ever gratefulness is to "Almightly" for directing our intellect along the right path.

Suggestions for improvement are welcome, which may please be sent to the first author at dr.krishnagarg@gmail.com

Authors

Contents

Preface to Fifth Edition   v

1. Cell   1
Electron Microscopic Structure   1
Multiple Choice Questions   5

2. Epithelial Tissue   6
Functions and Special Features   6
Characters   8
Simple Epithelium   9
Pseudostratified Epithelium   16
Compound Epithelium   16
Multiple Choice Questions   24

3. Connective Tissue   25
Cells   25
Fibres   28
Ground Substance   30
Loose Connective Tissue   32
Dense Ordinary Connective Tissue   36
Multiple Choice Questions   38

4. Skeletal Tissue: Cartilage and Bone   39
Cartilage Cells   39
Hyaline Cartilage   40
Elastic Cartilage   40
Fibrocartilage   42
Comparison of Cartilages   42
Bone   44
   Cells   44
   Matrix   46
Comparison of Cartilage and Bone   46
Microscopic Structure   47
   Compact Bone   47
   Spongy Bone   47

Ossification	47
Intramembranous	47
Intracartilaginous	50
Multiple Choice Questions	*52*

5. Muscular Tissue — 53

Skeletal Muscle	53
Smooth Muscle	56
Cardiac Muscle	58
Comparison of Muscles	60
Multiple Choice Questions	*61*

6. Nervous Tissue — 62

Neuron	62
Neuroglia	64
Nerve Fibres	69
Spinal Cord	72
Comparison of Grey Matter and White Matter	72
Ganglia	74
Comparison of Ganglia	74
Cerebrum	74
Cerebellum	78
Types of Neurons and Connections of Neurons	80
Multiple Choice Questions	*81*

7. Blood Vessels — 82

Arteries	82
Elastic	82
Muscular	84
Arterioles	84
Capillaries	86
Sinusoids	88
Veins	88
Differences between Arteries and Veins	90
Multiple Choice Questions	*91*

8. Lymphatic System — 92

Lymph Node	92
Spleen	94
Thymus	98
Palatine Tonsil	101
Comparison of Lymphatic Organs	102
Multiple Choice Questions	*104*

9. The Glands — 105

    Salivary Glands — 106
        Parotid — 106
        Submandibular — 106
        Sublingual — 108
    Multiple Choice Questions — *112*

10. Integumentary System — 113

    Epidermis — 113
    Dermis — 114
    Appendages of Skin — 114
        Hair Follicle — 114
        Sebaceous Gland — 116
        Sweat Gland — 116
    Types of Skin — 116
    Comparison of Thick Skin and Thin Skin — 118
    Multiple Choice Questions — *122*

11. Respiratory System — 123

    Nose — 123
    Nasopharynx — 124
    Larynx — 124
    Trachea — 124
    Bronchial Tubes — 126
    Respiratory Part — 128
    Features of Various Parts — 130
    Multiple Choice Questions — *134*

12. Digestive System: Oesophagus and Stomach — 135

    Digestive System — 135
    Oral Cavity — 135
    Teeth — 136
    General Plan of Gastrointestinal Tract — 137
    Nerve Supply — 138
    Oesophagus — 140
    Stomach — 142
    Multiple Choice Questions — *149*

13. Small and Large Intestines — 150

    Small Intestine — 150
    General Plan — 150
    Duodenum — 154
    Jejunum — 156

Ileum	156
Differences between Three Parts of Small Intestine	156
Large Intestine	158
Differences between Small and Large Intestines	158
Colon	160
Vermiform Appendix	160
Rectum	164
Anal Canal	164
Multiple Choice Questions	*166*

14. Liver, Gall Bladder and Pancreas — 167

Liver	167
Gall Bladder	172
Pancreas	172
Differences between Pancreas and Parotid Gland	176
Multiple Choice Questions	*176*

15. Urinary System — 177

Kidney	177
Differences between Proximal and Distal Convoluted Tubules	180
Ureter	182
Urinary Bladder	184
Female Urethra	184
Multiple Choice Questions	*186*

16. Male Reproductive System — 187

Testis	187
Epididymis	191
Ductus Deferens	191
Prostatic Gland	194
Seminal Vesicle	196
Penis	196
Male Urethra	198
Multiple Choice Questions	*200*

17. Female Reproductive System — 201

Ovary	201
Fallopian Tube	204
Uterus	206
Cervix	212
Vagina	212
Mammary Glands	214
Comparison of Lactating Mammary Gland and Prostate Gland	218

Placenta	219
Umbilical Cord	220
Multiple Choice Questions	*224*

18. Endocrine Glands — 225

Hypophysis Cerebri	225
Thyroid Gland	230
Parathyroid Gland	232
Suprarenal Gland	234
Pineal Gland	236
Multiple Choice Questions	*238*

19. Organs of Special Senses — 239

Olfactory Epithelium	239
Tongue	240
Taste Buds	242
Eyeball	246
Internal Ear	256
Multiple Choice Questions	*259*

20. Histological Techniques—Staining: Haematoxylin-Eosin — 260

Purpose of Fixation	260
Commonly Used Fixatives	261
Dehydration	263
Clearing	264
Tissue Embedding	264
Sectioning	264
Staining	264
Some Commonly Used Stains	266
Staining: Haematoxylin-Eosin	268

Index *271*

Cell

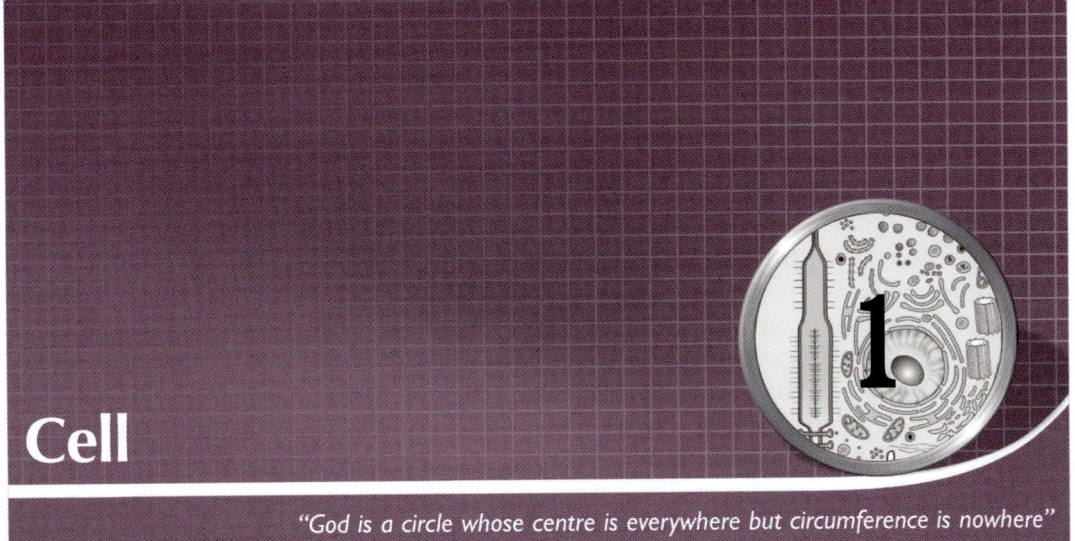

"God is a circle whose centre is everywhere but circumference is nowhere"

The basic unit of a tissue is the living cell. It consists of a cell membrane enclosing the cytoplasm with a nucleus usually in the centre. Its electron microscopic structure is described below.

ELECTRON MICROSCOPIC STRUCTURE

CELL MEMBRANE

Cell membrane limits the cell and acts as a barrier between the tissue fluid and the cytoplasm. Under the electron microscope it shows three layers, a lighter lipid layer in between the two darker layers of protein. The total thickness of the cell membrane is 7.5 nanometre. Some variation in the overall thickness is encountered from one cell type to another, but the basic trilaminar structure is found in all cell membranes and is referred to as the *unit membrane*. In its structure and chemical organisation lies the key to the selective permeability and its capacity to conduct impulses (Fig. 1.1).

CYTOPLASM

Control of the development and function of a cell resides mainly in the nucleus, while most of the responding metabolic synthetic activities are located in the cytoplasm. The cytoplasm consists of a cytoplasmic matrix with organelles and inclusions suspended in it. Organelles are living units while the inclusions are non-living entities.

Various cytoplasmic organelles seen with the electron microscope are the endoplasmic reticulum, Golgi apparatus, mitochondria, lysosomes, ribosomes and centriole.

Endoplasmic Reticulum

Endoplasmic reticulum may be in the form of rough surface or smooth surface vesicles/cisterns. Granular or rough surface endoplasmic reticulum forms a network of membrane bound organelles spread in the whole of the cytoplasm. In its typical form, it consists of an irregular network of branching and anastomosing flattened tubules and semi-flattened vesicles which form lamellar systems of parallel flat cavities. In addition to tubules, there are isolated vesicles which are also considered part of the endoplasmic reticulum. The basophilia of these structures does not reside in the canalicular system of reticulum but in small particles of ribonucleoproteins called *ribosomes*. These are found in great numbers adhering to the outer surface of their limiting membranes and are found free in the cytoplasm as well as attached to the membranes. The ribosomes are the sites of synthesis of new proteins in the cell. In protein secreting cells such as those of the pancreas, the endoplasmic reticulum is always of the granular type (Fig. 1.1).

Agranular or smooth endoplasmic reticulum is seen in some cell types. The tubules comprising the endoplasmic reticulum lack the associated ribosomes. In such cells the cytoplasm is usually acidophilic. Agranular endoplasmic reticulum is usually a close meshwork of tubules. In muscle, the endoplasmic reticulum is mainly of the smooth surface variety and is concerned with release and recapture of calcium ions in the cycle of contraction and relaxation. In liver, both rough and smooth surface endoplasmic reticulum are present and are involved in cholesterol and lipid metabolism.

Golgi Apparatus

Golgi apparatus can be seen in routine histological preparations. However, in tissues subjected to impregnation with osmium or silver, it can be demonstrated as a blackened network usually in the juxtanuclear region. Electron microscopically it is seen to consist of a lamellar membranous structure consisting of curved arrays of flattened saccules often expanded at each end. These are usually present between the nucleus and the apical part of the cell. The Golgi apparatus is concerned with aggregation, condensation and elaboration of the secretion of the cell. It also actively participates in synthesis of secretory products rich in complex polysaccharides, the carbohydrate moiety, which replenishes the cell membranes as and when required. The secretory vesicles leave the apical aspect of the cell in the form of zymogen granules (Fig. 1.1).

Mitochondria

Mitochondria can be seen in light microscopy as minute granules or filaments spread throughout the cytoplasm and can be stained in the living cell by the supravital dye, e.g. Janus green. The mitochondria show brownian movements and symbiosis. They divide by binary fission and are self replicating.

With the electron microscope, they are seen to have a complex sausage shaped structure being enclosed by two membranes. The outer membrane is a smooth continuous limiting membrane and the inner membrane is thrown into folds called **cristae**. The interior of the mitochondria have a dense fluid called the mitochondrial matrix which may show granules of iron or calcium in it. The mitochondria contain the enzymes responsible for oxidation of food-stuffs which give energy to the cell. The enzymes **flavoprotein** and **cytochromes** are attached to the membrane and are important for respiratory processes of the cell. The **dehydrogenase enzymes** which are responsible for Krebs citric acid cycle and for protein and lipid synthesis, are present in the mitochondrial matrix.

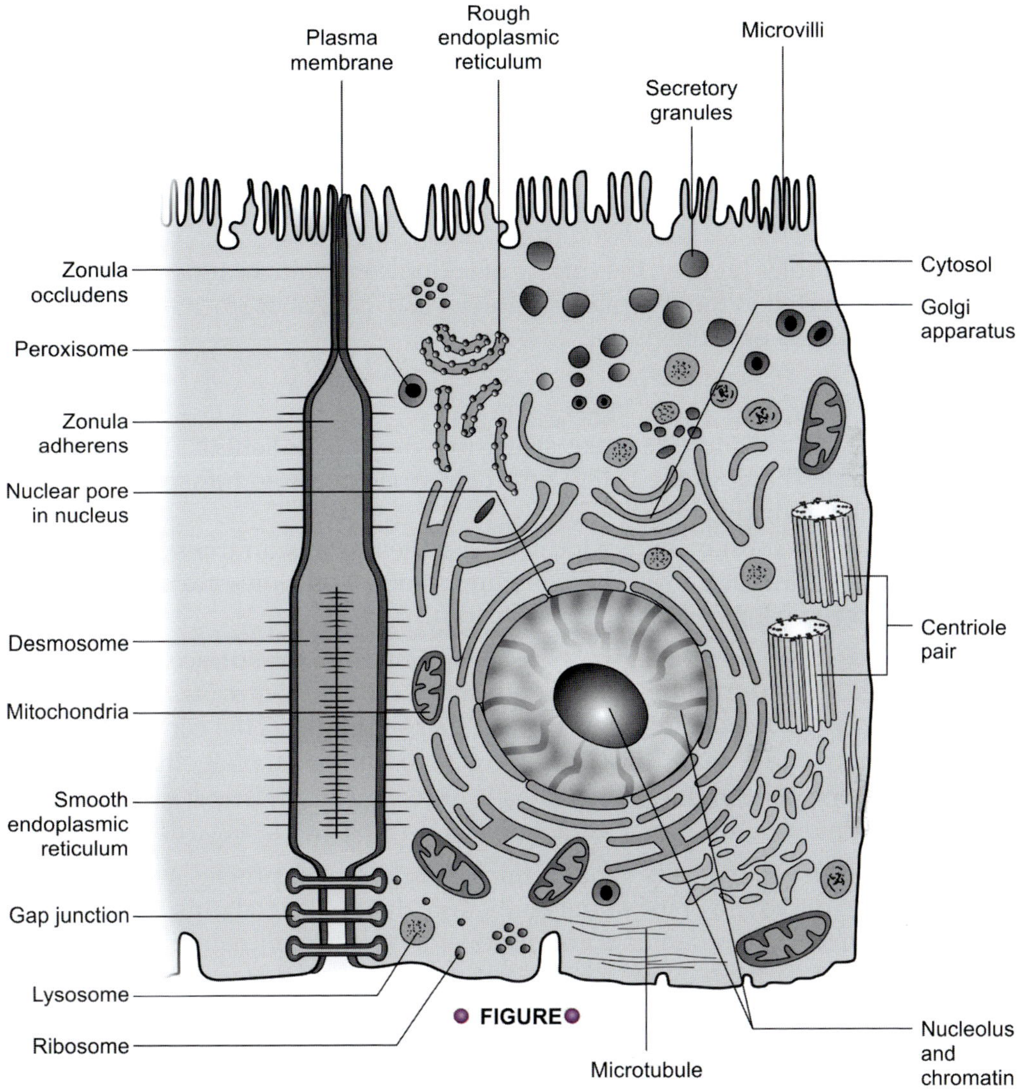

FACTS TO REMEMBER

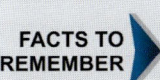

1. The cell membrane is a lipid bilayer
2. The cell organelles are mitochondria, endoplasmic reticulum, Golgi apparatus and lysosomes, etc. Nucleus is surrounded by nuclear membrane
3. The adjacent cells are joined together by zonula occludens, zonula adherens, desmosome and gap junctions

Fig. 1.1: *Electron microscopic structure of cell with cell junctions*

Lysosomes

Lysosomes are dense bodies, limited by a membrane containing a number of hydrolytic enzymes termed *acid hydrolases*. The enzymes play a role in the breakdown of an injured cell. These also take part in the intracellular digestion of foreign matter. The lysosomes are rich in glycoproteins.

Ribosomes

Ribosomes are granules lying on the surface of endoplasmic reticulum, making it rough. They are also collected in the cytoplasm in the form of polyribosomes which are active sites for the synthesis of proteins.

The Cytoskeleton

Microtubules: These are pipe/rod like structures of variable length. These are rigid bodies which give shape to the cell. These help in axoplasmic transport in neurons and also in melanin dispersion.

The centrioles are short cylinders located near the nucleus. In transverse section of centriole, 9 triplets are seen around the circumference. Centrioles are concerned with movement of chromosomes during cell division.

Flagella and cilia: These are motile processes extending from the surfaces of the cells. In their cores are the microtubules. Flagellum or cilium comprises nine pairs of microtubules around the circumference and a pair of tubule in the centre.

In human, only one type of cells, the spermatozoa contains a flagellum.

True cilia are present in the epithelial cells of respiratory mucous membrane. The cilia help in the movement of mucus laden with dust particles towards the larynx.

Microfilaments: Most of the cells contain microfilaments comprising of protein actin. These are seen in microvilli of intestinal epithelium. In the skeletal muscle the presence of actin and myosin microfilaments are responsible for the contraction of muscle.

Cytoplasmic Inclusions

Cytoplasmic inclusions are non-living entities and do not take part in the metabolism of the cell, e.g. stored food which may be seen in the form of glycogen and fat. Pigments may be of exogenous origin like dust, tattoo marks or endogenous origin which include haemoglobin of blood, melanin pigment of skin, hair, iris and lipofuscin pigment found in the heart muscle and in some nerve cells.

NUCLEUS

It is an essential component of nearly all cell types. Its components are:
   i. *Nuclear membrane*: It consists of two cell layers enclosing a narrow perinuclear space. The outer layer may have ribosomes adherent to its surface. The inner layer may have peripheral chromatin adherent to it. The nuclear membrane has small circular openings called *nuclear pores* 8 Angstrom in diameter closed by a thin membrane around which the two membranes fuse. This area of fusion is referred to as the *nuclear pore complex*. One of the **X-chromosomes** of the females is seen adherent to the nuclear membrane and is known as the **Barr body**.

ii. *Nuclear sap*: It is semifluid and lies within the nucleus. It stains poorly and is rich in proteins.
iii. *Nucleolus*: It is present in most of the nuclei. The number of nucleoli varies from one to five in each nucleus. The nucleolus consists of a dark and light component. The light component forms the canals which course through the dark substance. The dark components form the granular or fibrillar material in the nucleolus. It acts as an **auxiliary chromosome** and is rich in RNA (Fig. 1.1).
iv. *Chromatin*: It forms the bulk of the nucleus. In interphase some chromatin is adherent to the surface of the inner layer of nuclear membrane and is called *peripheral chromatin*. Some chromatin is distributed as strands in the nuclear sap. The rest of the chromatin surrounds the nucleolus. During the prophase of mitosis, chromatin gets collected into small rod-like bodies known as the *chromosomes*.

MULTIPLE CHOICE QUESTIONS

1. Which of the following cell organelle provides energy for functions of the cell?
   a. Lysosomes   b. Centriole
   c. Cilia   d. Mitochondria
2. Intracellular digestion is done by one of the following organelles:
   a. Centriole
   b. Lysosome
   c. Endoplasmic reticulum
   d. Golgi apparatus
3. Steroid synthesis is done by:
   a. Golgi apparatus
   b. Lysosome
   c. Smooth endoplasmic reticulum
   d. Mitochondria
4. Microtubules are not present in:
   a. Centriole
   b. Flagella
   c. Cilia
   d. Microvilli

ANSWERS

1. d   2. b   3. c   4. d

Epithelial Tissue

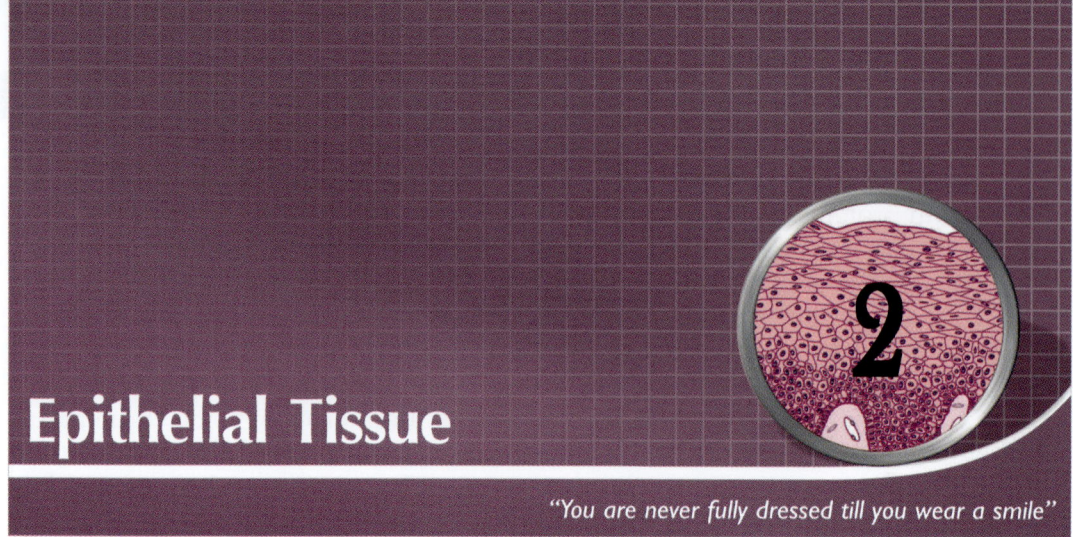

"You are never fully dressed till you wear a smile"

Histology is the microscopic study of various tissues of the body. A tissue is made up of groups of cells performing the same function. The cell is the basic structural unit of the body (Fig. 2.1).

The various tissues are:
- Epithelial tissue
- Connective tissue
- Muscular tissue
- Nervous tissue

FUNCTIONS OF EPITHELIAL TISSUE/EPITHELIUM

Epithelial tissue described below covers outer aspect of the body and lines various tubes and tracts.

a. *Protective*: The stratified squamous keratinised epithelium of skin offers mechanical protection including conservation of moisture.
b. *Secretory*: The glands which are derivatives of the epithelium secrete useful chemical substances.
c. *Absorptive*: Epithelia of small intestine and of proximal convoluted tubules of kidney are modified to specialise in absorptive functions.
d. *Excretory*: Epithelium of distal convoluted tubules and collecting ducts of kidney function as excretory organs.
e. *Sensory*: The rods and cones of retina and hair cells of olfactory mucous membrane are specialised sensory cells.

SPECIAL FEATURES OF EPITHELIUM

a. *Junctional complexes*: These are ultramicroscopic structures joining the adjacent sides of two epithelial cells. The important junctional complexes from apical end to the basal end of cells are:
   i. Zonula occludens

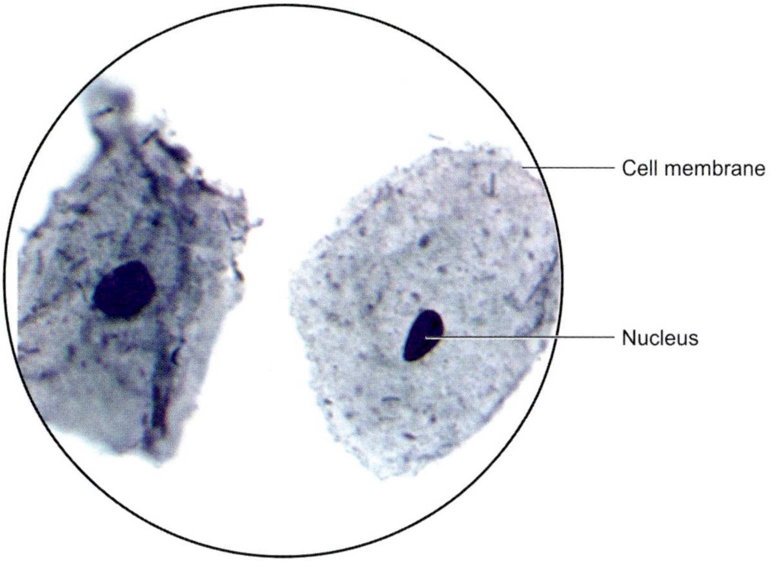

Epithelial Tissue

|PHOTOMICROGRAPH|

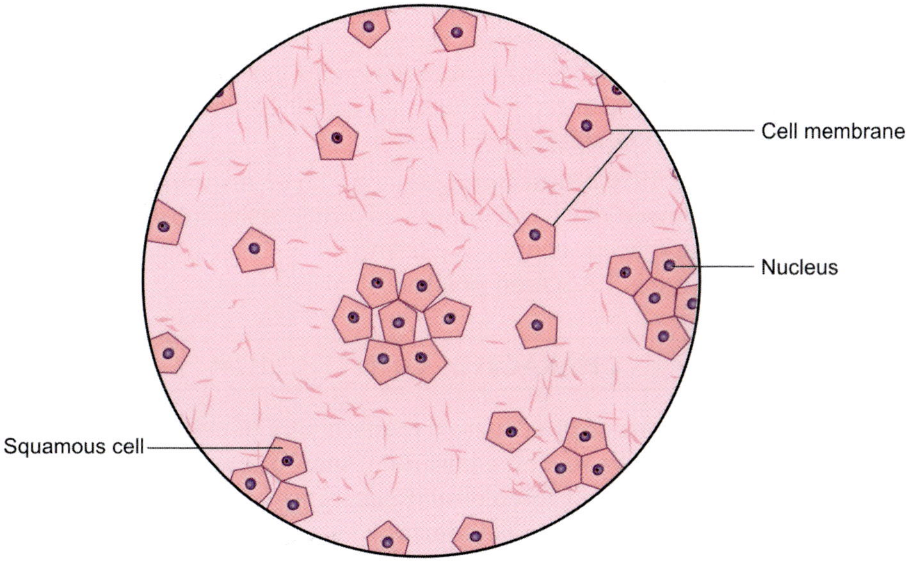

● FIGURE ●

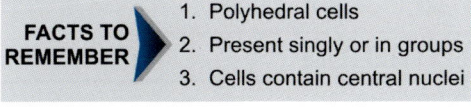

FACTS TO REMEMBER
1. Polyhedral cells
2. Present singly or in groups
3. Cells contain central nuclei

Fig. 2.1: *Desquamated squamous cells: Cheek mucosa. Stain: Haematoxylin-eosin, 100X*

ii. Zonula adherens
iii. Desmosome
iii. Gap junction (*see* Fig. 1.1)
   i. **Zonula occludens/tight junctions:** These are seen in the epithelia of renal tubules, gall bladder and intestines. Near the apical margin, the two cell membranes fuse completely over a short distance. Tight junction help to bind the adjacent cells to each other. These prevent movement of molecules and ions across the intercellular spaces.
   Zonula adherens: The plasma membranes below the apical parts are separated by a little gap.
   ii. **Desmosome:** These occur as belt desmosomes, and hemidesmosomes. These are characterised by local thickening of the adjacent cell membrane of the two epithelial cells. Radiating from the thickened cell membrane are cytoplasmic fibrils which pass into the cytoplasm. Desmosomes are bands present below and parallel to the tight junctions. These strongly anchor one epithelial cell to the next one.
   Hemidesmosomes are present at the basal border of the epithelial cells. These help to attach the epithelial cells firmly to the underlying basement membrane.
   iii. **Gap junctions** are typically seen in cardiac muscle and smooth muscle. These consists of proteinaceous tubes, which permit ions to travel from one cell to the next adjacent cell without passing through the cell membrane. These tubes are called 'connexons'. Gap junctions are areas with very low electrical resistance. So electrical impulses or action potentials can easily spread from one cell to the next cell through the gap junctions.
b. *Basement membrane*: It is a thin homogeneous layer on which the basal epithelial cells rest. It is comprised of a basal lamina, product of the cells and a reticular lamina derived from the subjacent connective tissue.
Basement membrane is PAS stain positive.

CHARACTERS OF EPITHELIUM

1. Epithelium may consist of one layer or many layers of cells.
2. The deepest layer of cells rest on a basement membrane.
3. There is minimal amount of intercellular substance.
4. Epithelium may develop from ectoderm, e.g. skin; from mesoderm, e.g. urinary system; from endoderm, e.g. gastrointestinal system.
5. Nutrition of epithelium is by diffusion from the underlying capillaries.
6. Epithelium covers the exterior of body surface and lines the interior of cavities/passages.

CLASSIFICATION OF EPITHELIUM

1. Simple epithelium
2. Pseudostratified epithelium
3. Compound epithelium

Epithelial Tissue

SIMPLE EPITHELIUM

It can be of the following types:

a. *Squamous (scale like) or pavement epithelium:* Seen in alveoli of lungs (Fig. 2.2), endothelium of blood vessels and mesothelium of serous membranes. The epithelium in sections is seen to consist of a single layer of thin cells with flattened nuclei.

b. *Cuboidal epithelium:* Seen in thyroid gland acini during resting phase (Fig. 2.3), small ducts of the glands. The cells have equal width and height with the round central nuclei.

c. *Columnar epithelium:* The cells are almost three times taller than their width. Nucleus is basal and oval in shape. Its modifications are as follows:

   i. *Simple columnar epithelium:* Lining of stomach (Fig. 2.4) and lining of cervical canal of uterus. This epithelium is secretory.

   ii. *Columnar cells with microvilli or brush border:* Seen in gall bladder (Fig. 2.5), lining of entire small intestine. The free margin of the cell shows bright red membrane. Electron microscope depicts the free margin of the cell thrown in the form of projections, seen as faint vertical striations, to increase the surface area for absorption.

   Some cells have large regular microvilli or stereocilia. These are present at the free surfaces of cochlear and vestibular receptor cells and in the epithelial cells of the epididymis.

   iii. *Ciliated columnar epithelium:* Seen in epithelium of fallopian tube (Fig. 2.6) and olfactory mucosa. Some of these columnar cells have hair-like processes projecting from their surfaces. The movement of the cilia propels the fluid.

   iv. *Goblet cells:* Plenty in large intestine (Fig. 2.7), small intestine, trachea, bronchi. These are unicellular glands and appear empty with haematoxylin and eosin staining, as the mucus contained in these cells gets dissolved during the staining procedure. The columnar cell assumes the shape of a goblet. The cell full of mucus with flattened nucleus close to the base is seen with special stains. Mucus is expelled from the cells by a process involving the dissolution of the apical part of the cell (apocrine nature).

Functional Aspect

a. *Squamous epithelium*
- Simple squamous epithelium of alveoli permits efficient exchange of gases between the alveoli and the capillaries. Endothelium of blood vessels permits passage of nutrients, fluids across the capillary wall.
- Mesothelium of the peritoneum, pleura or pericardium allows friction free movement of the organs.

b. *Cuboidal epithelium*
- The epithelium lines the ducts of the gland. Large cuboidal cells with microvilli line proximal convoluted tubules. These absorb glucose and water from the filtrate.
- The cells lining thyroid gland acini synthesise thyroxine from amino acid tyrosine and iodine.

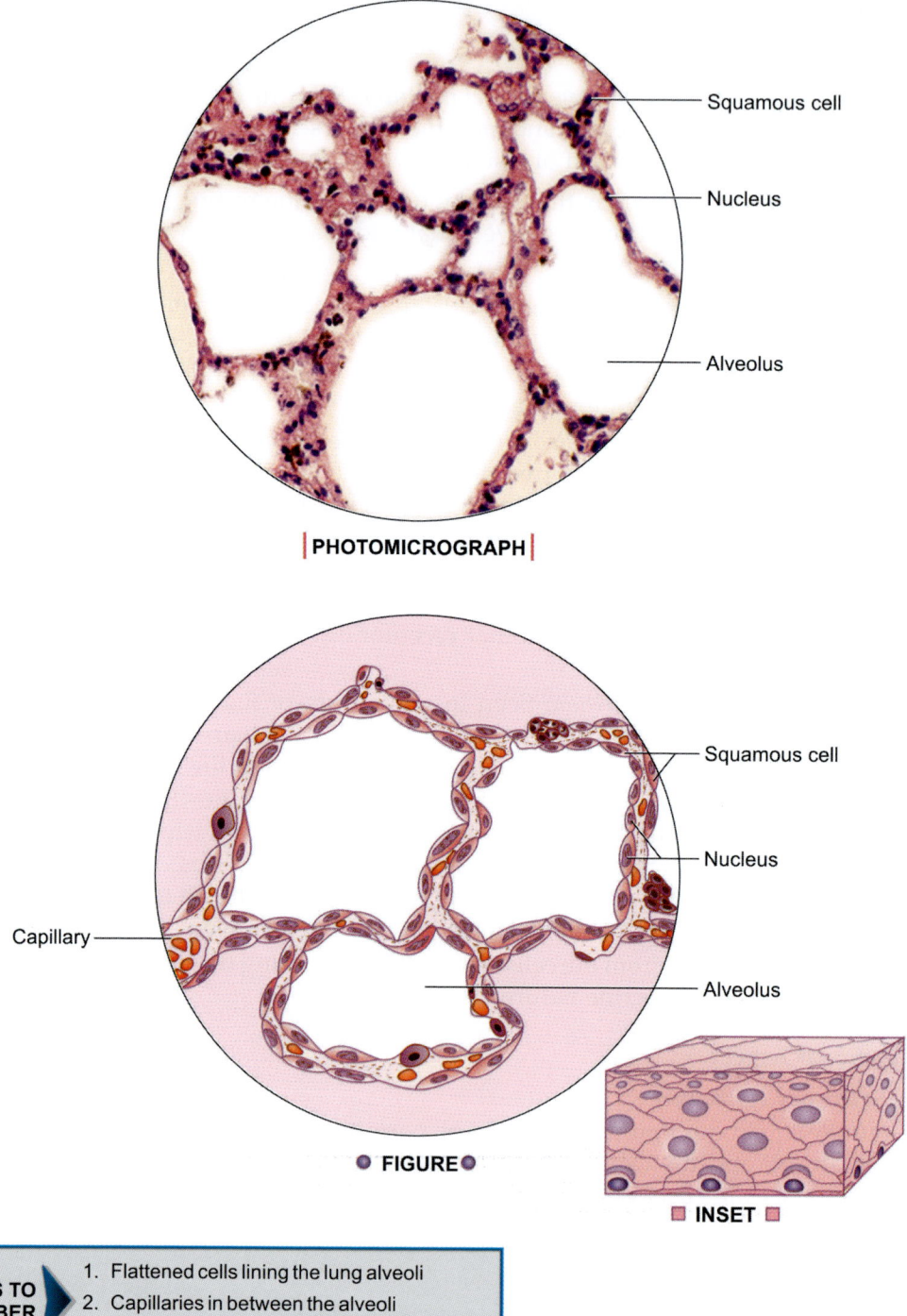

Fig. 2.2: *Squamous epithelium: Lung parenchyma. Stain: Haematoxylin-eosin, 400X*

FACTS TO REMEMBER
1. Flattened cells lining the lung alveoli
2. Capillaries in between the alveoli
3. Squamous cells permit exchange of gases

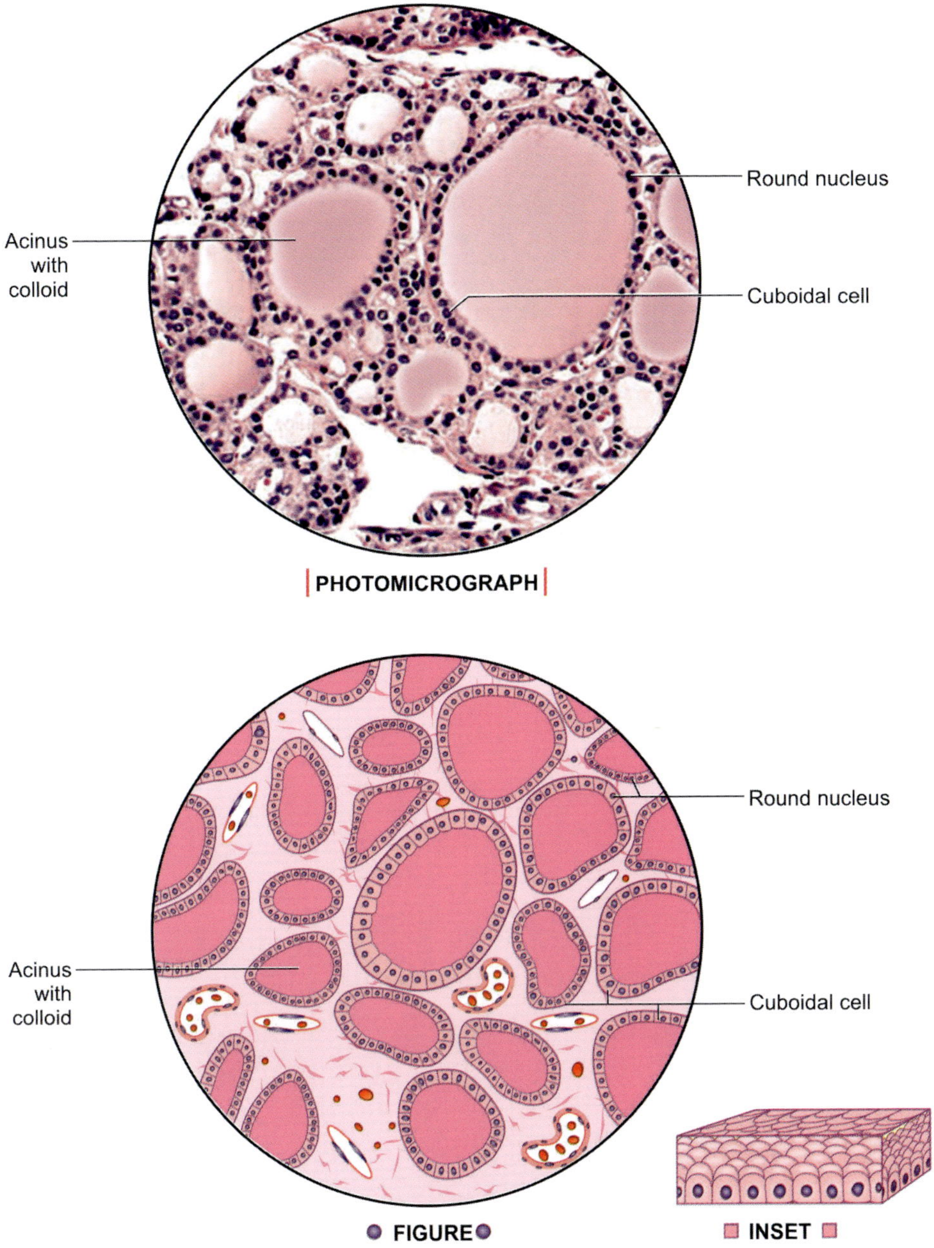

Epithelial Tissue

| PHOTOMICROGRAPH |

- Acinus with colloid
- Round nucleus
- Cuboidal cell

● FIGURE ●   ■ INSET ■

- Acinus with colloid
- Round nucleus
- Cuboidal cell

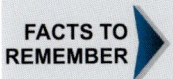
FACTS TO REMEMBER
1. The cells have same width and height
2. The cells contain a central nucleus
3. All the cells rest on the basement membrane

Fig. 2.3: *Cuboidal epithelium: Thyroid gland. Stain: Haematoxylin-eosin, 400X*

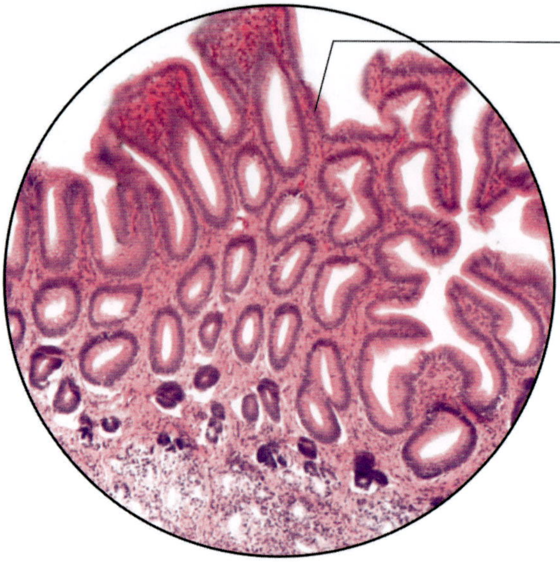

Tall columnar cell

|PHOTOMICROGRAPH|

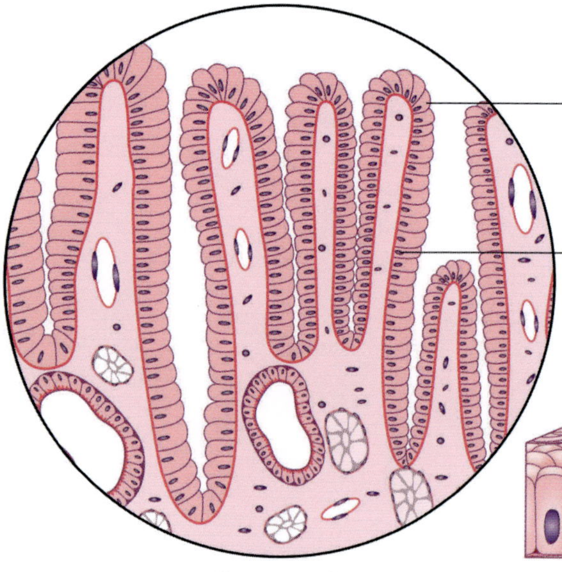

Tall columnar cell

Oval nucleus

● FIGURE 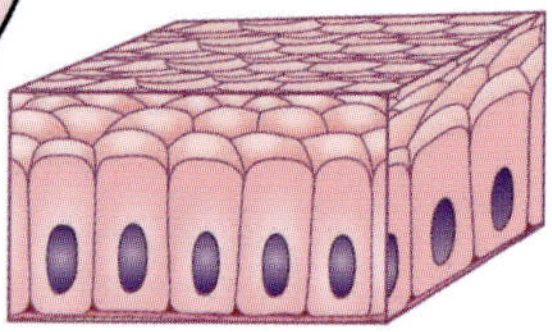 ●   ■ INSET ■

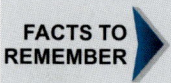

FACTS TO REMEMBER
1. The cells are three times taller than their width
2. Nucleus is basal and oval in shape
3. All the cells look alike

Fig. 2.4: *Simple columnar epithelium stomach. Stain: Haematoxylin-eosin, 400X*

Epithelial Tissue

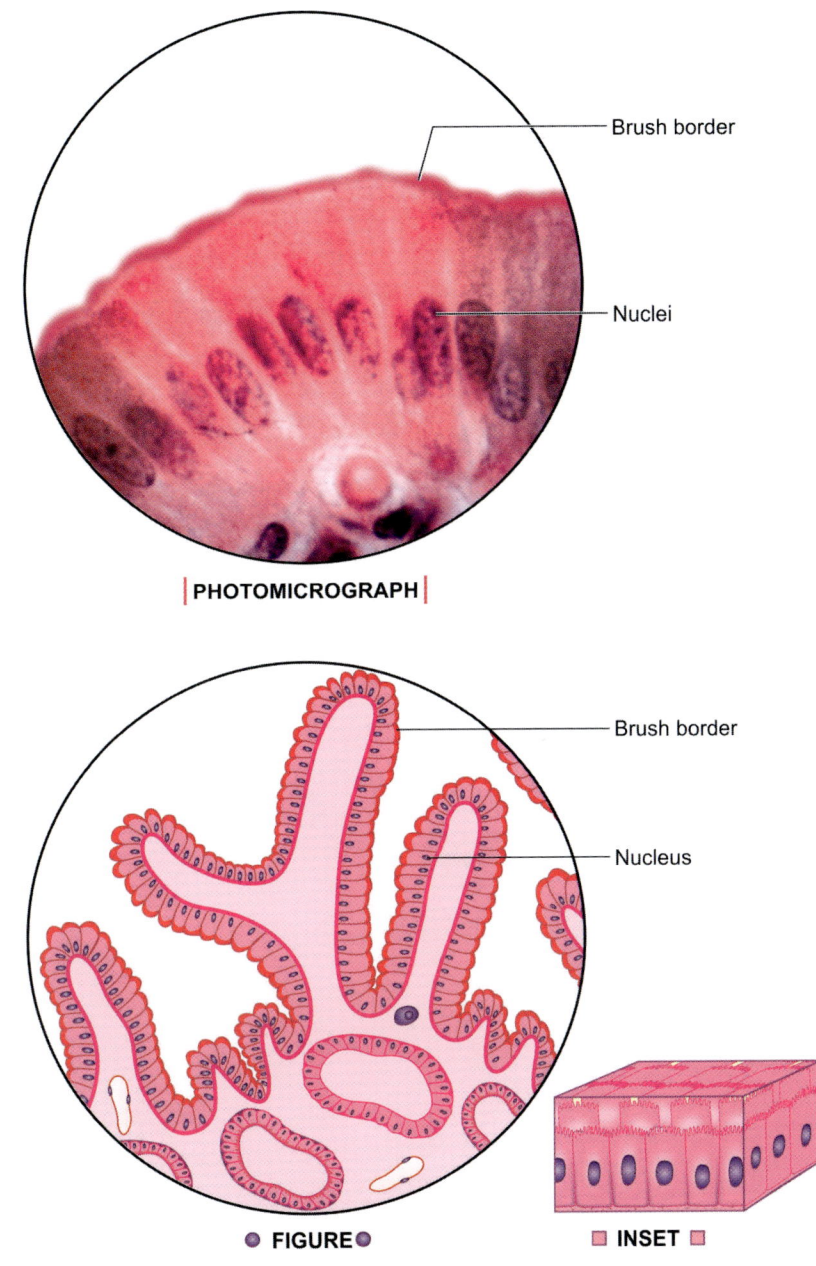

|PHOTOMICROGRAPH|

FACTS TO REMEMBER
1. The cells are columnar in shape
2. The free margin shows a bright red membrane called the brush border
3. The brush border is due to invaginations of the surface membrane

Fig. 2.5: *Columnar epithelium with brush border: Gall bladder. Stain: Haematoxylin-eosin, 400X*

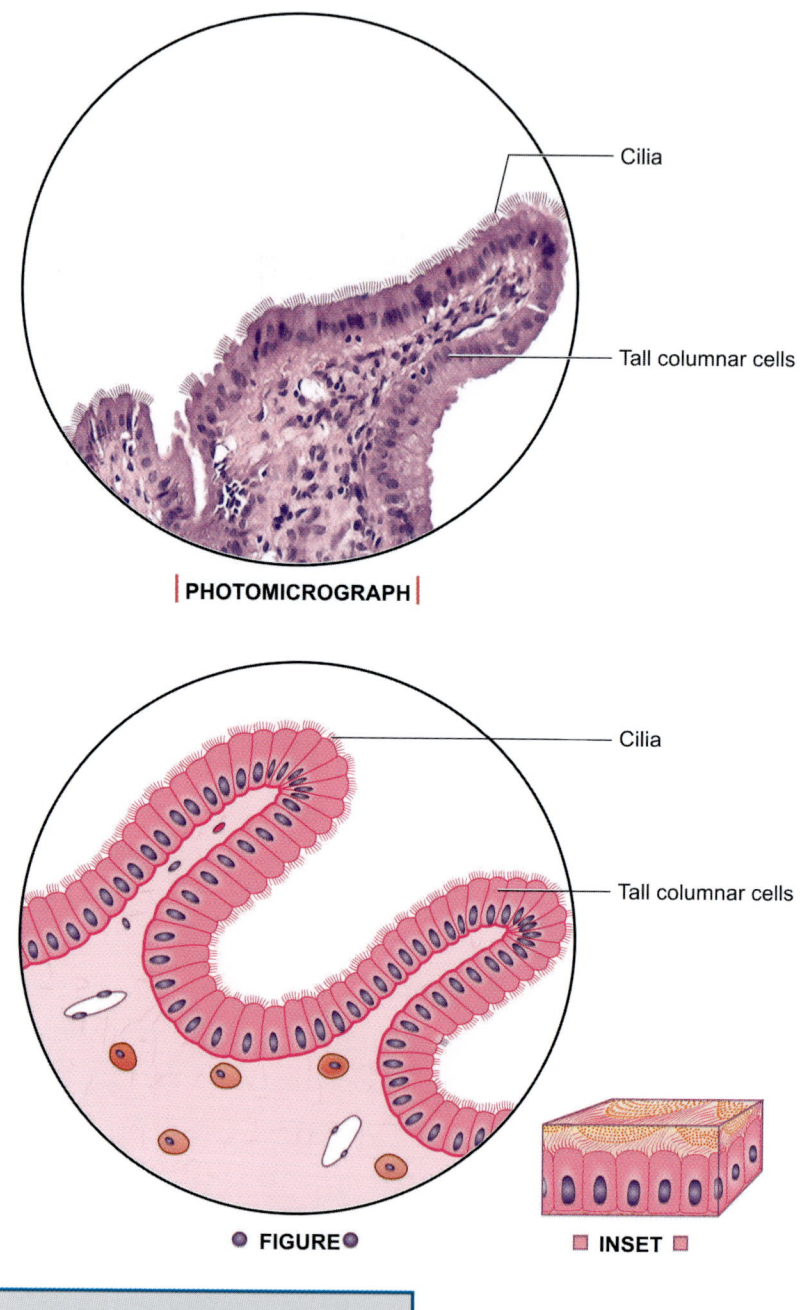

Fig. 2.6: *Ciliated columnar epithelium: Fallopian tube. Stain: Haematoxylin-eosin, 400X*

FACTS TO REMEMBER
1. The cells are columnar in shape
2. Some cells show hair-like projections called cilia
3. Cilia help in the movement of small particles/fluid

Epithelial Tissue

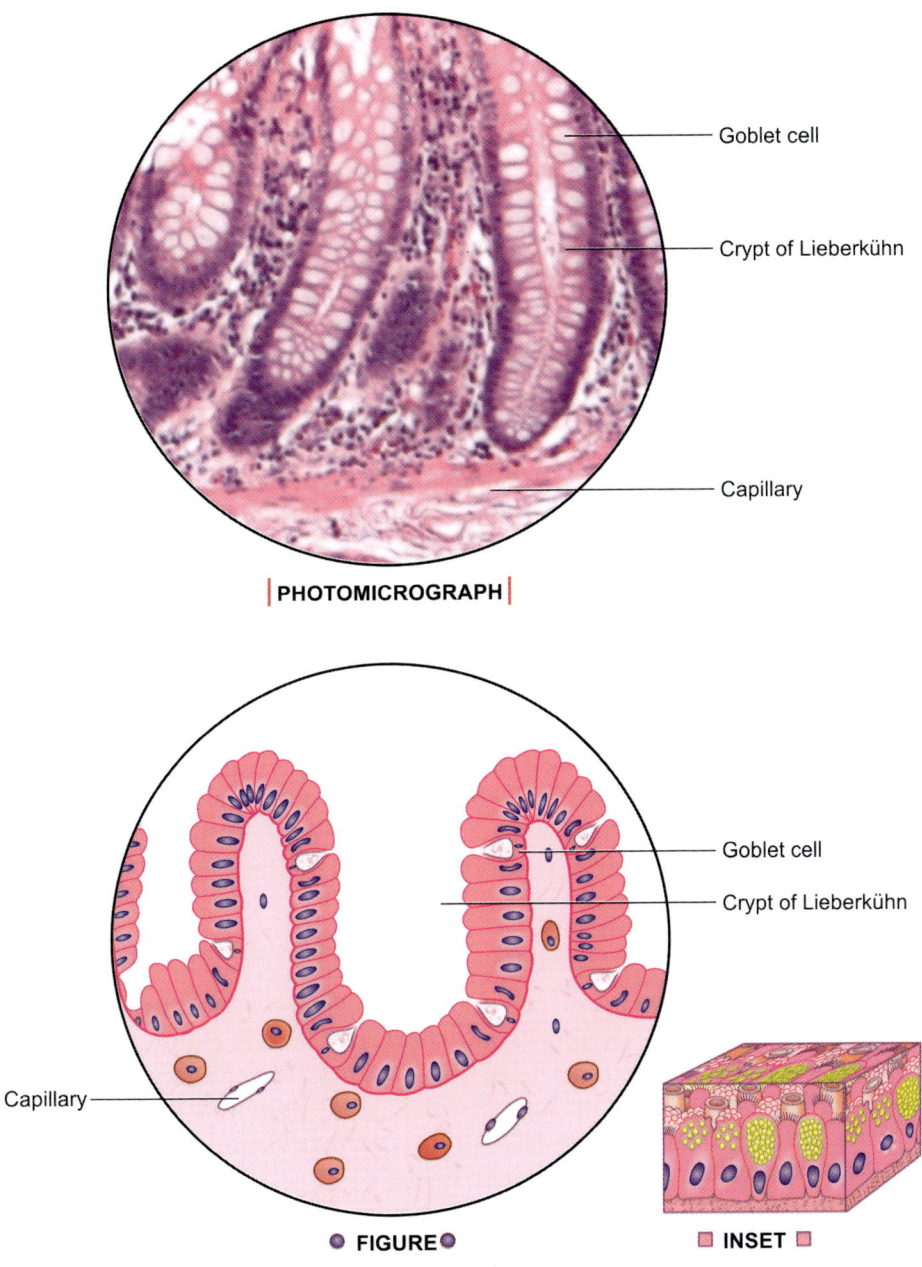

Fig. 2.7: *Goblet cells: Large intestine. Stain: Haematoxylin-eosin, 400X*

c. *Columnar epithelium*
  i. *Simple columnar epithelium*: This type of epithelium secretes mucus. The soft coating of mucus protects the layers of stomach from the harsh chemicals required for digesting the various components of food.
  ii. *Columnar epithelium with microvilli or brush border*
     - The chief function of small intestine is absorption. The microvilli situated on each of the columnar cells lining the villi enhance the absorptive surface area many times. The microvilli absorb fluids and nutrients from the contents of intestine.
     - Gall bladder receives and stores the bile from the liver. It also concentrates the bile by absorption of fluids. The absorption is aided by the microvilli. As the bile gets concentrated, at times the salts may crystallize to form the "gall stones".
  iii. *Ciliated cells and cells with stereocilia*
     - The cilia in the epithelium of fallopian tube help to move the fluid and provide oocyte/zygote with nutrients.
     - The larger regular cilia or stereocilia in epididymis absorb fluids produced by the testis.
     - Cilia on the olfactory cells, cochlear and vestibular receptor cells are components of the respective sense apparatus.
  iv. *Goblet cells*
     - The goblet cells of intestine secrete mucus, which protects the epithelial lining from the harsh chemicals that enter the intestine.
     - As the faecal matter hardens, mucus secreted by goblet cells prevents abrasion of the epithelial lining by the firm faecal matter. Mucus also facilitates passage of hardened faeces.

PSEUDOSTRATIFIED EPITHELIUM

This type of epithelium is one cell thick, but cells are of varying heights. So it is a type of simple epithelium. Some cells are short, not reaching the surface, others are tall columnar and a few are goblet cells. Thus, the nuclei of these cells lie at different levels giving a false appearance of many layers. This epithelium is columnar and ciliated, e.g. trachea (Fig. 2.8), olfactory epithelium, epithelium of membranous cochlea, saccule, utricle, semicircular canals and of taste buds.

Functional Aspect

- The short cells are precursors of the other cells. Columnar ciliated cells prevent particulate matter passing towards the lungs. The cilia beat upwards and push particulate matter towards the oropharynx.
- Goblet cells secrete mucus to humidify the dry air.

COMPOUND EPITHELIUM

This type of epithelium is protective in nature. Various types of compound epithelium are:

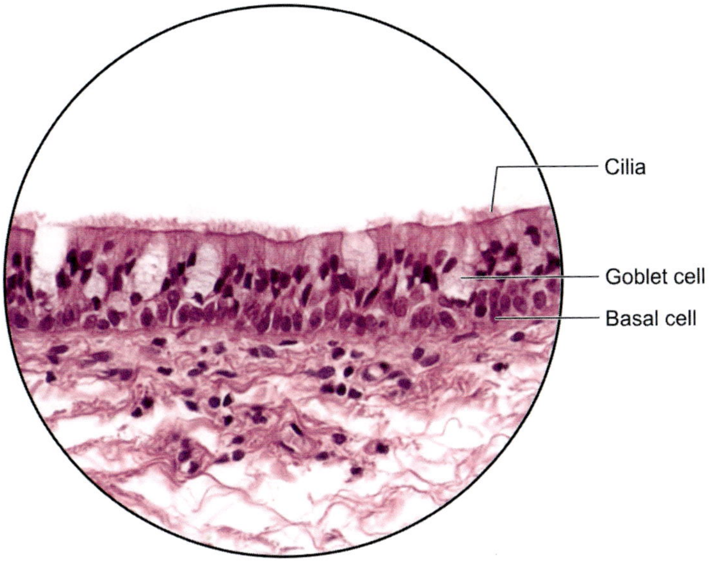

Epithelial Tissue

PHOTOMICROGRAPH

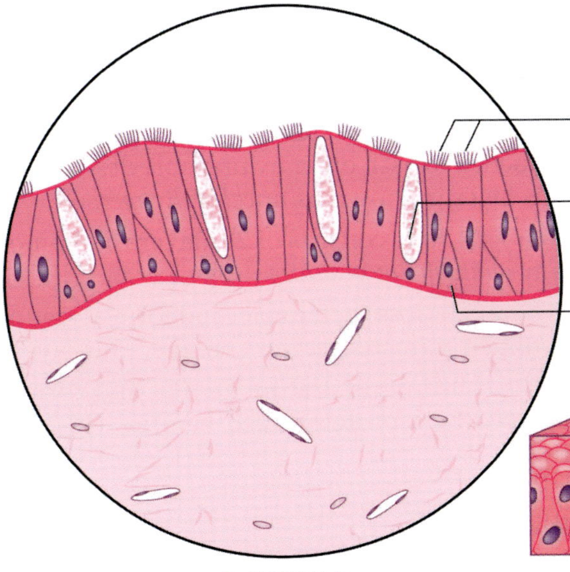

- Cilia
- Goblet cell
- Basal cell

FIGURE 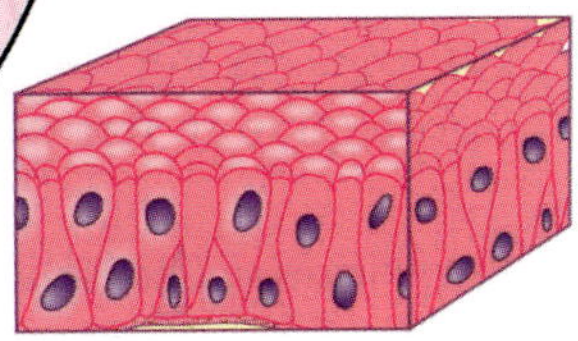   **INSET**

- Cilia
- Goblet cell
- Basal cell

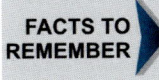

FACTS TO REMEMBER
1. All the cells rest on the basement membrane
2. Some cells are short and basal, others are tall ciliated columnar
3. A few empty-looking goblet cells are seen

Fig. 2.8: *Pseudostratified columnar ciliated epithelium: Trachea. Stain: Haematoxylin-eosin, 400X*

a. Stratified Columnar Epithelium

Seen in moderate sized ducts of glands, e.g. salivary glands (Fig. 2.9) and transition zone of epithelium of anal canal. It is usually made up of two layers of cells, a deeper layer of cuboidal cells and a superficial layer of columnar cells.

b. Stratified Squamous Non-keratinised Epithelium

Example is oesophagus (Fig. 2.10); oral cavity and vagina. The cells occur in three layers or zones as follows:
  i. The deepest single layer of cells resting on the basement membrane is of columnar type and is called stratum basale.
  ii. The intermediate zone is of 3–6 layers of polyhedral cells.
  iii. The superficial zone is of 2–5 layers of flattened or squamous cells.

  The epithelium of oesophagus in lower animals shows keratinisation.

c. Stratified Squamous Keratinised Epithelium

Seen in skin (Fig. 2.11). The layers or zones are as follows:
  i. *Stratum basale or stratum germinativum*: The cells are columnar, resting on the basement membrane. Varying number of pigment cells called melanocytes are also present here. These cells send dendritic processes amongst the next zone of cells. The melanocytes are derived from the neural crest.
  ii. *Stratum spinosum*: The zone is made up of 3–7 rows of cells. The cells are polygonal in shape and are attached to each other by unstable desmosomes, giving it a prickly appearance. So this layer is known as *prickle cell layer*.
  iii. *Stratum granulosum:* This zone consists of 2–3 layers of diamond shaped elongated cells which contain *keratohyalin granules*.
  iv. *Stratum lucidum:* These cells lose their nuclei and form a zone of flattened ill-defined cells. These cells contain refractile *eleidin granules*. This layer looks unstained.
  v. *Stratum corneum:* The cells in this stratum are flat and cornified. The nucleus and cytoplasm get replaced by a protein called keratin. This zone is waterproof and protective in nature.

d. Transitional Epithelium

It is a form of stratified epithelium capable of considerable distension. It is not a transition between two types of epithelium, as its name implies. Examples are in the epithelium of ureter (Fig. 2.12); urinary bladder and proximal urethra.

The epithelium is made up of 4–6 layers of cells loosely applied to each other. The luminal cells are rounded or large cuboidal with a convex luminal border which stains more deeply than the cells of other layers. These cells are also called *umbrella-shaped* cells. The surface membrane, called *cuticle* is seen as a thin eosinophilic band which makes the cells impermeable to urine present in the lumen. These cells may contain 2 nuclei and have depressions on their under surfaces to fit on the pear shaped cells of the underlying layer. The intermediate zone of cells of 2–4 rows are pear shaped or

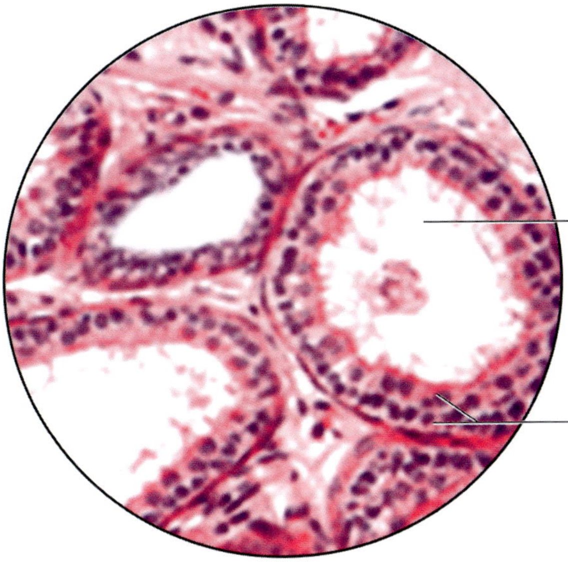

Epithelial Tissue

|PHOTOMICROGRAPH|

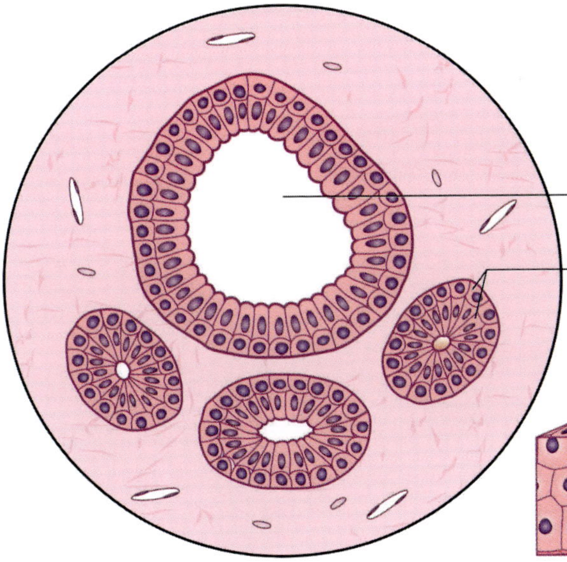

- Lumen of the duct
- Bilaminar epithelium

● FIGURE ●

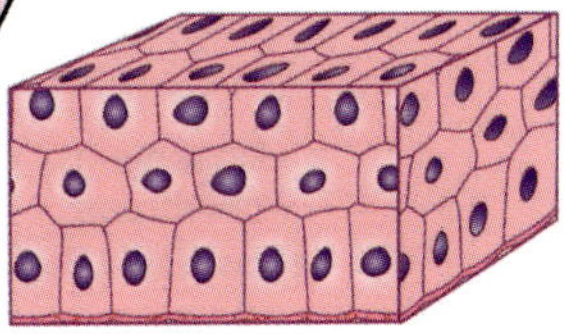

- Lumen of the duct
- Bilaminar epithelium

■ INSET ■

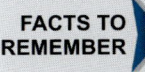 **FACTS TO REMEMBER**
1. Only the basal cells rest on the basement membrane
2. The basal cells are cuboidal
3. The luminal cells are columnar

Fig. 2.9: *Stratified columnar epithelium: Large duct. Stain: Haematoxylin-eosin, 400X*

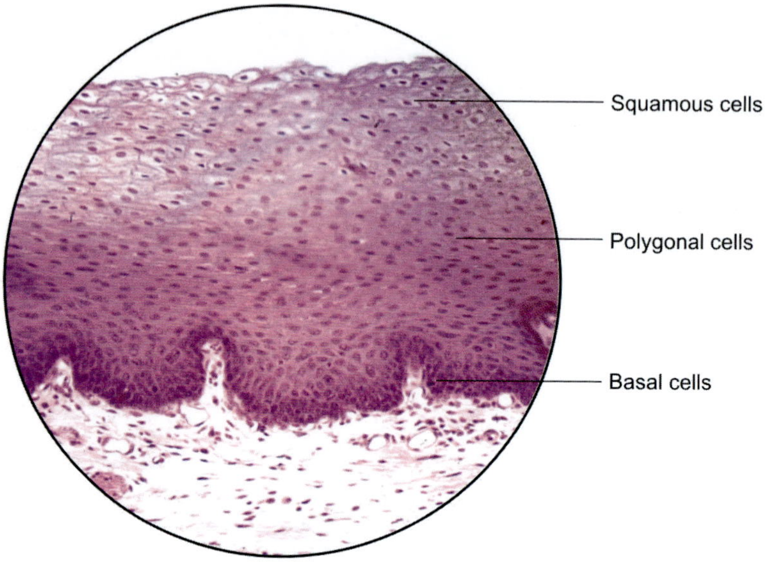

PHOTOMICROGRAPH

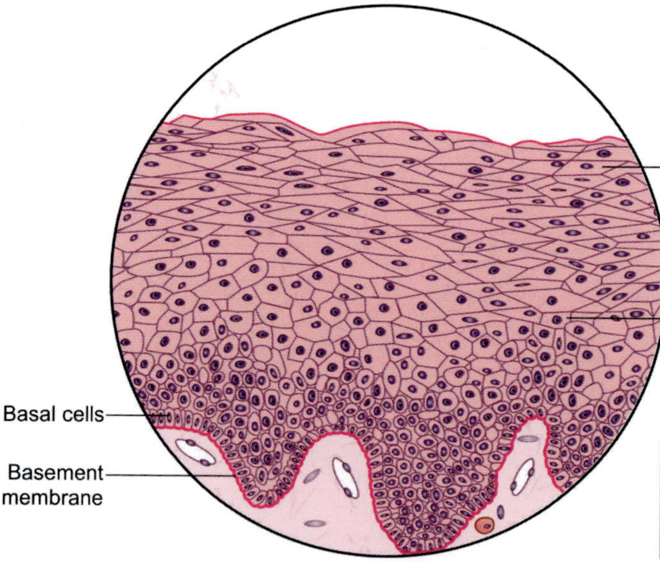

- Squamous cells
- Polygonal cells
- Basal cells

FIGURE

- Squamous cells
- Polygonal cells
- Basal cells
- Basement membrane

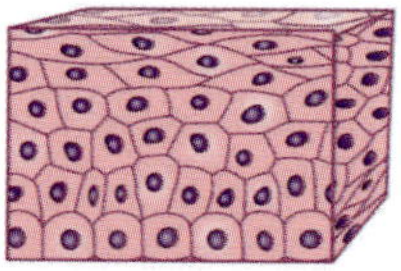

INSET

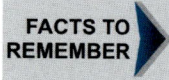

FACTS TO REMEMBER
1. Basal layer formed of columnar cells
2. Intermediate layers formed of polygonal cells
3. Superficial layers formed of squamous cells

Fig. 2.10: *Stratified squamous non-keratinised epithelium: Oesophagus. Stain: Haematoxylin-eosin, 400X*

Epithelial Tissue

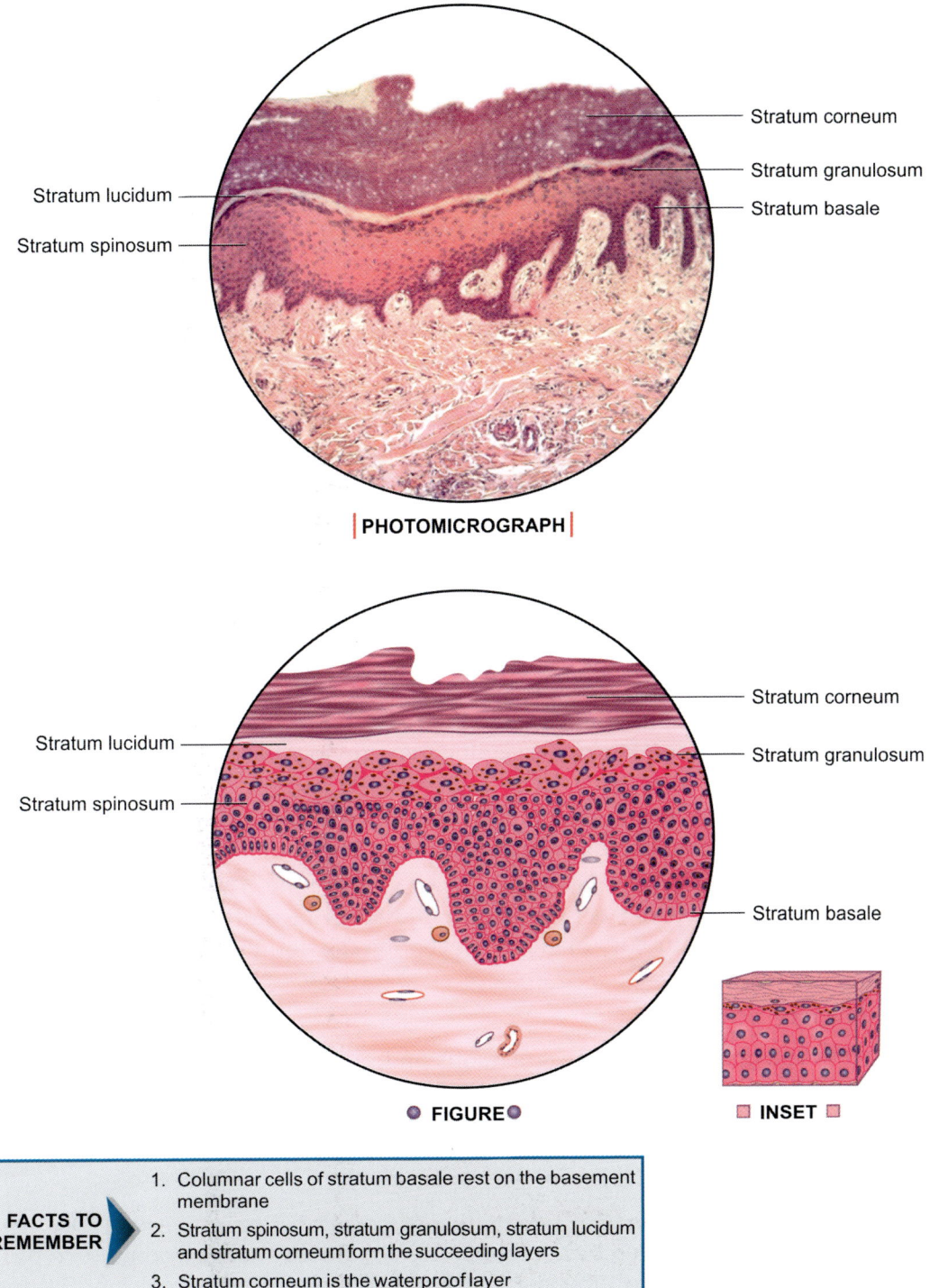

Fig. 2.11: *Stratified squamous keratinised epithelium: Skin. Stain: Haematoxylin-eosin, 400X*

FACTS TO REMEMBER
1. Columnar cells of stratum basale rest on the basement membrane
2. Stratum spinosum, stratum granulosum, stratum lucidum and stratum corneum form the succeeding layers
3. Stratum corneum is the waterproof layer

irregularly polyhedral in shape. The basal cells layer is made up of cuboidal cells. The number of cell layers decrease with distension of the organ and relatively increase when the organ is contracted or empty.

MEMBRANES

Membranes are sheets of epithelial tissue and their supporting connective tissue that lines/covers the cavities or internal structures. The membranes are of following types:

- *Mucous membrane/mucosa:* Lines the digestive tract, respiratory tract, genital tract. The epithelial cells forming mucous membrane secrete mucus, which protects the underlying cells from mechanical or chemical injury.
- *Serous membrane/serosa:* Lines the outer aspects of the viscera. Serous membrane consists of a double layer of loose areolar tissue lined by simple squamous epithelium. Visceral layer surrounds the organ within the cavity while parietal layer lines the cavity. The two layers are separated by a thin layer of serous fluid. Serous membrane is seen in pleura, pericardium, peritoneum and tunica vaginalis of the testis. Small amount of serous fluid allows the organ free and frictionless gliding within the cavity.
- *Synovial membrane:* Lines the joint cavity. The synovial membrane secretes a clear sticky oily synovial fluid, which acts as a lubricant to the joint. The membrane consists of a thin flattened epithelial cells resting on a layer of connective tissue.

Functional Aspect

- Stratified columnar epithelium provides protection to the contents of the ducts. Stratified squamous non-keratinised epithelium provides the protection these organs deserve.
- Stratified squamous keratinised epithelium present in the epidermis gives extra protection from abrasion. This also acts as a first line of defense against bacteria.
- The transitional epithelium lines the urinary system only. This special epithelium acts as an osmotic barrier between concentrated urine and the capillaries in the underlying layers of urinary bladder, preventing the dilution of urine.

Applied Aspect

- *Dysplasia* is a condition seen in squamous and glandular epithelia where the cell maturation is abnormal. It is characterized by nuclear enlargement and persistent mitotic activity even in maturing superficial layers of epithelium. Metaplastic cervical and bronchial epithelia and regenerating colonic epithelium in ulcerative colitis are the common sites of development of dysplasia.
- *Metaplasia* is the alteration in differentiation of the basal or primitive cells. One type of mature tissue is replaced by another in this condition. The most common type is squamous metaplasia of urothelial transitional epithelium or tracheobronchial and endocervical columnar epithelium in response to chronic irritation and inflammation. Other types are intestinal metaplasia in gastric mucosa and osseous metaplasia in scars. Metaplastic cells may develop into cancer cells.

Epithelial Tissue

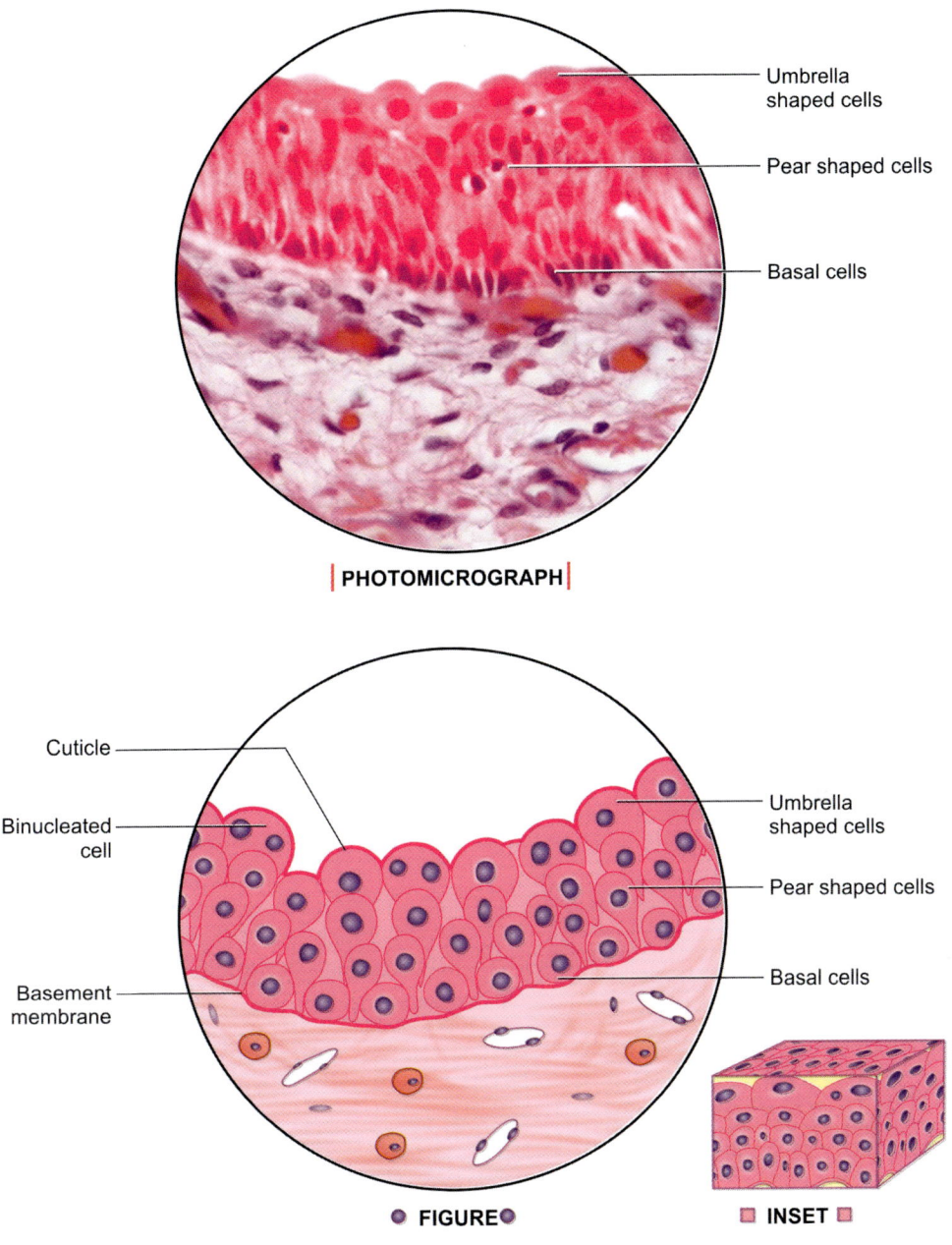

Facts to Remember
1. The bright active luminal cells are umbrella shaped, some are binucleated
2. The pear shaped cells form intermediate layer
3. The basal cells are cuboidal in shape

Fig. 2.12: *Transitional epithelium: Ureter. Stain: Haematoxylin-eosin, 400X*

MULTIPLE CHOICE QUESTIONS

1. **Which of the following is not a simple epithelium?**
   a. Stratified squamous
   b. Pseudostratified
   c. Columnar
   d. Squamous

2. **Goblet cells are not present in:**
   a. Duodenum
   b. Colon
   c. Stomach
   d. Ileum

3. **Urothelium is one of the following type of epithelium:**
   a. Cuboidal
   b. Columnar
   c. Transitional
   d. Squamous

4. **Lining of visceral pleura is:**
   a. Columnar
   b. Squamous
   c. Cuboidal
   d. Stratified cuboidal

5. **Which nerve endings are present in epithelium of skin?**
   a. Meissner's
   b. Paccinian
   c. Krause's end bulb
   d. Free nerve endings

6. **Which one is not a stratified epithelium?**
   a. Stratified cuboidal
   b. Transitional
   c. Stratified squamous keratinised
   d. Pseudostratified

ANSWERS

| 1. a | 2. c | 3. c | 4. b |
| 5. d | 6. d | | |

Connective Tissue

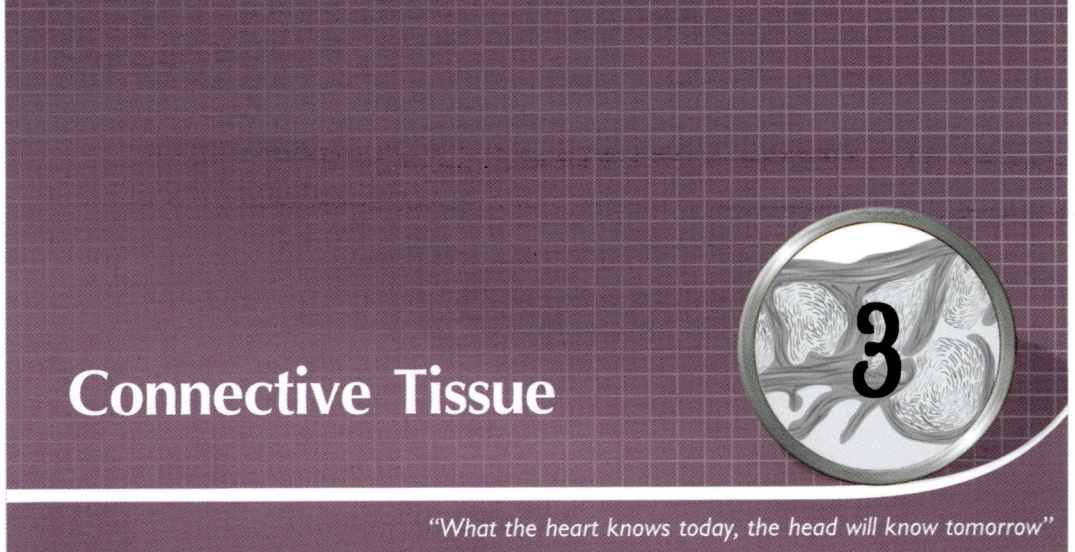

"What the heart knows today, the head will know tomorrow"

As the name suggests, the connective tissue binds and weaves through diverse tissues of the body. It provides them mechanical support for withstanding stresses and strains to which the tissues are subjected in life. Mostly the connective tissue develops from mesoderm or mesenchyme except some types of neuroglia and certain pigment cells which arise from neural crest cells. Connective tissue is composed of cells, fibres and ground substance.

CELLS

The cells may be
1. Fixed, e.g. fibroblasts, adipose cells, mesenchymal cells and pigment cells; or
2. Wandering, e.g. macrophages, plasma cells, mast cells and white blood cells.

FIXED CELLS

a. Fibroblasts

i. *Function*: These cells are responsible for the production and long-term maintenance of extracellular components, e.g. fibres and ground substance (Fig. 3.1).

ii. *Morphology*: These are stem cells with multiple processes, basophilic cytoplasm, and large rounded vesicular nuclei. In the resting phase, these cells appear spindle shaped with long tapering ends and are called fibrocytes.

iii. *Staining properties*: The cytoplasm takes up deep basic stain and appears homogeneous. Nucleus is light staining. The fibrocytes contain a deeply basophilic nucleus but the cytoplasm is sparse and faintly basophilic.

iv. *Situation:* These cells are found in all types of connective tissues.

b. Adipose or Fat Cells

i. *Function*: Specialised cells for the synthesis and storage of fat (Fig. 3.1).
ii. *Morphology*: These cells are spherical/oval in shape. Each of the cells accumulate lipid to such an extent that the nucleus gets flattened and displaced to 'one side'

and cytoplasm becomes so thinned that it is resolved only as a thin line around the rim of the single large droplet. The cells may appear singly or in groups, the resulting tissue is then called adipose tissue.

iii. *Staining properties*: In freshly stained connective tissue, adipose cells appear as large glistening drops of oil. In the usual histological preparations, fat is dissolved during processing of the tissue and there remains only a thin layer of cytoplasm, slightly thickened in one area to accommodate the nucleus. Fat cells can be stained with Sudan III and Scharlach Red which impart these cells orange and red colour respectively.

iv. *Distribution*: In the subcutaneous tissue, in the mesentery and posterior abdominal wall.

c. Mesenchymal Cells

i. *Function*: These cells have great potentialities and can change into any type of cell under a proper stimulus. Thus, mesenchymal cells are the precursors of all types of cells.

ii. *Morphology and staining properties*: These cells are often smaller than fibroblasts but have the same general appearance and staining characteristics.

iii. *Distribution*: They are usually arranged along the blood vessels particularly along the capillaries.

d. Pigment Cells

i. *Function*: The pigment cells of skin and uveal tract protect these tissues against the harmful effects of ultraviolet light rays. Melanocytes produce the melanin and melanophores store it. Some pigment cells increase with age (Fig. 3.1).

ii. *Morphology*: These are stellate cells with branching processes. The cytoplasm contains dark brown/black pigment granules which are usually of melanin. These cells are of neural crest origin.

iii. *Staining properties*: DOPA (dihydroxyphenyl alanine) is a special reagent to visualise the melanin granules in melanocytes.

iv. *Distribution*: In the epidermis of skin, including the hair follicles, a few areas of nervous tissue and the middle coat of the eyeball.

WANDERING CELLS

a. Macrophages/Histiocytes

i. *Function*: Phagocytic (phage—to eat) in nature, i.e. they phagocytose and digest bacteria and foreign bodies, damaged and dead tissues.

ii. *Morphology*: These cells may be fusiform, stellate or spheroidal in shape. The nucleus tends to be smaller, darkly stained, usually indented and lies at one end of the cell. The cytoplasm often contains a variety of granules and vacuoles.

iii. *Staining properties*: Macrophages are specially stained by vital staining. If a colloidal dye such as trypan blue is injected into loose connective tissue, these cells show the injected dye as accumulations in their cytoplasm.

iv. *Distribution*: Most numerous in loose connective tissue, also in the connective tissue of various organs.

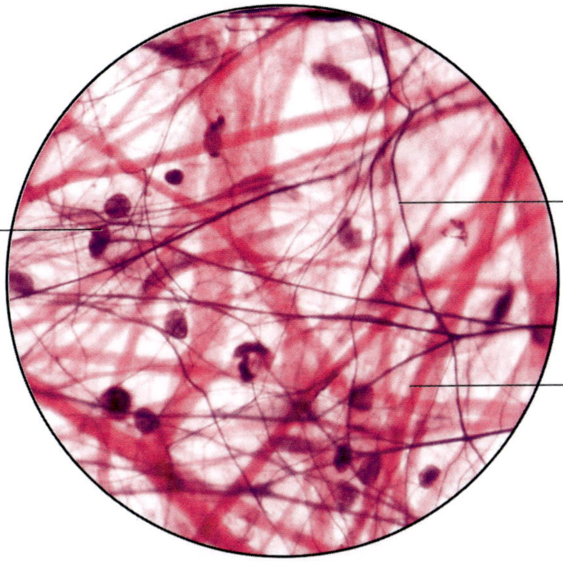

Connective Tissue

PHOTOMICROGRAPH

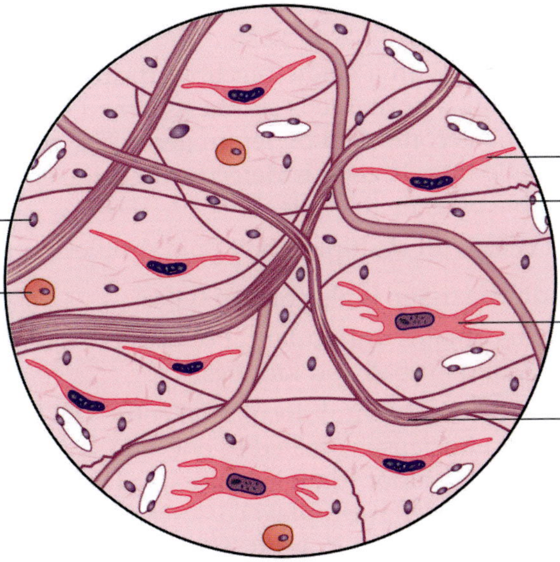

Labels: Plasma cell, Elastic fibres, Collagen fibres

FIGURE

Labels: Lymphocyte, Plasma cell, Fibrocyte, Elastic fibres, Fibroblast, Collagen fibres

FACTS TO REMEMBER
1. Bundles of collagen fibres
2. Scattered elastic fibres
3. Various types of connective tissue cells

Fig. 3.3: *Areolar tissue: Superficial fascia. Stain: Haematoxylin-eosin, 100X*

non-sulphated. The former are comprised of *chondroitin sulphate* and keratosulphate, while the latter group belongs to hyaluronic acid.

Hyaluronic acid binds down water to the tissues and controls permeability of the ground substance. Hyaluronidase, an enzyme, dissolves the hyaluronic acid and increases tissue permeability. Thus, bacteria producing the enzyme hyaluronidase tend to spread the infection quickly.

Depending upon the relative proportion of cells, fibres and ground substance, the connective tissue is classified as follows:

I. LOOSE CONNECTIVE TISSUE

1. *Areolar tissue*, e.g. superficial fascia (Fig. 3.3). It shows collagen fibres in bundles and elastic fibres dispersed singly. The nuclei seen belong to fibroblasts. Various other cell types may be seen scattered among the connective tissue fibres.
2. *Adipose tissue*, e.g. mesentery (Fig. 3.4). Adipose tissue contains fat cells (adipose cells). The fat cells synthesise and store large amounts of lipids. The fat cell is round shaped with a flattened peripheral nucleus. The cytoplasm forms only a thin rim around the lipid which occupies the whole cell. The adipose cells do not undergo mitosis. These cells stain orange with Sudan III stain. With haematoxylin and eosin stain the lipid gets dissolved and the cell looks empty with a peripheral flattened nucleus. Adipose cells may be of two types:
    a. Unilocular, i.e. fat cell with a single big lipid droplet. These are seen in white adipose tissue. Leptin, a hormone is synthesised and secreted by white adipose tissue. The hormone is controlled by leptin gene. The gene controls food intake and basal metabolic rate. If gene is defective or deficient, the person becomes obese. It is treatable by gene therapy.
    b. Multilocular fat cells with multiple small lipid droplets in their cytoplasm.

    Accordingly the adipose tissue is also of two types:
    - *White adipose tissue:* It contains unilocular fat cells. It is present in superficial fascia, in the mesentery, around eyeball and kidneys.
    - *Brown adipose tissue:* It contains multilocular fat cells. The lipid is in form of small droplets and the round nucleus is pushed to one side. It is seen in newborn babies in some regions like the posterior triangle of neck and posterior abdominal wall. As the child grows the multiple fat droplets coalesce to form single fat droplet thus reducing the brown adipose tissue in adult. The brown adipose tissue is also seen in hibernating animals.

    The brown colour of fat is because of presence of huge amounts of cytochrome oxidase present in mitochondria. This type of fat maintains the normal body temperature. The protein thermogenin of mitochondria regulates the temperature.
3. *Reticular tissue*, e.g. spleen (Fig. 3.5), liver, lymph node. Reticular tissue contains reticular fibres which get stained with silver stains.
4. *Myxomatous tissue*, e.g. umbilical cord (Fig. 3.6), vitreous humour of eye. This tissue shows fine collagen fibres with stellate-shaped cells and their nuclei. The matrix is mucoid in nature.

Connective Tissue

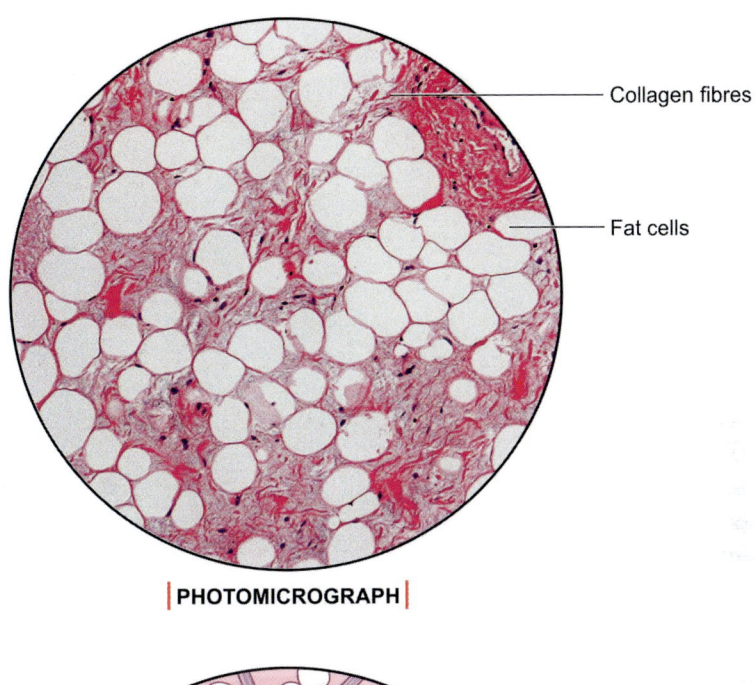

|PHOTOMICROGRAPH|

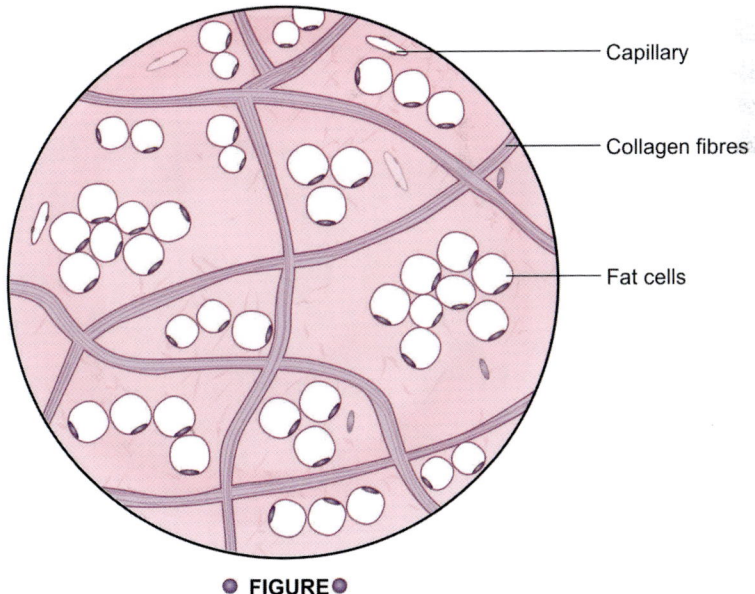

● FIGURE ●

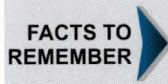

FACTS TO REMEMBER
1. Bundles of collagen fibres
2. Groups of fat cells
3. Fat cells contain peripheral flattened nuclei

Fig. 3.4: *Adipose tissue: Mesentery. Stain: Haematoxylin-eosin, 100X*

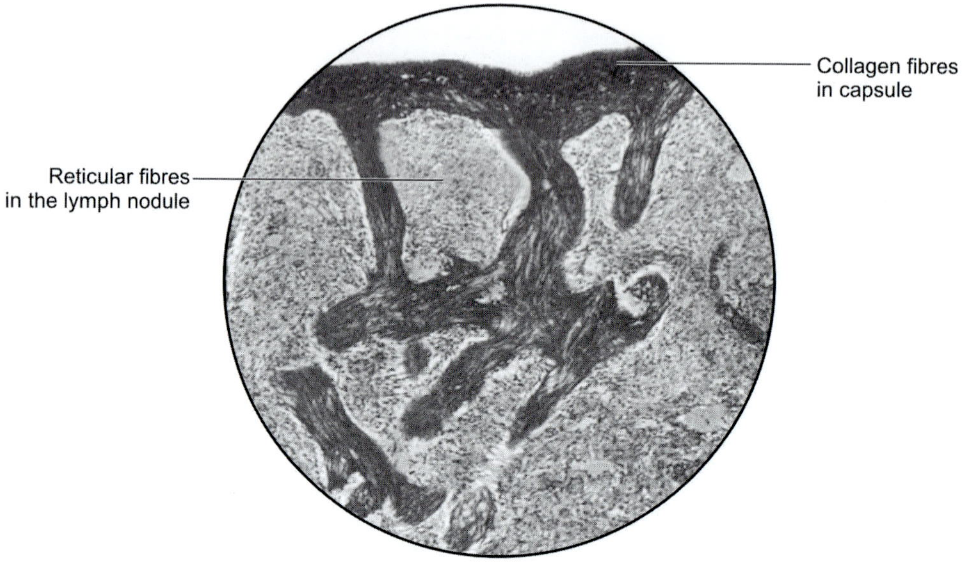

|PHOTOMICROGRAPH|

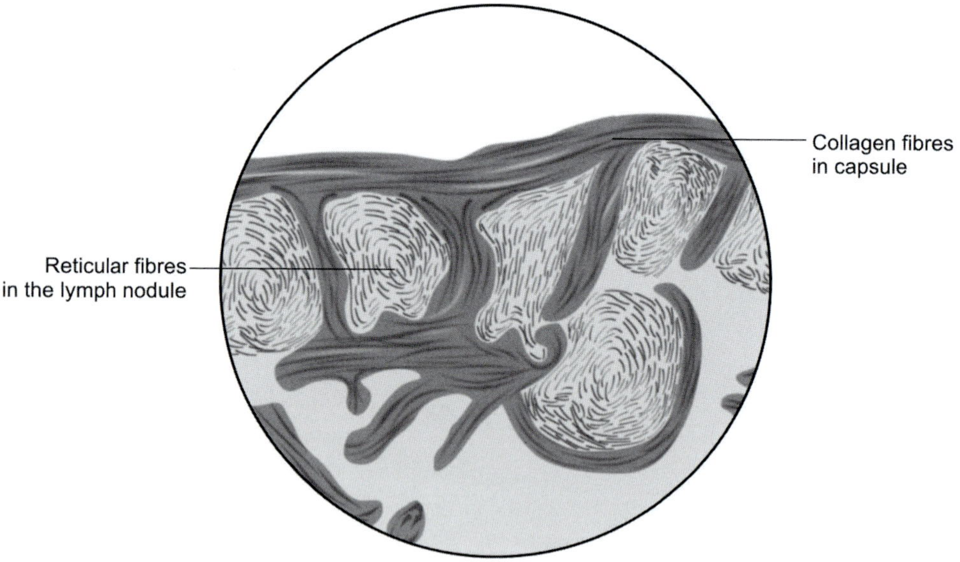

- Collagen fibres in capsule
- Reticular fibres in the lymph nodule

●FIGURE●

- Collagen fibres in capsule
- Reticular fibres in the lymph nodule

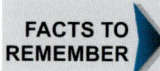
FACTS TO REMEMBER
1. Collagen fibres present in capsule and trabeculae
2. Reticular fibres are thin and curved
3. Reticular fibres support the cellular elements

Fig. 3.5: *Reticular tissue: Spleen. Stain: Haematoxylin-eosin, 100X*

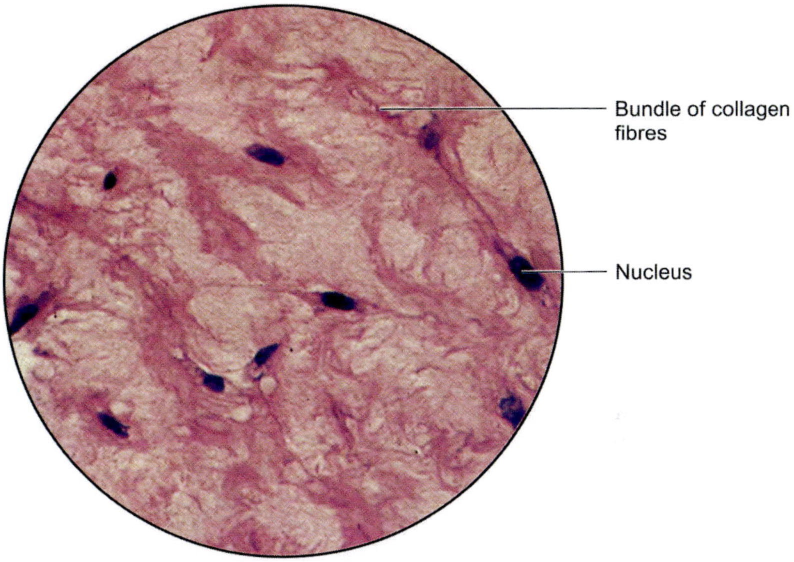

Connective Tissue

| PHOTOMICROGRAPH |

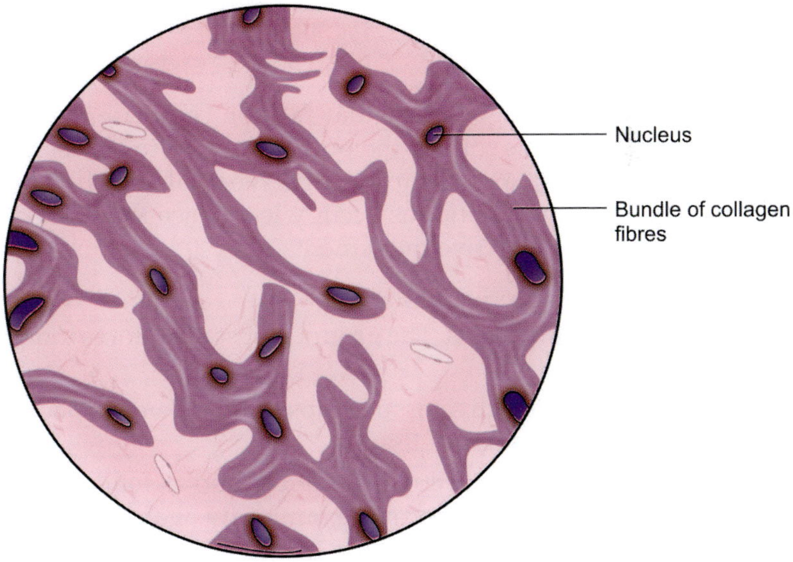

- Bundle of collagen fibres
- Nucleus

| FIGURE |

- Nucleus
- Bundle of collagen fibres

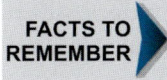
FACTS TO REMEMBER
1. Bundles of collagen fibres
2. Stellate-shaped cells
3. Seen in umbilical cord and vitreous humour

Fig. 3.6: *Myxomatous tissue: Umbilical cord. Stain: Haematoxylin-eosin, 100X*

II. DENSE CONNECTIVE TISSUE

Dense connective tissue: The dense connective tissue is of following 2 types:

1. *Dense ordinary connective tissue*
- *Ordinary irregular dense connective tissue:* It is seen in the dermis of skin as papillary and reticular layers. The connective tissue is irregular in its disposition (see Fig. 10.1).
- *Ordinary regular dense connective tissue:* The collagen fibres are arranged in a closely packed bundles in regular parallel manner with fibroblast nuclei which get pressed due to pressure of fibres. This type of tissue is seen in tendons of the muscles as these cross the joints. Tendons are easily visible on the dorsum of hands and feet (Fig. 3.7).

Even in aponeurosis, like bicipital aponeurosis of cubital fossa, palmar aponeurosis of palm and plantar aponeurosis of sole, the tissue is of regular dense connective tissue type. These provide strength to the areas which are sites of mechanical stress.

Retinacula: Flexor, extensor of wrist, superior, inferior extensor, flexor and superior, inferior peroneal retinacula around the ankle joint comprise dense regular connective tissue. Ligaments of the joints also comprise regular dense connective tissue.

2. *Specialised regular dense connective tissue*, e.g. cartilage and bone, described in Chapter 4.

Functional Aspect

The collagen fibres arranged in regular fashion comprise the tendon. Tendon shows tensile strength. Tendons convey the pull of muscles to the respective bones. Tendons while crossing the joint are covered by the synovial sheath, which prevent wear and tear of the tendon fibres. Tendons occupy less space than muscles, so many tendons can cross the joint for effective movements.

More functions of connective tissue:
- *Storage:* Fat cells store lipids. The ground substance stores inorganic materials, water and ions.
- *Packing material:* Connective tissue helps to fill up small spaces between tissues. It is done by areolar and adipose tissues.
- *Defense:* The cells of connective tissue try and defend the body against harmful substances. These cells also provide immunity against the antigens.
- *Strength:* Connective tissue supports the tissue wherever it is present.

Applied Aspect

- *Scleroderma* is a slowly progressive rheumatic disease accompanied by vascular lesions, especially in the skin, lungs and kidneys. It is characterised by deposition of fibrous tissue in the skin. This leads to thickness and firmness of the affected areas. It is an autoimmune disease of connective tissue.
- *Dupuytren's contracture*: Occurs due to contraction of fibrous tissue of palmar aponeurosis. The disease results in flexion deformities of fingers especially ring finger and little finger.

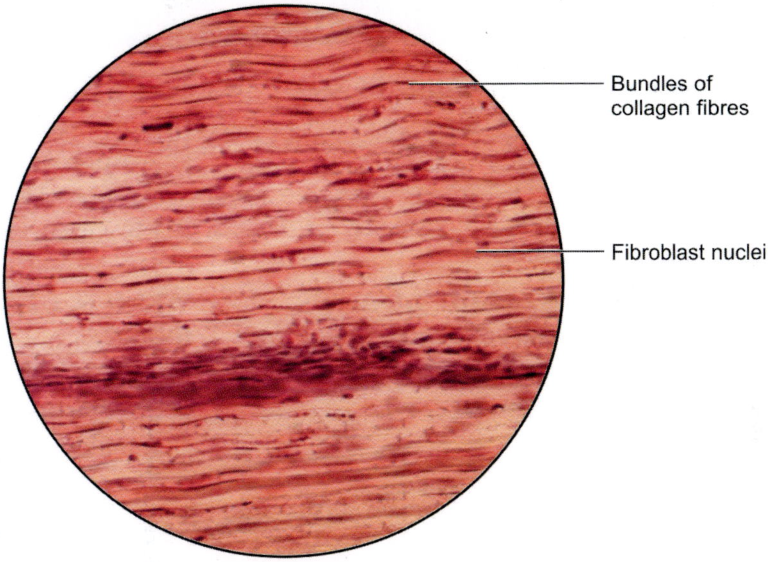

Connective Tissue

| PHOTOMICROGRAPH |

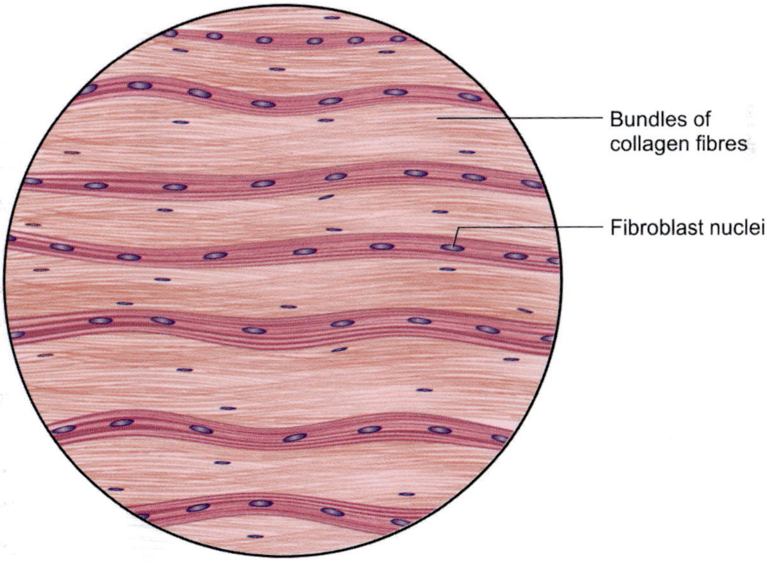

Bundles of collagen fibres

Fibroblast nuclei

● FIGURE ●

Bundles of collagen fibres

Fibroblast nuclei

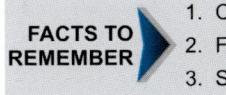

1. Collagen fibres bundles
2. Fibroblast nuclei
3. Seen in tendons

Fig. 3.7: *Dense connective tissue: Tendon. Stain: Haematoxylin-eosin, 100X*

MULTIPLE CHOICE QUESTIONS

1. **The wandering cell of the connective tissue is:**
   a. Fibroblast
   b. Adipose cell
   c. Plasma cell
   d. Mast cell

2. **Which is an example of dense irregular connective tissue?**
   a. Tendon
   b. Myxomatous tissue
   c. Areolar
   d. Dermis

3. **Which connective tissue is present in umbilical cord?**
   a. Adipose
   b. Areolar tissue
   c. Myxomatous/mucoid tissue
   d. Dense regular

4. **Which is a specialised connective tissue?**
   a. Adipose tissue
   b. Areolar tissue
   c. Cartilage
   d. Dense connective tissue

ANSWERS

1. d   2. d   3. c   4. c

Skeletal Tissue: Cartilage and Bone

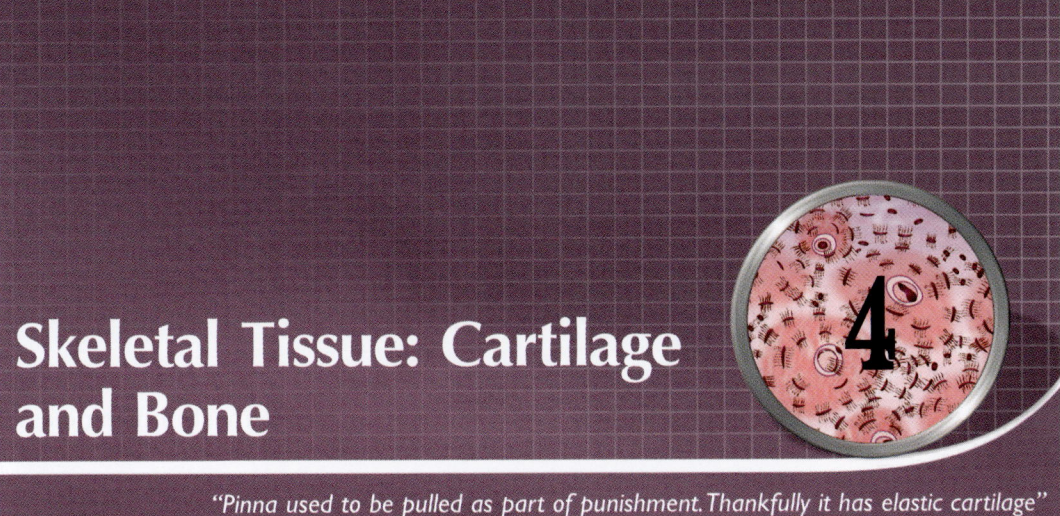

"Pinna used to be pulled as part of punishment. Thankfully it has elastic cartilage"

CARTILAGE

Cartilage is a specialised dense connective tissue.

Functions
i. It bears the weight of the body and plays an important role during the growth in length of long bones.
ii. Gives support to developing organs.
iii. Cartilage helps in withstanding bending and torsional forces.

Composition
The cartilage comprises cells, ground substance and fibres. The latter two, i.e. ground substance and fibres, together are termed as intercellular substance. The cartilages are usually covered with a fibrovascular membrane called perichondrium, comprised of an outer dense vascular connective tissue with type I collagen layer and an inner chondrogenic layer which gives rise to chondroblasts which secrete cartilaginous matrix. Articular hyaline cartilage and fibrocartilage are not covered by periochondrium. Growth in cartilage occurs by:
a. Appositional growth: By surface deposition from the cells of inner perichondrial layer.
b. Interstitial growth: By the multiplication of cells situated within the matrix of the cartilage.

1. CELLS OF THE CARTILAGE
The mature cartilage consists of cells called chondrocytes, situated in spaces of the matrix known as lacunae.

Single cells are spherical in shape but the small groups of 2–4 cells are rounded with flat opposing surfaces (D-shaped). These group of cells are termed as 'cell nests'.

The nuclei of the cartilage cells are large and round with 1–2 nucleoli and the cytoplasm is basophilic. The stained sections of the cartilage show the cytoplasm shrunken from the sides of the lacunae. This is a shrinkage artefact. During fixation and dehydration the cartilage cells retract from the lacunar wall and leave a gap between them and the lacunae. Main function of chondrocytes is to maintain cartilage matrix. The young cartilage cells are known as chondroblasts. These are smaller in size and irregular in shape due to branched cytoplasmic processes.

2. FIBRES

Fibres are type I/type II thick collagen fibres or branching and anastomosing elastic fibres.

3. GROUND SUBSTANCE

It is an amorphous gel-like substance.

It is stained by basic dyes due to the presence of a glycoprotein, the chondromucoprotein which on hydrolysis yields chondroitin sulphates and keratosulphates.

The ground substance which surrounds the chondrocytes usually stains more deeply than elsewhere. The deep basophilic rim is called the capsular territorial matrix and stains darker than the interterritorial matrix. The basophilic stain is due to strongly acidic sulphate groups of chondroitin sulphate A and C.

Ground substance is produced and maintained by chondrocytes.

It is greatly hydrated for the diffusion of nutrients as cartilage is avascular.

CLASSIFICATION OF CARTILAGE

The classification is based on the visibility and nature of fibres in the ground substance. Accordingly the cartilage is classified as:
1. Hyaline cartilage containing thin (invisible) bundles of collagen fibres.
2. Elastic cartilage with branching elastic fibres.
3. Fibrocartilage containing thick bundles of collagen fibres.

HYALINE CARTILAGE

It is most common and further subdivided into two varieties, i.e.
a. Costal cartilage present as epiphyseal plates permitting growth of bone in length at the ends of growing bones, anterior ends of ribs and in respiratory passages. It is covered by the perichondrium (Fig. 4.1).
b. Articular cartilage present at the articular ends of the bones. There is no perichondrium covering the articular cartilage.

Features

i. Cells are encapsulated in groups of 2–6 "Cell nests" .
ii. The matrix appears homogeneous and has affinity for basic dyes.
iii. The type II collagen fibrils are not seen as a distinct entity in hyaline cartilage since the refractive index of fibres and ground substance is same.

ELASTIC CARTILAGE

This type of cartilage has elasticity, i.e. it comes back to its natural size after being stretched, i.e. it is highly flexible. It is present in pinna (external ear), epiglottis, external

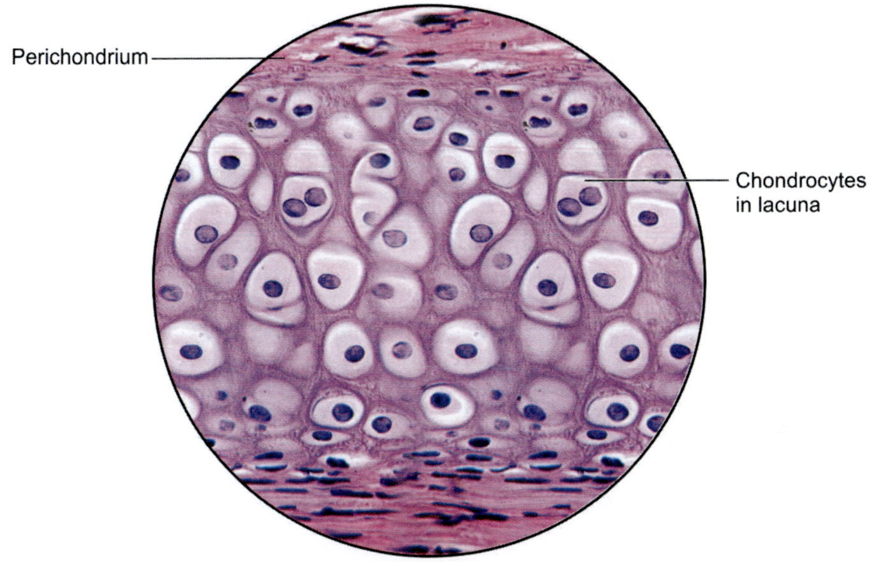

Skeletal Tissue: Cartilage and Bone

Perichondrium

Chondrocytes in lacuna

|PHOTOMICROGRAPH|

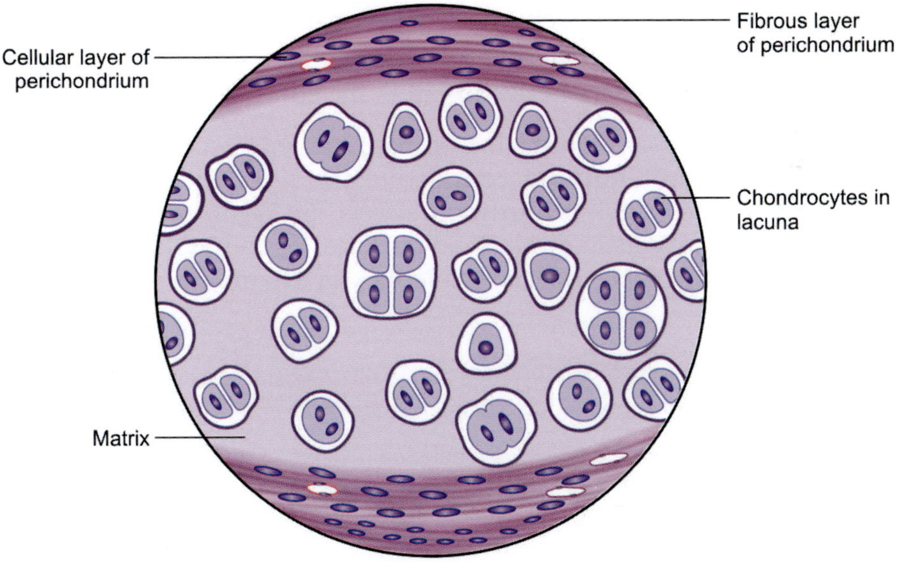

Cellular layer of perichondrium

Fibrous layer of perichondrium

Chondrocytes in lacuna

Matrix

● FIGURE ●

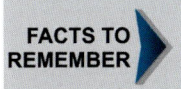

FACTS TO REMEMBER
1. Perichondrium seen all around
2. Ground substance appears homogeneous
3. Chondrocytes in lacuna lie in groups of 2–4 cells

Fig. 4.1: *Hyaline cartilage: Trachea. Stain: Haematoxylin-eosin, 100X*

auditory meatus, part of arytenoid, corniculate and cuneiform cartilages. In fresh state this cartilage is yellowish in colour (Fig. 4.2).

Features

i. Chondrocytes are larger than those of hyaline cartilage and are present singly or in small groups.
ii. The ground substance contains abundance of branching and anastomosing elastic fibres.
iii. Perichondrium is present and is comprised of an outer fibrous and an inner chondrogenic and vascular layer.

FIBROCARTILAGE

It is also termed as white fibrocartilage and is present in intervertebral discs, pubic symphysis, intra-articular discs (Fig. 4.3). It provides tensile strength, resists compression and bears weight.

Features

1. Most of the chondrocytes lie singly and are in smaller numbers. These are squeezed and aligned in narrow rows between the thick parallel bundles of type I collagen fibres situated in the ground substance.
2. Perichondrium is characteristically absent in the adult fibrocartilage (Table 4.1).

Nutrition of all cartilages: The nutrition of mature cartilage is derived by diffusion from capillaries in the adjoining connective tissue or by means of synovial fluid from joint cavities. Lack of nutrition affects the cartilage adversely. Lack of vitamins and proteins results in diminished thickness of epiphyseal plate. Deficiency of vitamin C causes improper matrix, while lack of vitamin D results in excessive

TABLE 4.1: Comparison of types of cartilages

	Hyaline cartilage	Elastic cartilage	Fibrocartilage
Perichondrium	Present, comprising of an outer fibrous layer and inner chondrogenic vascular layer	Present, comprising of an outer fibrous layer and inner chondrogenic vascular layer	Absent
Fibres	Thin collagen fibres	Elastic fibres branching and anastomosing	Thick bundles of collagen fibres
Cells	Chondroblasts and chondrocytes	Chondroblasts and chondrocytes	Fibroblasts and chondrocytes
Ground substance	Glycoprotein—the chondromucoprotein	Glycoprotein—the chondromucoprotein	Minimal ground substance
Calcification	Occurs in old age	Does not occur	Occurs only during bone repair
Sites	Most of the respiratory system, ossifying bones	External ear, epiglottis, cuneiform and corniculate cartilages of larynx	Intervertebral discs, menisci of knee joint and intra-articular discs of the joints

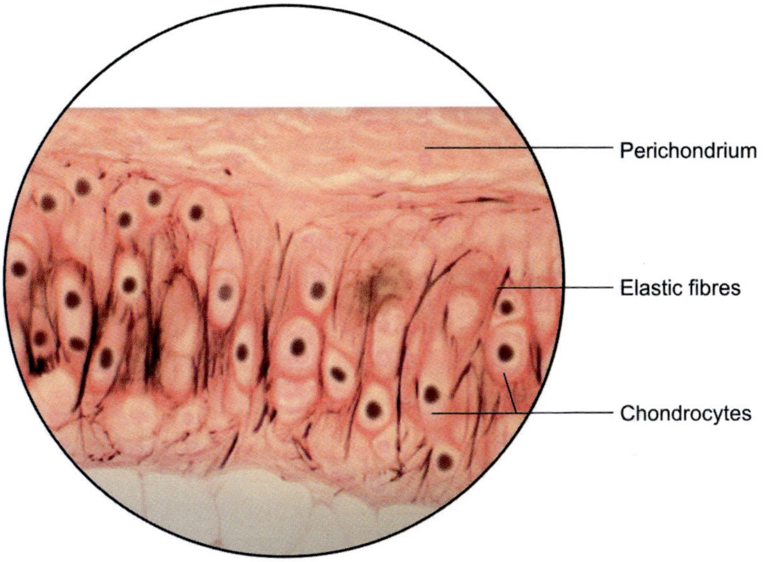

Skeletal Tissue: Cartilage and Bone

PHOTOMICROGRAPH

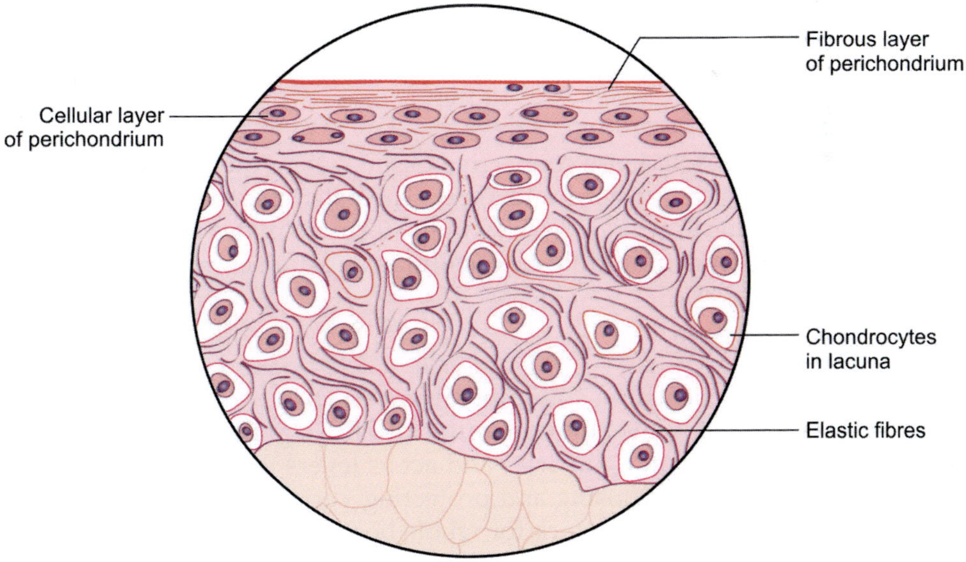

- Perichondrium
- Elastic fibres
- Chondrocytes

FIGURE

- Fibrous layer of perichondrium
- Cellular layer of perichondrium
- Chondrocytes in lacuna
- Elastic fibres

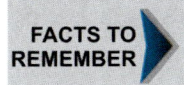

FACTS TO REMEMBER
1. Perichondrium seen
2. Short yellow elastic fibres
3. Single chondrocytes seen in lacuna

Fig. 4.2: *Elastic cartilage: Epiglottis. Stain: Haematoxylin-eosin, 100X*

proliferation of cartilage with diminished ossification, leading to deformity of bones.

Functional Aspect

- Cartilage is a flexible regular dense tissue. The chondroblasts lie in the perichondrium surrounding the cartilage. These cells lay down ground substance and fibres and later mature to become chondrocytes.
- Hyaline cartilage is for support, elastic cartilage is for flexibility and fibrocartilage is essential for weight-bearing strength.

Applied Aspect

- *Osteoarthritis*: Arthritis is the inflammation of one or more large joints characterised by warmth, redness of overlying skin, swelling, pain in the involved areas and restriction of movements. Osteoarthritis is the most common form of arthritis. It causes fibrillation in the centre of articular cartilage and osteophyte formation at the periphery of articualr cartilage. Weight-bearing joints like hips, lower back, knees and feet are mostly affected.
- *Rheumatoid arthritis* is another form of arthritis that also causes inflammation of joints. It is an autoimmune disease. The synovial membrane becomes thickened with subchondral necrosis and may cause warmth, swelling and pain in the joint. Joints affected are small joints of hands on the both sides of the body.

BONE

Bone is another specialised dense connective tissue, where the matrix is impregnated with calcium salts making it hard and rigid. The calcium salts exist in the form of hydroxyapatite crystals [$Ca_{10}(PO_4)_6(OH)_2$] in the form of 'plates or rods'. Matrix is the complex of organic and inorganic intercellular substances which surrounds the osteocytes in a bone.

FUNCTIONS

a. It is the storehouse of calcium and minerals
b. Bone marrow present in the bones manufacture RBC, granular WBC and platelets
c. Bones provide attachment to muscles and act as levers for movements
d. Bones form cavities for enclosing and protecting various viscera
e. Bones form supporting framework for whole body and transmit the body weight.

CHARACTERISTIC FEATURES

Bone has an organised canalicular mechanism and is highly vascular. Bone is composed of cells and intercellular substances. It is covered by a fibrovascular osteogenic membrane called the periosteum. Bone only grows by surface accretions, i.e. by appositional growth. It is a vascular tissue (Table 4.2).

CELLS OF BONE

a. *Osteogenic cells*: These are the precursors of other cell types and are found in the inner layer of the periosteum.

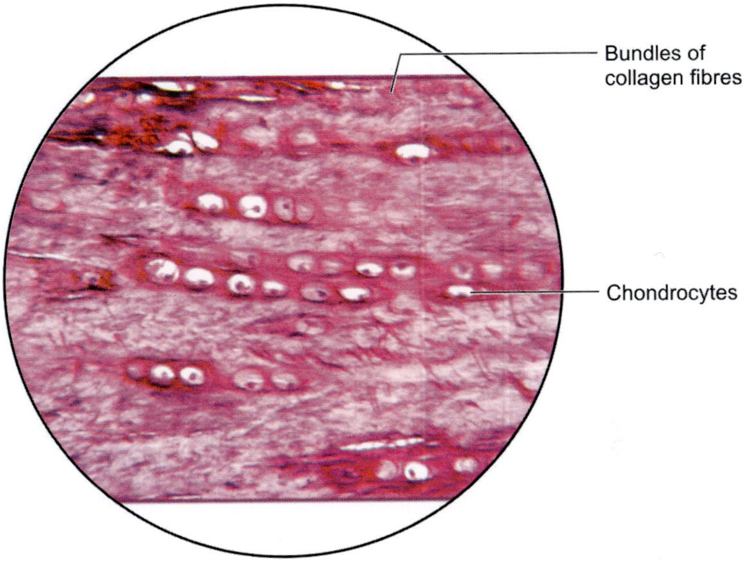

Skeletal Tissue: Cartilage and Bone

Bundles of collagen fibres

Chondrocytes

|PHOTOMICROGRAPH|

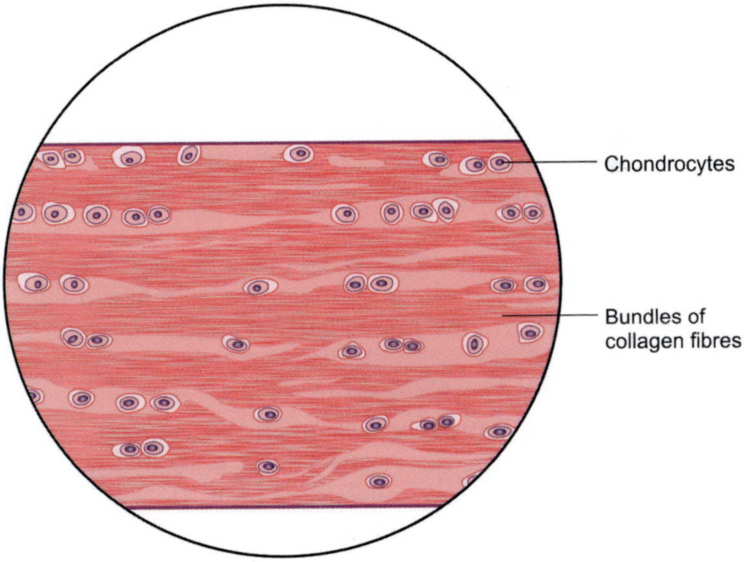

Chondrocytes

Bundles of collagen fibres

● FIGURE ●

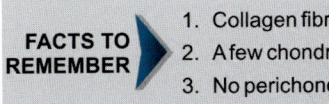

1. Collagen fibres in bundles
2. A few chondrocytes in between
3. No perichondrium

Fig. 4.3: *White fibrocartilage: Intervertebral disc. Stain: Haematoxylin-eosin, 100X*

TABLE 4.2: Comparison of the structure of cartilage and bone

Features	Cartilage	Bone
Nature	Firm	Hard
Ground substance	High concentration of proteoglycans	Low concentration of proteoglycans
Fibres and lamellae	Fibres vary according to nature of cartilage, lamellae not seen	Only collagen fibres organised as lamellae and other minerals are deposited on the lamellae
Mineral salts	Nil	Calcium, phosphate and other minerals are deposited
Cells	Chondrocytes in lacunae	Osteocytes in lacunae with processes
Nourishment	By diffusion through the matrix	Canaliculi of the osteocytes help in passage of nutrients
Growth	Both by appositional and interstitial	Only by appositional growth

b. *Osteoblasts*: These are found where active bone is being formed. These are large basophilic cells with large rounded eccentric nuclei. These cells lay down fibres and matrix in the areas of bone formation.

c. *Osteocytes*: These are resting cells enclosed in the bony matrix. Osteocytes lie in spaces/lacunae in the matrix. Radiating in all directions from the lacunae are exceedingly slender branching tubular passages called the canaliculi. The canaliculi anastomose with similar canaliculi of the neighbouring lacunae. The processes of osteocytes occupy these canaliculi. The cytoplasm of osteocytes is less basophilic.

d. *Osteoclasts*: These are large/giant cells present where bony resorption is required. The cytoplasm is eosinophilic and nuclei are 5–15 in number. All the four types of bony cells work in harmony under normal circumstances.

INTERCELLULAR SUBSTANCES/MATRIX

a. *Inorganic matter*: It is comprised of calcium hydroxyapatite crystals [$Ca_{10}(PO_4)_6(OH)_2$]. The inorganic matter provides rigidity to the bone. If bone is put in strong acids, the salts get dissolved, and bone becomes flexible. Then it can be tied as a knot.

b. *Organic matter*: Formed by dense bundles of collagen fibres embedded in amorphous ground substance comprised of protein polysaccharides and hyaluronic acid. All these elements are secreted by osteoblasts. Organic matter can be destroyed by burning when the bone becomes brittle though its shape is retained.

HISTOLOGICAL CLASSIFICATION OF BONE

I. Compact or Dense

Bone is harder and denser, e.g. shaft of long bones.

II. Cancellous or Spongy

Bone has bigger marrow spaces and is relatively less hard, e.g. the ends of long bones.

MICROSCOPIC STRUCTURE OF COMPACT BONE

1. Bone is covered by the periosteum, consisting of an outer fibrous layer and an inner osteogenic and vascular layers. Collagen fibres from this layer penetrate into the outermost lamellae of bone nailing the two together. These are termed Sharpey's fibres.
2. Characteristic histologic feature of compact bone is haversian system or osteon. Each haversian system comprises the following:
   a. A centrally situated haversian canal containing fine vessels, nerves and lymphatics. The haversian canal is surrounded by 6–12 concentric lamellae (Fig. 4.4).
   b. Haversian lamella or matrix is composed of collagen fibres and the deposited calcium salts. The collagen bundles run spirally along the long diameter of the bone. The pitch and direction vary in the adjacent bundles. The variation in pitch and direction causes the lamellar appearance.
   c. Between the lamellae or on the lamellae are small spaces/lacunae imprisoning the osteocytes. Canaliculi from the adjacent lacunae communicate with each other. These canaliculi are occupied by the processes of the osteocyte. Through these processes the nourishment reaches the distantly placed osteocytes.
   d. Haversian canals are connected with one another and communicate with the marrow cavity via canals called Volkmann's canals.
   e. Interstitial lamellae lie in the angles between the adjoining haversian lamellae. These lamellae belong to the relatively older bone. These lamellae also contain lacunae and canaliculi.
   f. Subjacent to the periosteum are the outer circumferential lamellae.
   g. Similarly next to the endosteum are the inner circumferential lamellae.

MICROSCOPIC STRUCTURE OF CANCELLOUS/SPONGY BONE

a. Haversian systems are absent in spongy bone.
b. Bone tissue is arranged as thin plates or trabeculae (Fig. 4.5).
c. Between the adjoining trabeculae are large irregular spaces containing red bone marrow.
d. At the margin of trabeculum are osteoblasts and osteoclasts and in the lacunae of trabeculum are present the osteocytes.
e. Cancellous bone is covered with the periosteum.

OSSIFICATION OF BONES

- Intramembranous ossification
- Intracartilaginous ossification (Fig. 4.6)

Intramembranous Ossification

The replacement of membrane directly to bone without the intervening stage of cartilage is called intramembranous ossification. It occurs in bones of vault of the skull and in some facial bones. It is a quicker process than the intracartilaginous ossification.

Some **mesenchymal** cells get converted into **osteoblasts** with capillaries in specific region of the membrane, called the **"centre of ossification"**. Osteoblasts lay down the

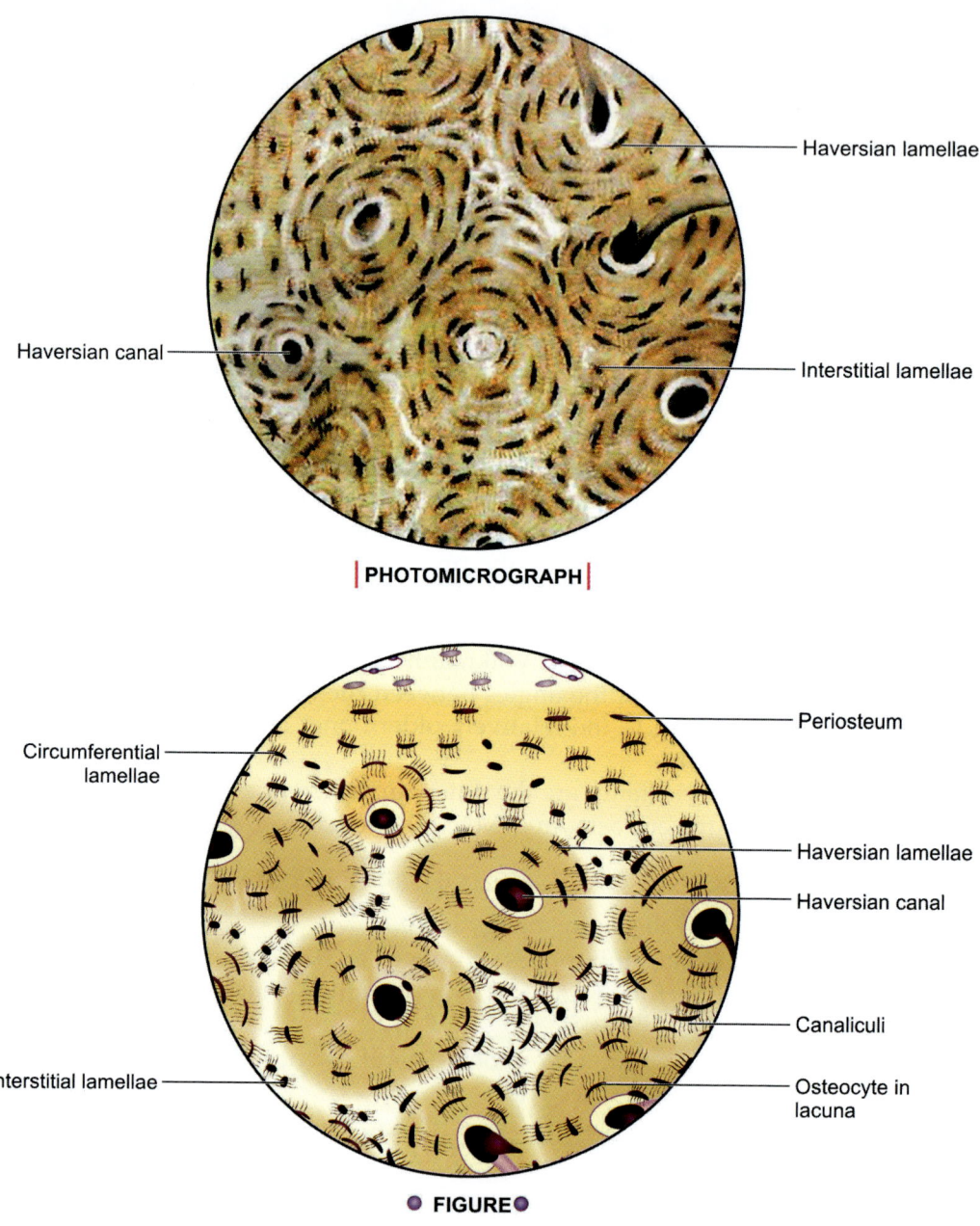

Facts to Remember
1. Outer periosteum seen
2. Three types of lamellae seen: haversian, interstitial and circumferential
3. In between lamellae are osteocytes in the lacuna with canaliculi

Fig. 4.4: *Shaft of a long bone. Stain: Haematoxylin-eosin, 100X*

Skeletal Tissue: Cartilage and Bone

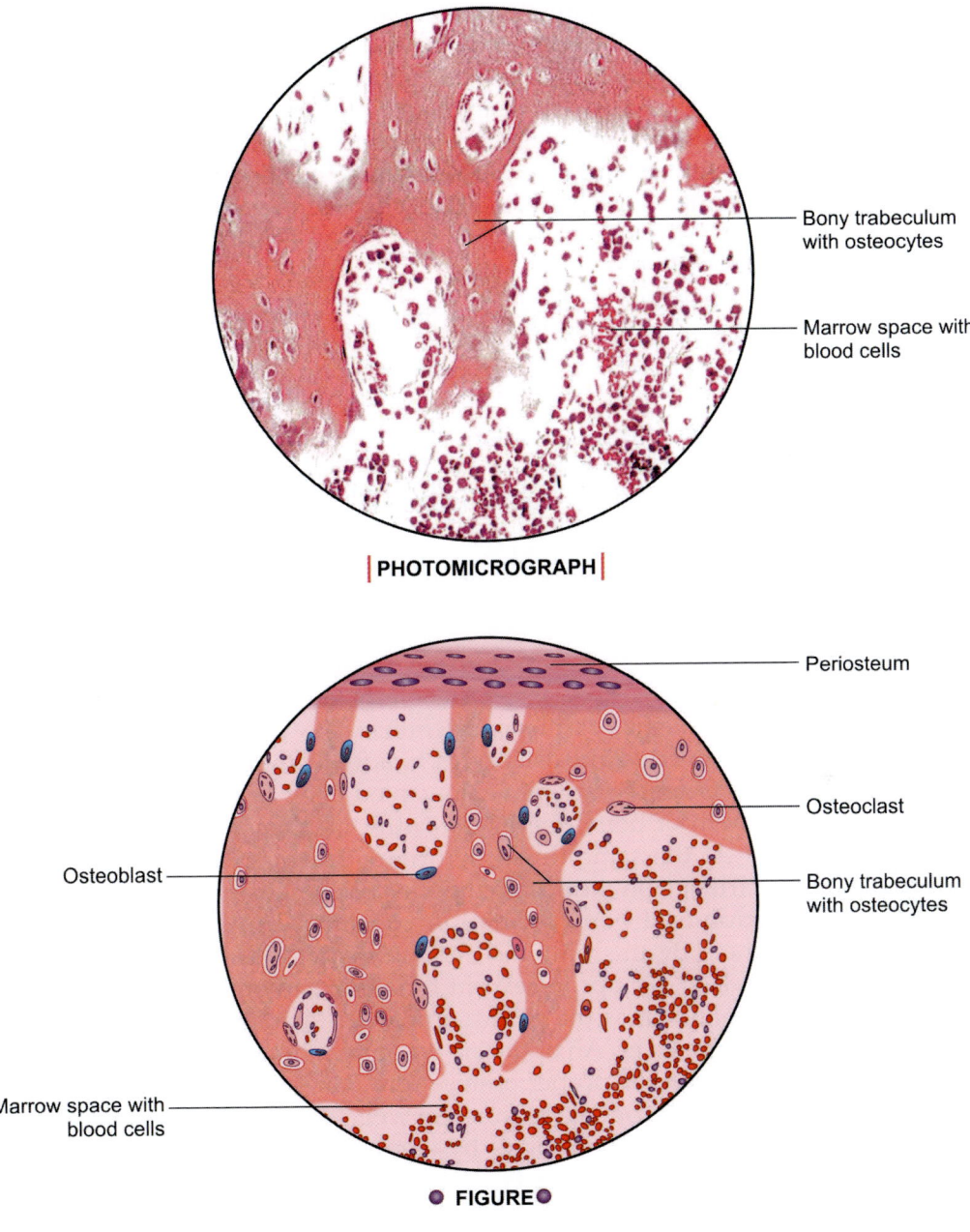

Fig. 4.5: *Cancellous bone. Stain: Haematoxylin-eosin, 100X*

organic bony matrix on which calcium hydroxyapatite crystals are deposited. Some of the cells get incorporated into the bony spicules and these are then called **osteocytes**. The first laid bone is cancellous in nature, i.e. bony trabeculae which anastomose and enclose irregular marrow spaces in between them. Later the bone becomes compact in nature by the reduction in size of the marrow spaces and concentric arrangements of the bony trabeculae. A few **osteoclasts** which are large multinucleated cells, have the task of removing unwanted trabeculae and thus shaping the growing bone tissue.

Intracartilaginous Ossification

The long and short bones of the skeleton are ossified in cartilage. From the connective tissues of the embryo, a model of the bone is first laid down in hyaline cartilage. The first sign of ossification is that the cartilage cells or chondrocytes arrange themselves in columns as follows:

1. Zone of resting cartilage cells (Fig. 4.6).
2. Zone of proliferating cartilage cells.
3. Zone of hypertrophied maturing cartilage cells. The cells increase in size and secrete alkaline phosphatase.
4. Zone of calcification: Calcium salts are deposited in the matrix of the cartilage, thus converting it into the calcified cartilage. Due to lack of nutrition, chondrocytes die, leaving lacunae.
5. Zone of ossification: Blood vessels grow into the region from the periosteum, bringing with them osteoblasts and osteoclasts. Osteoblasts lay down the matrix along the sides of the column of calcified cartilage. Calcium salts get precipitated on the matrix and osteoblasts get converted into osteocytes. Gradually the entire calcified cartilage is replaced by bone. Osteoclasts remove unwanted bony spicules.

In subsequent growth of bone, there is steadily increasing core of bone in the cartilaginous model. At the same time, the original cartilage is itself growing by deposition of more cartilage on the surface by the perichondrium. The two processes of cartilage deposition and bone formation continue, until the adult stage of development is reached. By this time the bone formation has outstripped cartilage formation so that cartilage disappears, except for a thin rim on articular surface. The perichondrium now is known as the periosteum and is made up of an outer fibrous layer and inner osteogenic layer. An optimum amount of proteins, minerals, vitamins and hormones are required for proper ossification. Bones maintain normal calcium levels in blood, helping other organs to function well.

Parathormone increases calcium levels by stimulating osteoclasts. Hormones of follicular cells of thyroid gland counteract parathormone. Calcitonin inhibits osteoclasts, decreases, calcium resorption and enhances calcium excretion in kidneys.

Functional Aspect

- Bones are living tissues, getting ossified, remodelled, renewed according to the needs of the body, calcium is extremely important for development and maintenance of ideal bony architecture. Lack of bony tissue results in osteoporosis with vulnerability for fracture of the bones.
- Osteogenic cells are the stem cells present in periosteum outside and in the endosteum lining the marrow cavity.

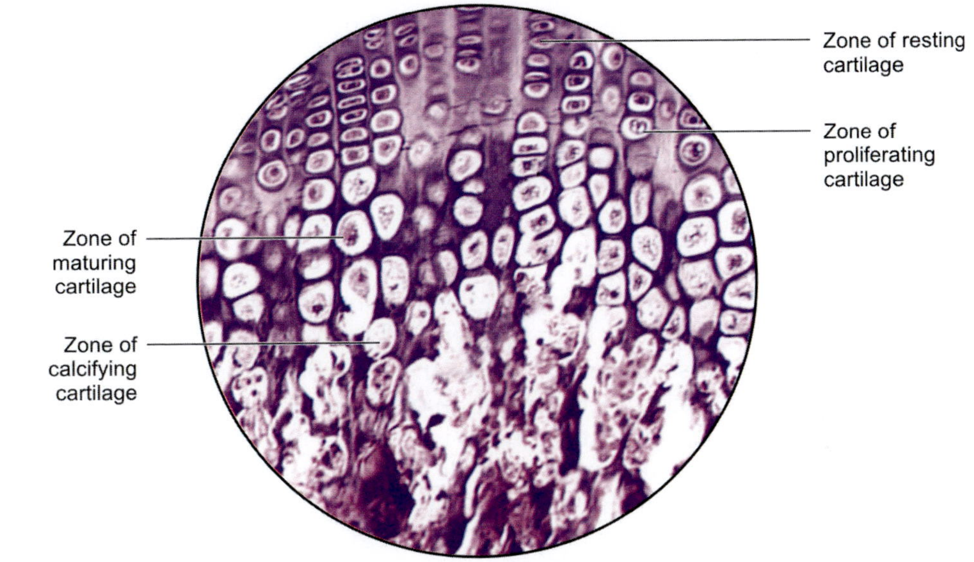

Skeletal Tissue: Cartilage and Bone

| PHOTOMICROGRAPH |

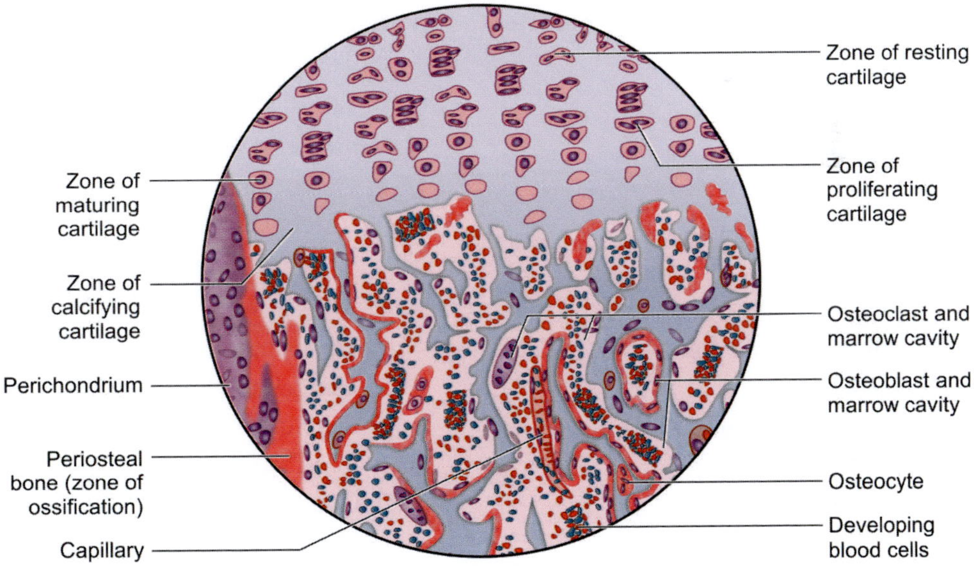

Labels (photomicrograph):
- Zone of resting cartilage
- Zone of proliferating cartilage
- Zone of maturing cartilage
- Zone of calcifying cartilage

● FIGURE ●

Labels (figure):
- Zone of resting cartilage
- Zone of proliferating cartilage
- Zone of maturing cartilage
- Zone of calcifying cartilage
- Perichondrium
- Periosteal bone (zone of ossification)
- Capillary
- Osteoclast and marrow cavity
- Osteoblast and marrow cavity
- Osteocyte
- Developing blood cells

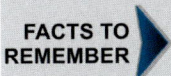 **FACTS TO REMEMBER**
1. Zones of resting, proliferating, maturing and calcifying cartilage cells
2. Zone of ossification with capillaries, osteoclast and osteoblast cells
3. Osteoblasts lay down the bone and then change to osteocytes

Fig. 4.6: *Ossifying bone: Articular end of a bone. Stain: Haematoxylin-eosin, 100X*

- Osteoblasts are multinucleated cells for resorption of bone required in bone remodelling.
- The osteoblasts secrete the organic components of bone—the osteoid. The osteoid gets mineralised to become bone.
- Osteocytes are surrounded by bony matrix.

Applied Aspect

- *Osteoporosis* is a disease of bone. It results in thinness of the bone and weakens the bone to the point that they become fragile and breaks easily. Hip, spine and wrist are the most affected bones in both women and men with osteoporosis.
- *Osteogenesis imperfecta* is a genetic disorder in which bones break easily. This is due to a genetic defect, which affects formation of collagen, a protein that make bones strong. Any individual with osteogenesis imperfecta inherits faulty gene from one parent. It also causes weak muscles, brittle teeth, curved spine and hearing loss.
- Fracture of bone may occur due to a fall or being hit by a strong object.

MULTIPLE CHOICE QUESTIONS

1. Which of the following has the hyaline cartilage?
   a. Intervertebral disc
   b. Glenoidal labrum
   c. Epiphyseal plate
   d. Menisci

2. Which is not a white fibrocartilage?
   a. Menisci
   b. Intra-articular disc
   c. Intervertebral disc
   d. Tracheal ring

3. Haversian system is characteric feature of:
   a. Cartilage
   b. Bone
   c. Tendon
   d. Epidermis

4. Which cell is not a bone cell?
   a. Osteoclast
   b. Osteocyte
   c. Chondrocyte
   d. Osteoblast

5. Where is haversian system present?
   a. Cancellous bone
   b. Cartilage
   c. Tendon
   d. Cortical bone

ANSWERS

1. c   2. d   3. b   4. c   5. d

Muscular Tissue

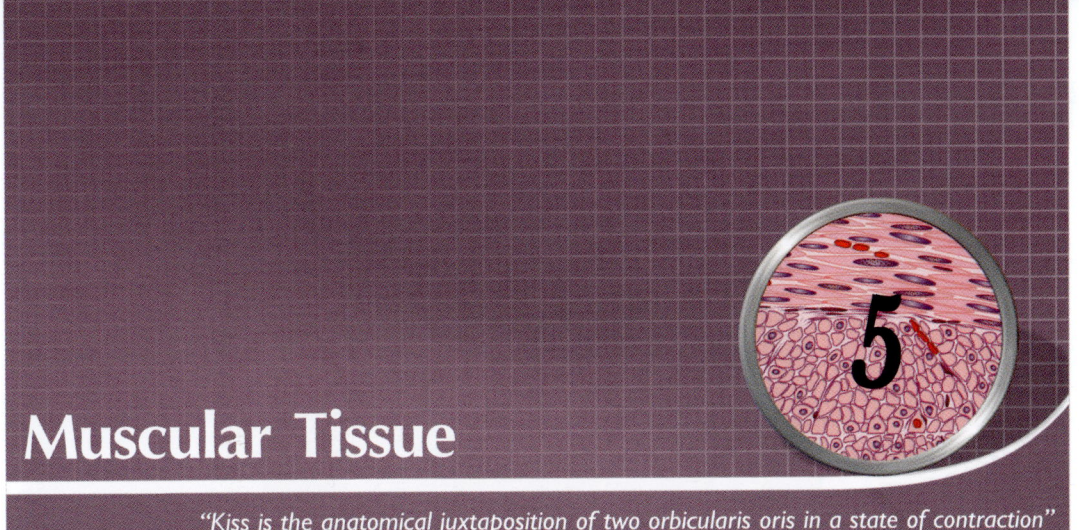

"Kiss is the anatomical juxtaposition of two orbicularis oris in a state of contraction"

Muscular tissue is responsible for movement of various parts of body with respect to one another. All muscles comprise elongated cells called fibres. The cytoplasm of muscle fibre is sarcoplasm, and the cell membrane is sarcolemma. The fibre contains myofibrils made of proteins myofilaments actin and myosin.

TYPES

1. Striated or skeletal or striped or voluntary.
2. Smooth or unstriated or unstriped or involuntary.
3. Cardiac or striated and involuntary.

SKELETAL MUSCLE

SKELETAL OR STRIATED MUSCLE

It is present in muscles of the limbs and trunk, e.g. deltoid and rectus abdominis. The muscle as a whole is enclosed in a connective tissue layer called *epimysium*. Septa extend inwards from the epimysium dividing the muscle into various fasciculi. Thus, each fasciculus is surrounded by *perimysium* from which extend fine septa called *endomysium* that invest individual muscle fibres (Fig. 5.1). This type of muscle is under conscious control.

STRUCTURE OF SKELETAL MUSCLE

With haemotoxylin and eosin stain, skeletal muscle fibres are seen as highly eosinophilic cylinders with multiple peripheral nuclei taking up a basic stain. Each fibre is surrounded by an outer limiting membrane called *sarcolemma* (Fig. 5.2).

The cytoplasm or sarcoplasm contains extensive sarcoplasmic reticulum, mitochondria and glycogen granules as well as large number of longitudinally running myofibrils. Under high power, the myofibrils depict alternate dark and light bands. These dark and light bands in all the myofibrils are "in register", providing a continuous cross striations in the muscle fibre. These well marked transverse/cross striations are a diagnostic and characteristic feature of the striated muscle.

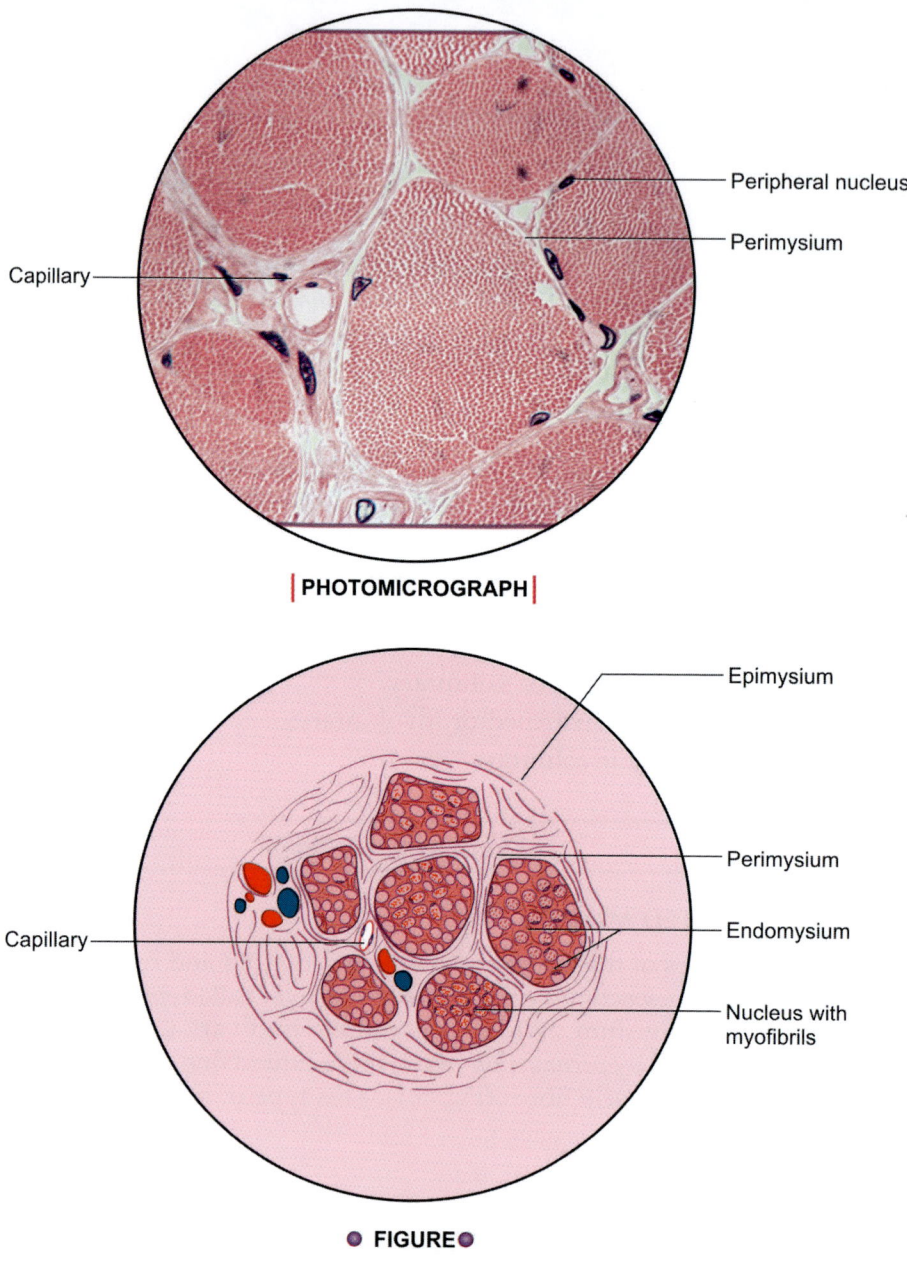

Fig. 5.1: *Deltoid muscle of a limb (transverse section). Stain: Haematoxylin-eosin, 100X*

Muscular Tissue 55

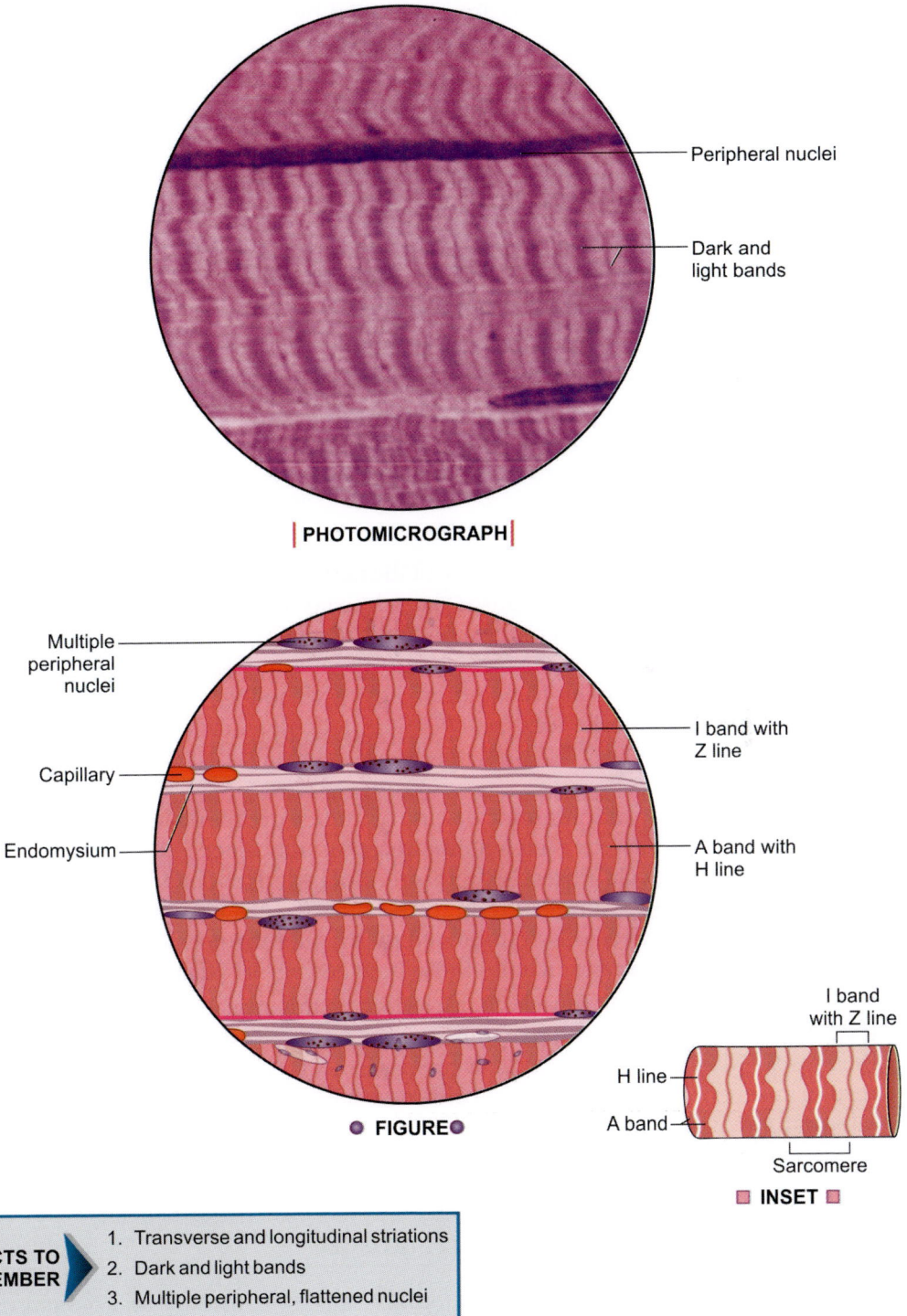

Fig. 5.2: *Striated muscle (longitudinal section): Deltoid. Stain: Haematoxylin-eosin, 400X*

Each of the dark and light bands are intersected by lines:

Dark band or A band contains a light zone called H zone. Light band or I band is similarly bisected by a dark transverse line, the Z line. The functional unit of a muscle fibre is known as the **sarcomere** which is the segment between two successive Z lines, and therefore includes one A band and half of two contiguous I bands.

During phases of contraction, length of 'A' band remains constant while length of H band and I band is shortened. Sarcomere shortens during muscle contraction.

Neuromuscular spindles are specialised stretch receptors seen in all muscles. The spindle contain intrafusal fibres and nerve endings. Stretching of muscle produces stretch reflex and movement to shorten the muscle.

Motor end plates are sites of innervations and transmission of stimuli to muscles.

Length of I band is greatest in stretched muscle, shorter in resting muscle. The nuclei of skeletal muscle fibres are flattened, multiple and peripheral. These are mostly seen beneath the sarcolemma at the periphery of the fibre. Some nuclei appearing in the central part of the fibre belong to the connective tissue around the muscle fibres.

Functional Aspect

The skeletal muscle contracts only because of the nerve impulse sent from the respective axon. The arrival of the impulse causes the release of acetylcholine into the synaptic cleft, which is small gap between the axon and the muscle fibre. The acetylcholine on combining with its receptor on the muscle fibre membrane stimulates the muscle fibre resulting in its contraction. This transmitter, the acetylcholine is inactivated by another enzyme, the acetylcholinesterase.

Applied Aspect

- *Myasthenia gravis* is an autoimmune disease of muscle of unknown origin. Antibodies are produced that bind to acetylcholine receptor and block it. The nerve impulse transmission to muscle fibres is therefore blocked. This leads to extensive and progressive muscle weakness although the muscles are normal. Extraocular and eyelid muscles are affected first, followed by those of the neck and limbs. It affects more women that men and usually those between age of 20 and 40 years.
- *Polymyositis* is a disease of muscle characterised by inflammation of the muscle fibres. It starts when white blood cells (immune cells of inflammation) spontaneously invade the muscle. Muscles close to trunk or torso are mostly affected by polymyositis that results in severe weakness. Polymyositis associated with skin rash is referred to as "dermatomyositis".
- *Hypertrophy:* Increase in size of the skeletal muscle fibres by weight lifting exercises.

SMOOTH MUSCLE

Smooth muscle is present in muscle of stomach, intestine, urinary and genital tracts, and in walls of blood vessels. A smooth muscle fibre or myocyte is an elongated spindle shaped or fusiform cell, which contains a single centrally placed nucleus (Fig. 5.3). The cell membrane is called the plasmalemma, and its cytoplasm is termed as the

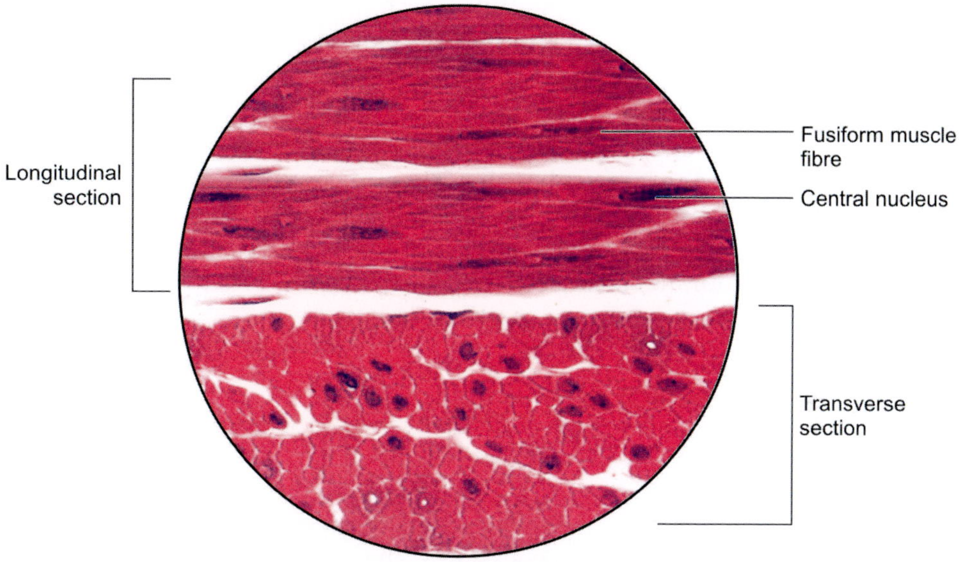

Muscular Tissue

| PHOTOMICROGRAPH |

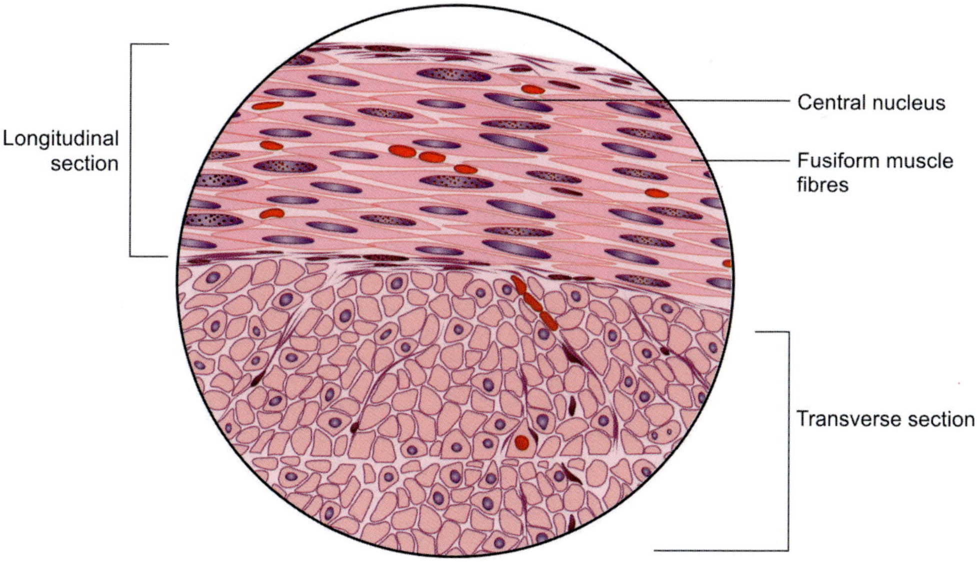

Longitudinal section — Fusiform muscle fibre, Central nucleus
Transverse section

| FIGURE |

Longitudinal section — Central nucleus, Fusiform muscle fibres
Transverse section

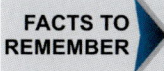

FACTS TO REMEMBER
1. Longitudinal striations
2. Single central nucleus
3. Transverse section shows round/oval fibres

Fig. 5.3: *Smooth muscle: Stomach. Stain: Haematoxylin-eosin, 100X*

sarcoplasm. The sarcoplasm is eosinophilic and homogeneous. There are no transverse striations. However, longitudinal striations are visible.

Fibres in the smooth muscle are arranged in bundles. The thick segment of one fibre lies opposite the thin segment of the adjacent fibre and the nuclei are contained in the central thick segments only. The transverse section of the muscle would show fibres of varying sizes. Only the larger fibres have round central nuclei.

There is minimal connective tissue between the adjacent fibres. The smooth muscle fibres appear as sheets as these are connected to each other through nexus which is fusion of plasma membranes of adjacent myocytes (Fig. 5.3). Actin and myosin filaments are present, but lack regular arrangement or striations.

Functional Aspect

- These muscle fibres show slow sustained automatic contraction throughout the muscle. There are specialised cell junctions called gap junctions between the muscle fibres. The visceral muscle fibres are also innervated by postganglionic neurons of sympathetic and parasympathetic nerves with opposing actions. When the muscle fibres contract, nuclei acquire a cockscrew shape. These muscles are regulated by autonomic nervous system and hormones.
- If each smooth muscle fibres receive its separate nerve supply, it is called "multi-unit type" as in muscle of iris, ciliary body, vas deferens, arrector pili muscle of hair follicles. If nerve impulse reaches via gap junction from one muscle to other, it is called "unitary type" as in visceral smooth muscle fibres like uterus, urinary bladder, stomach, etc.

Applied Aspect

- *Hyperplasia*: Increase in number of smooth muscle fibres. Usually occurs in uterus during pregnancy.

CARDIAC MUSCLE

Example of cardiac muscle is the muscle of the heart and large vessels attached to the heart. Cardiac muscle resembles skeletal muscle partially. Cross striations of actin and myosin filaments form A band, I band. It consists of short/cylindrical muscle fibres, which branch and anastomose with each other. Each fibre contains a single oval centrally placed large nucleus. Some cells show a perinuclear clear space. The transverse striations are present but are not as conspicuous as in skeletal muscle (Fig. 5.4).

The muscle fibres are joined together by surface specialisations known as intercalated discs which contain gap junctions. These intercalated/intercalary discs or junctional complexes appear as zigzag transverse lines and are caused by the apposed plasma membranes of the two fibres. These intercalated discs are better visible by silver stains. The spaces between the branchings of muscle fibres are occupied by fine connective tissue and blood capillaries. With increasing age, lipofuscin pigment is, deposited around the nuclei of the muscle fibres. Mitochondria are more abundant and larger in cardiac muscle.

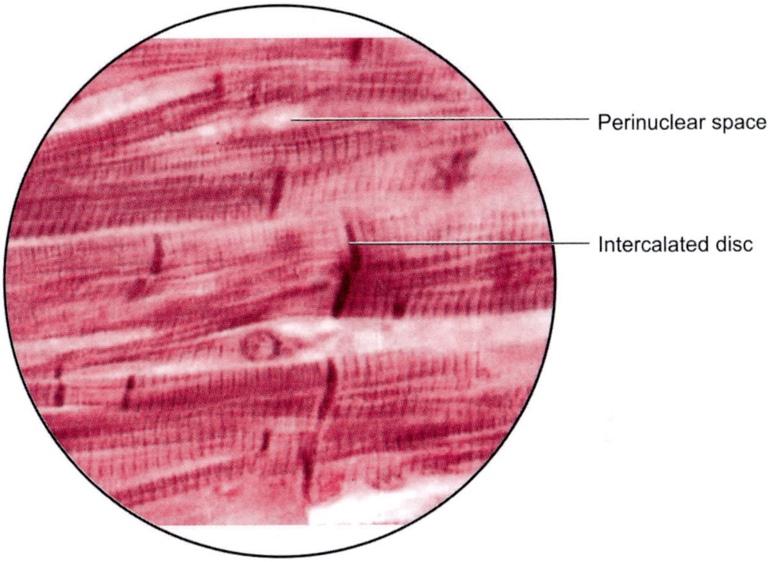

Muscular Tissue

| PHOTOMICROGRAPH |

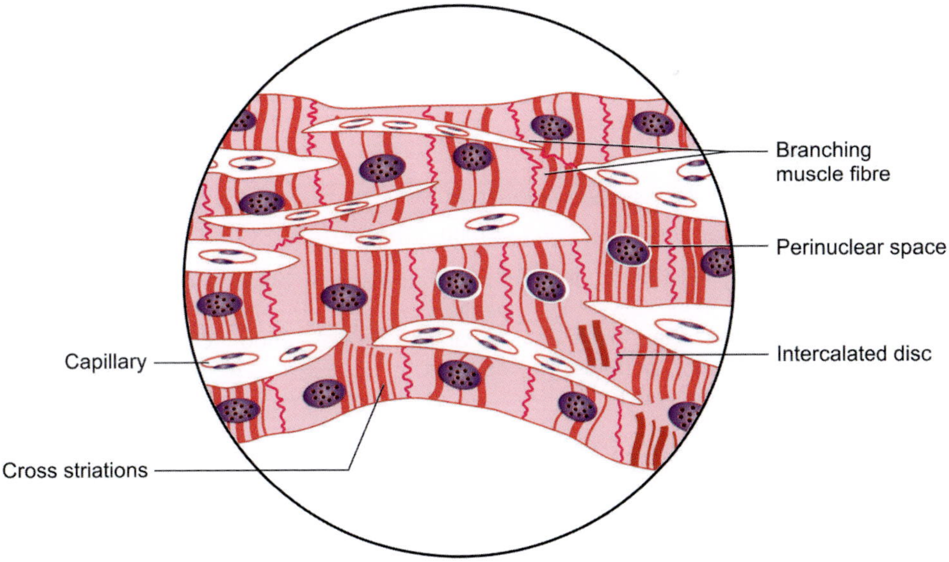

- Perinuclear space
- Intercalated disc

● FIGURE ●

- Branching muscle fibre
- Perinuclear space
- Intercalated disc
- Capillary
- Cross striations

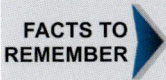
FACTS TO REMEMBER
1. Faint longitudinal and transverse striations
2. Branching muscle fibres
3. Presence of intercalated discs

Fig. 5.4: *Cardiac muscle. Stain: Haematoxylin-eosin, 400X*

Functional Aspect

- These muscle fibres also have gap junctions between adjacent fibres. The intercalated discs bind all cardiac muscle fibres, so that the myocardium contracts as a whole.
- Sympathetic nerves increase the heart rate and raise the blood pressure while parasympathetic nerves slow the heart rate and lower the blood pressure.

Applied Aspect

- *Fibrillation* is the abnormal contraction of cardiac muscle. The cardiac chambers do not contract as a whole resulting in the disruption of pumping action. In atrial fibrillation, there is rapid and uncoordinated contraction of atria, ineffective pumping and abnormal contraction of the AV node. Ventricular fibrillation is characterised by very rapid and disorganised contraction of ventricles. This leads to disruption of ventricular function.
- *Angina pectoris*: Episodes of chest pain due to temporary ischaemia of cardiac muscle. It is usually relieved by rest and nitrites.
- *Myocardial ischaemia*: Persistent ischaemia due to blockage of more than one arteries results in necrosis (death) of the cardiac muscle. Pain, not relieved by rest, gets referred to left arm, chest, and neighbouring areas.

The comparison between the three types of muscle fibres is shown in Table 5.1:

TABLE 5.1: Comparing various types of muscles

Features	Skeletal muscle	Smooth muscle	Cardiac muscle
Location	Mostly in limbs, trunk	In wall of viscera, blood vessels	Heart
Connective tissue	Encloses the muscle as epimysium, perimysium and endomysium	Organised as only endomysium	Organised as only endomysium
Fibre:			
Length	Very long	Up to 15–200 mm	50–100 mm
Width	Wide fibre	Small	Small
Striations	Transverse striations prominent	Not seen	Faint transverse striations
Nucleus	Peripheral and multi-nucleated	Central and single	Central and single
Shape	Cylindrical	Spindle shaped	Short cylinders with branches
Junctional complexes	Nil	Gap junctions	Intercalated discs with desmosome
Nerve supply	Cranial and spinal nerves	Autonomic nervous system	Autonomic nervous system
Activity	Voluntary contraction strong, discontinuous quick voluntary contraction	Slow, weak involuntary contraction	Quick, strong continuous involuntary contraction

MULTIPLE CHOICE QUESTIONS

1. Which is not a feature of skeletal muscle?
   a. Spindle shaped cell
   b. Striations
   c. Cylindrical cell
   d. Multiple peripheral nuclei
2. Smooth muscle fibres are present in all tissues *except*:
   a. Aorta
   b. Inferior vena cava
   c. Stomach
   d. Deltoid muscle
3. Intercalated disc is a feature of:
   a. Skeletal muscle
   b. Smooth muscle
   c. Cardiac muscle
   d. All of the above
4. Epimysium, perimysium and endomysium envelope the following structure:
   a. Cardiac muscle
   b. Smooth muscle
   c. Skeletal muscle
   d. Tendon
5. Cross striations are best seen in:
   a. Skeletal muscle
   b. Cardiac muscle
   c. Smooth muscle
   d. Cartilage

ANSWERS

1. a   2. d   3. c   4. c
5. a

6

Nervous Tissue

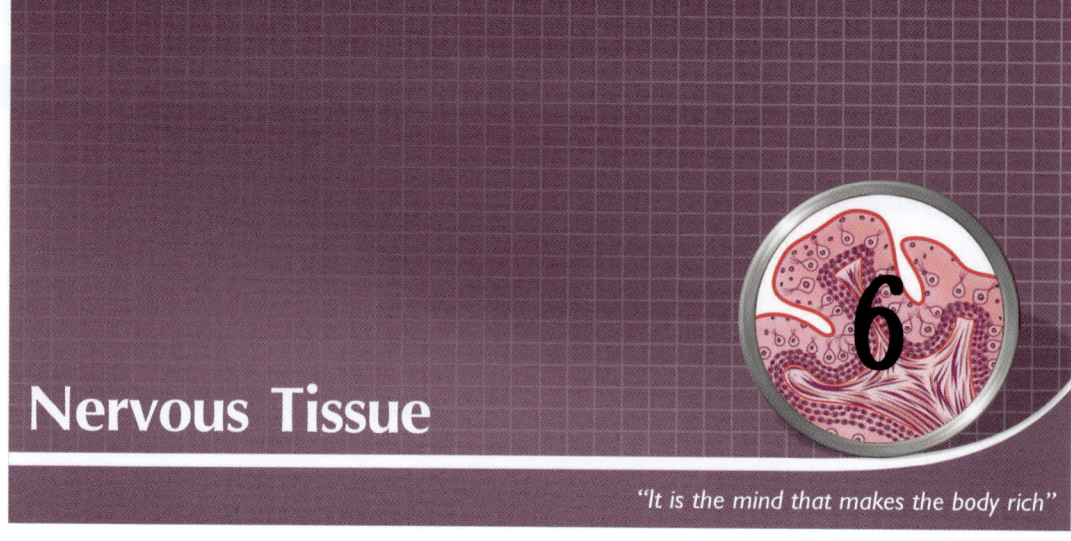

"It is the mind that makes the body rich"

Nervous tissue is the specialised tissue responsible for excitability and conduction of impulses. Nervous tissue comprises:

Neuron, i.e. nerve cells with its processes.

Neuroglia, the cellular connective tissue of the nervous system.

NEURON

Neuron is the structural and functional unit of nervous tissue.

Size: The size of a neuron varies from 4 to 20 microns. Motor neurons are larger than the sensory neurons.

Nucleus: It is large, pale, vesicular and usually central in position. It has a fine chromatin network and a large prominent nucleolus. The *sex chromatin* in the females is often visible as being attached to the nuclear membrane.

Cytoplasm: The cytoplasm is basophilic and contains usual cell organelles like Golgi apparatus and mitochondria. But the *centrosome* is conspicuously absent in mature neuron showing its inability to divide. The cytoplasm of neuron contains two specialised organelles, e.g. Nissl granules and neurofibrils (Fig. 6.1).

Nissl granules are chromophilic bodies which give a granular appearance to the neurons. These are easily stained by toluidine blue and cresyl violet. Nissl granules are the rough endoplasmic reticulum, responsible for synthesis of proteins. These are usually present around the nucleus and in the dendrites, but are absent from the axon hillock (the part of neuron which gives origin to the axon) and axon. Nissl granules degenerate due to fatigue/injury to the neuron and the process is called *chromatolysis*. Neurons synthesise neurotransmitters and neurohormones.

Neurofibrils are thread like structures easily stained with silver impregnation techniques. They form a plexiform pattern in the cell body and are arranged in parallel manner in both the dendrites and axon of the neuron. The neurofibrils give support to the body and processes of the neuron.

Nervous Tissue

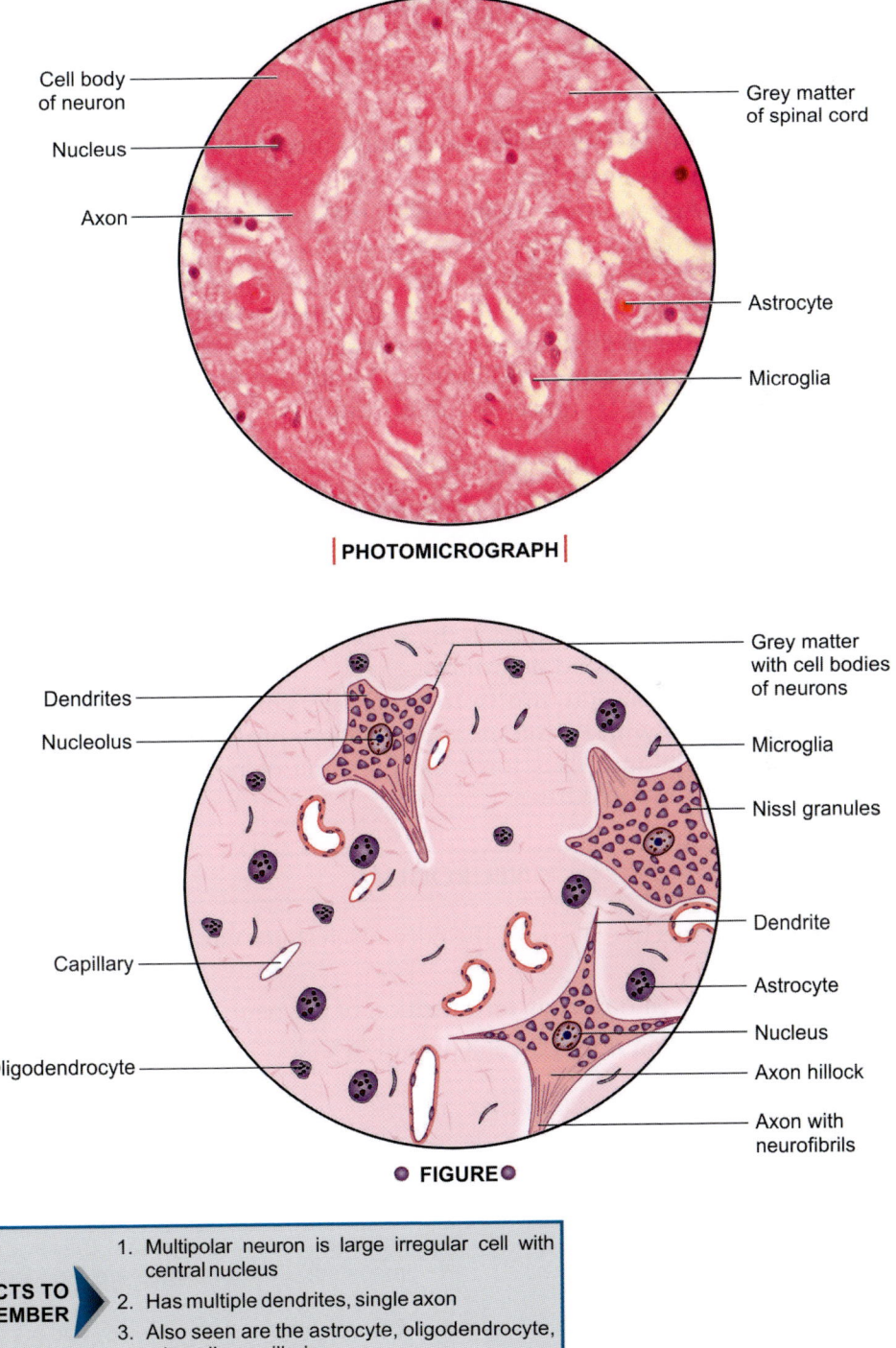

Fig. 6.1: *Grey matter of spinal cord. Stain: Haematoxylin-eosin, 400X*

Pigments as inclusions are also present in the neuron in the form of lipofuscin and melanin. These increase with age.

CLASSIFICATION

Depending upon the number of processes, the neurons are classified as:
  i. Unipolar, e.g. mesencephalic nucleus of trigeminal or V cranial nerve.
  ii. Pseudounipolar, e.g. dorsal root ganglia. A single process attached to the neuron divides into two; one is axon and other is dendrite.
  iii. Bipolar, e.g. olfactory neuroepithelium, spiral ganglia of cochlea, vestibular ganglia and bipolar cells of retina. Axon and dendron arise from opposite poles of neuron.
  iv. Multipolar, e.g. most of the neurons of cerebrum and cerebellum. One process is axon and rest of the processes are dendrites. Multipolar neuron may be pyramidal as in spinal cord (Fig. 6.1) and cerebrum or pear-shaped as in cerebellum.

CELL PROCESSES ARE AXON AND DENDRITES

a. *Axon*: Every neuron has only one long thin process or axon which arises from a special region or axon hillock, devoid of Nissl granules. It carries the impulse away from the cell body. The passage of impulse is always unidirectional, from dendrite: through cell body to the axon. This is known as "Law of forward conduction". The limiting membrane of axon is termed as the axolemma, containing the homogeneous substance called axoplasm and neurofibrils.

b. *Dendron/dendrites* are single/multiple processes containing the extension of cytoplasm of neurons with its cell organelles. These provide receptive surface for the neuron and carry impulses towards the soma of neuron. Table 6.1 shows comparison of axon and dendrites.

NEUROGLIA

This is the cellular connective tissue of the nervous system. Various cells of neuroglia are:

Astrocytes: Protoplasmic and fibrous for nutrition of the neuron (Fig. 6.2).

Oligodendrocytes: For laying down myelin sheath in CNS.

TABLE 6.1: Comparison of axon and dendrite

Axon	Dendrites
1. Only one axon is present in a neuron	Usually multiple in a neuron
2. Thin long process of uniform thickness and smooth surface	These are short multiple processes. Their thickness diminishes as these divide repeatedly. The branches are studded with spiny projections
3. The branches of axon are fewer and at right angles to the axon Golgi apparatus is present	The dendrites branch profusely and are given off at acute angles Golgi apparatus is absent
4. Axon contains neurofibrils and no Nissl granules	Dendrites contain both neurofibrils and Nissl granules
5. Forms the efferent component of the impulse	Forms the afferent component of the impulse

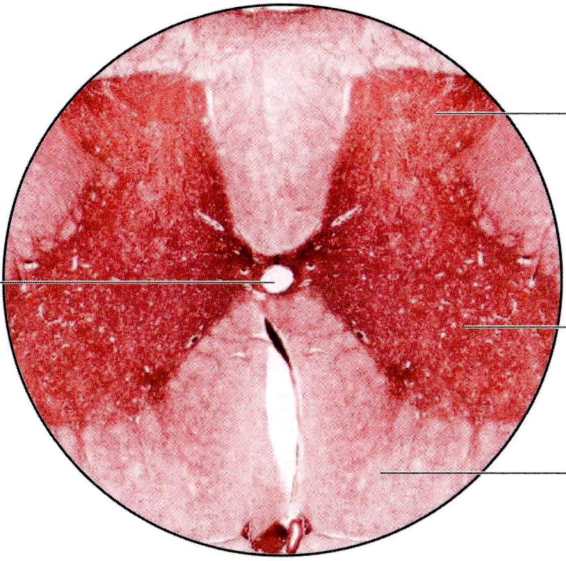

Nervous Tissue

| PHOTOMICROGRAPH |

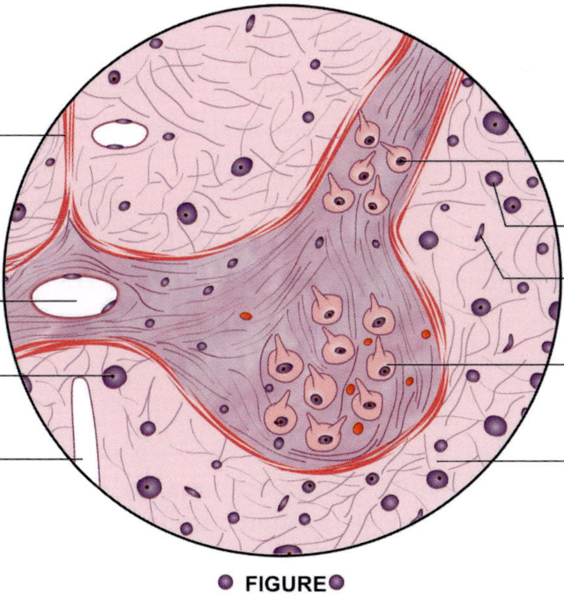

Labels: Central canal, Posterior horn, Grey matter of anterior horn cells, White matter

| FIGURE |

Labels: Posterior median septum, Central canal, Astrocyte, Anterior median fissure, Posterior horn with sensory neurons, Oligodendrocyte, Microglia, Anterior horn with motor neurons, White matter

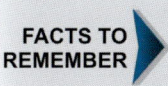

FACTS TO REMEMBER
1. Inner grey matter contains cell bodies of neurons
2. Outer white matter contains processes of neurons and neuroglial cells
3. Central canal lies in the grey commissure

Fig. 6.2: *Neuron and neuroglia: Spinal cord. Stain: Haematoxylin-eosin, 100X*

Microglia: Phagocytose cellular debris.

Ependymal cells: Line the central canal of spinal cord and ventricles of brain.

Satellite or capsular cells: Surround the neurons of the ganglia.

Schwann cells: Lay down myelin sheath on peripheral nerves.

ASTROCYTES

These are star-shaped cells with multiple processes. These cells are small with large vesicular indented nuclei, and cytoplasm drawn into number of processes. Development is from neural crest. These are of two types.

i. Protoplasmic astrocytes have thick processes with abundant granular cytoplasm. Some of the processes are attached to neighbouring capillaries by perivascular sucker feet. These sucker feet withdraw nutrition from them for transmission to the neuron. These are found in the grey matter (Figs 6.1 to 6.3).

ii. Fibrous astrocytes have long and straight processes which are seen only in the white matter.

Functions

Astrocytes form a supporting framework for the neurons.

They provide nourishment to the metabolically active neuronal processes.

These support metabolic exchange between the neurons and the capillaries of the central nervous system.

These also control chemical environment around neurons by removing excessive potassium ions and neurotransmitters like glutamate.

The astrocytes also contain glycogen and thus provide energy.

If brain is injured, these cells proliferate to form a scar.

OLIGODENDROCYTES

These cells have fewer and shorter processes, with no sucker feet. These make up three-fourth of the glial cells. These are smaller than astrocytes with deep basophilic round or oval nuclei, prominent nucleoli and abundant cytoplasm. Oligodendrocytes are present both in the grey and white matter. In the grey matter these are perineuronal in position. In the white matter these cells lie along the myelinated nerve fibre. These cells also develop from neural crest (Figs 6.2 and 6.3).

Function

The primary function of each cell is to lay down myelin sheath around the several axons within the central nervous system. Because of the myelin sheath formation these cells provide insulation and prevent formation of random synapses. Oligodendrocytes/oligodendroglia also support the neuronal network.

Nervous Tissue

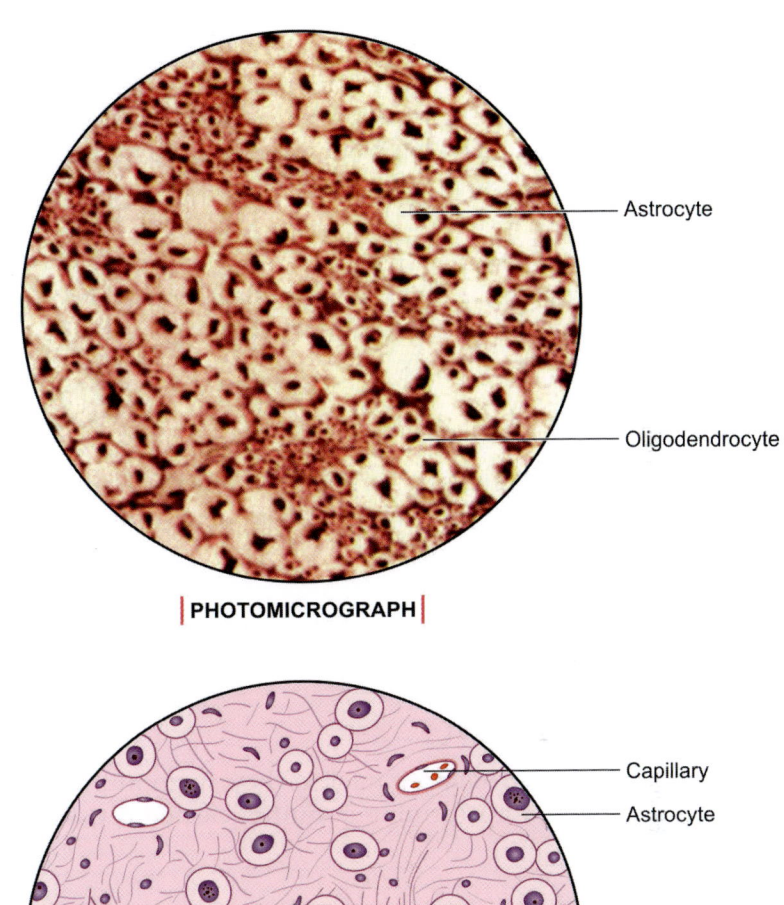

PHOTOMICROGRAPH

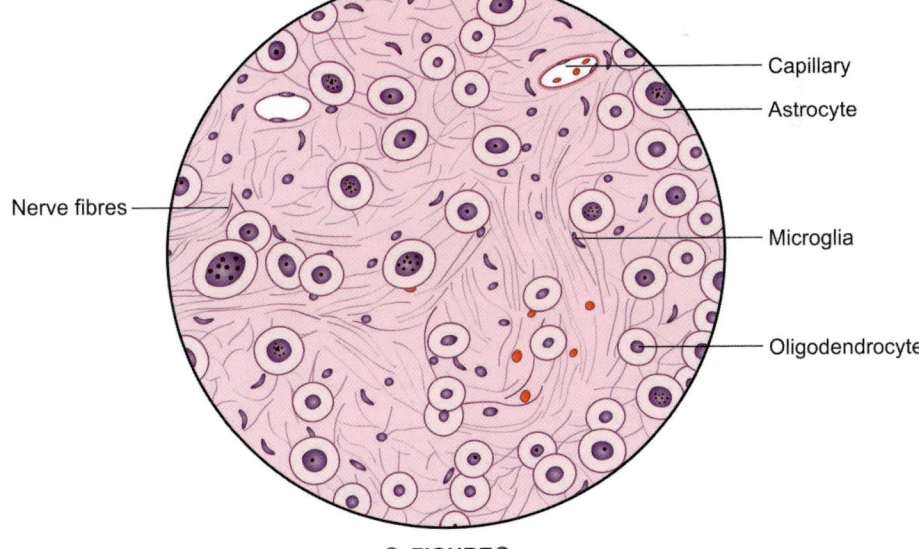

FIGURE

FACTS TO REMEMBER
1. Nerve fibres seen
2. Neuroglial cells, i.e. astrocytes, oligodendrocyte and microglial cells seen
3. Capillaries also seen

Fig. 6.3: *White matter of spinal cord. Stain: Haematoxylin-eosin, 100X*

MICROGLIA

These are smallest of the neuroglia and are present both in the grey and white matter. The nuclei of microglial cells are small, comma shaped, deeply stained and surrounded by scanty cytoplasm. They develop from mesoderm (Figs 6.1 to 6.3).

Function

These cells act as scavenger cells. In trauma or other destructive lesions of the central nervous system, the microglia show phagocytic activity. These form brains immune system. These also function as antigen-presenting cells. Also secrete cytokines which are immunoregulatory in function.

EPENDYMAL CELLS

These are tall columnar ciliated cells. These cells line the ventricles of the brain and the central canal of spinal cord. They develop from neural tube (Fig. 6.2).

Function

In the ventricles of brain the ependymal cells secrete cerebrospinal fluid. A small amount of CSF is also secreted by ependymal cells lining the central canal of spinal cord.

SATELLITE OR CAPSULAR CELLS

These are flat cells with prominent nuclei. They surround the neurons of the spinal and autonomic ganglia, thus forming a multinucleated capsule for these irreparable cells.

Function

Support and protect the neurons.

SCHWANN CELLS

These are derivatives of neural crest. The nucleus of a Schwann cell is flattened, surrounded by abundant cytoplasm.

It is responsible for laying down myelin sheath over a segment of a single axon after it indents into the Schwann cell. Myelin is stained with osmium tetroxide.

Function

These cells form myelin sheath in the peripheral nerves, thus protecting and insulating them. Due to the presence of myelin sheath the passage of impulse is faster as the rate of conduction is directly proportional to the thickness of the myelin.

Applied Aspect

- *Ependymomas*: Within the brain and spinal cord there are glial cells which support and protect the nerve cells. Tumor of these glial cells are called glioma. Ependymomas are rare type of glioma. These develop from the ependymal cells

which line the ventricles (fluid filled spaces in the brain) and from the central canal of the spinal cord. These can also be found in any parts of the brain, and are partially common in the cerebellum in children. They are the second most common spinal tumor.
- *Gliosis* is the diffuse proliferation of neuroglial cells.

NERVE FIBRES

A peripheral nerve fibre (Fig. 6.4) is an axon/dendron with its covering, i.e. myelin sheath and neurilemma. These fibres are myelinated. Each fibre consists of:
  i. A central axon/axis cylinder with axoplasm and neurofibrils contained within the axolemma.
  ii. Myelin sheath is composed of phospholipids, interrupted at intervals along with the length of the fibre. It is stained by osmic acid and not by H & E stain.
  iii. Thin neurilemma sheath is present outside the myelin sheath. The cells of neurilemma are also known as Schwann cells, which are neuroectodermal in origin. At the points of interruption of myelin sheath the neurilemma comes into intimate contact with the axon and such areas are known as Nodes of Ranvier. The impulse jumps from one node to the next node.
  iv. Endoneurium is a thin connective tissue layer of mesodermal origin. It supports the nerve fibres. The potential space between neurilemma and endoneurium contains tissue fluid for the nourishment of the nerve fibre.

NERVE TRUNK

Transverse section of nerve trunk shows that it is surrounded by connective tissue sheath called *epineurium*. It sends in septa dividing the nerve trunk into various fascicles, each of which is surrounded by a dense sheath, the *perineurium*. From the perineurium, numerous septa extend to form a sheath enclosing each nerve fibre. This sheath is known as *endoneurium*. This connective tissue skeleton supports the nerve fibres and carries capillaries with them.

In transverse sections stained with osmic acid (Fig. 6.5) myelin sheath is stained black and neurilemma as well as axis cylinder (axon) remain unstained. With haematoxylin and eosin stain (Fig. 6.6), the neurilemma and the axis cylinder are stained pink, whereas the area occupied by myelin sheath is observed as halo or unstained space.

Applied Aspect

- *Bell's palsy* is the compression of a facial nerve in or just outside stylomastoid foramen due to inflammation and oedema of the nerve. This causes paralysis of facial muscles and loss of facial expression on the affected side.
- *Acute idiopathic inflammatory polyneuropathy (Guillain-Barré syndrome)* is a sudden, acute and progressive bilateral ascending paralysis which starts at the lower limb and then spreads to arms, trunks and cranial nerves. It is characterised by widespread inflammation with some demyelination of spinal, peripheral and cranial nerves and the spinal ganglia.

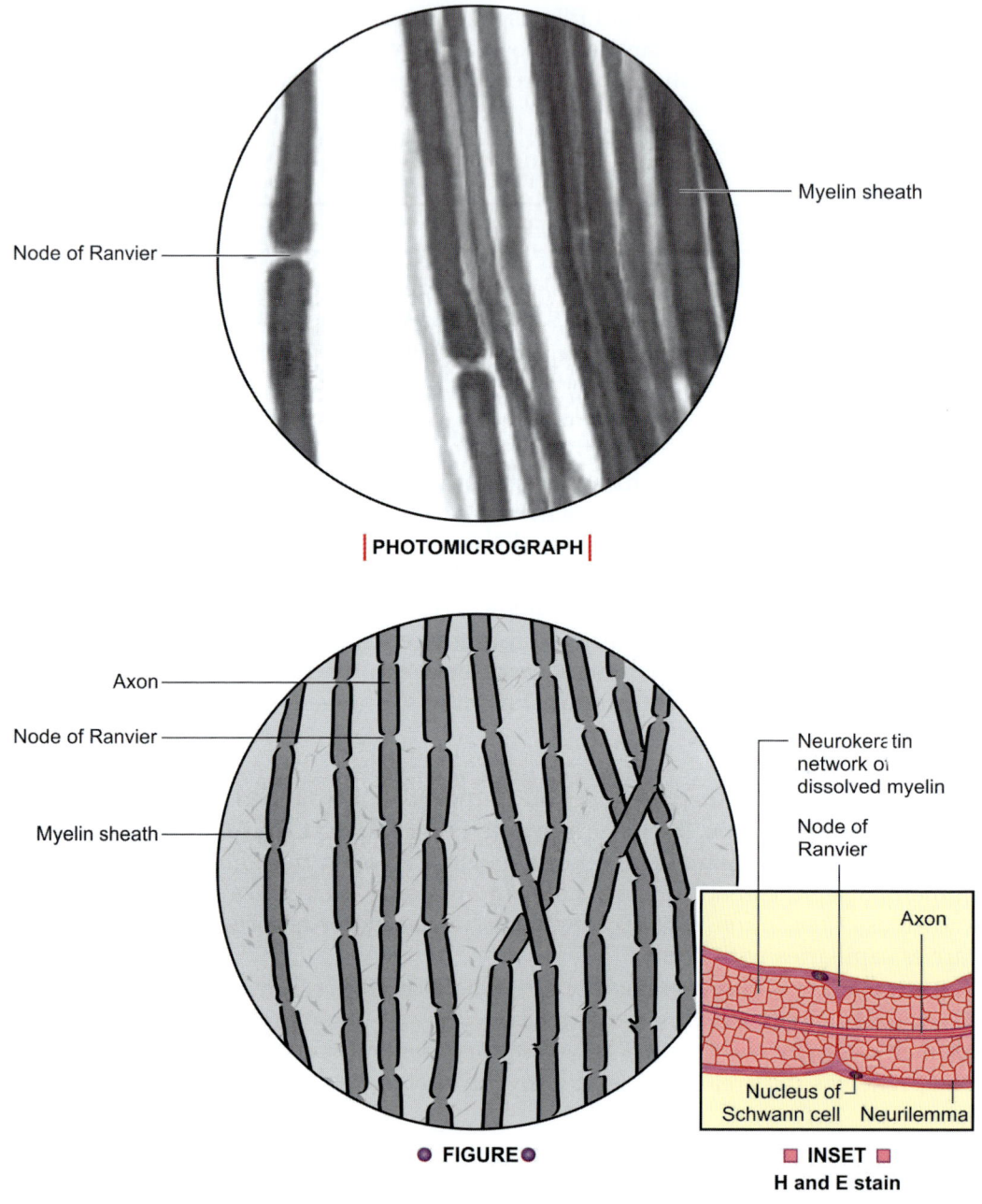

Fig. 6.4: *Longitudinal section of myelinated nerve fibres: Stain: Osmic acid, 100X*

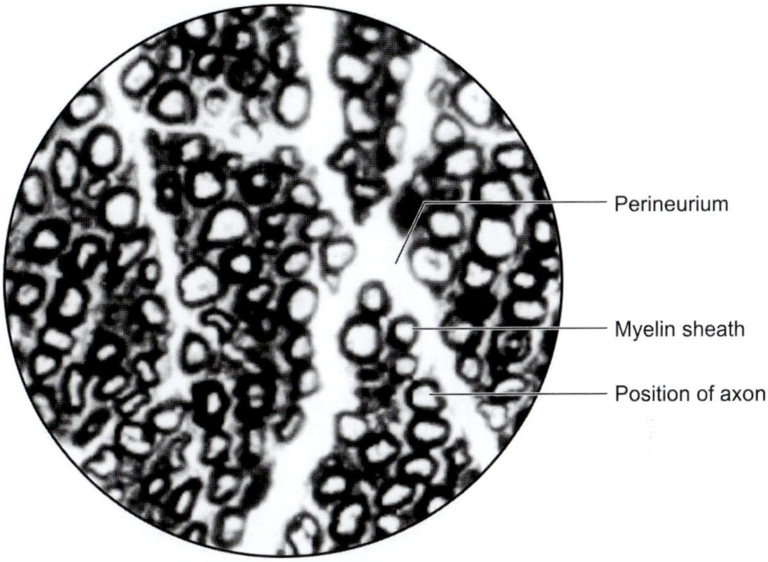

Nervous Tissue

PHOTOMICROGRAPH

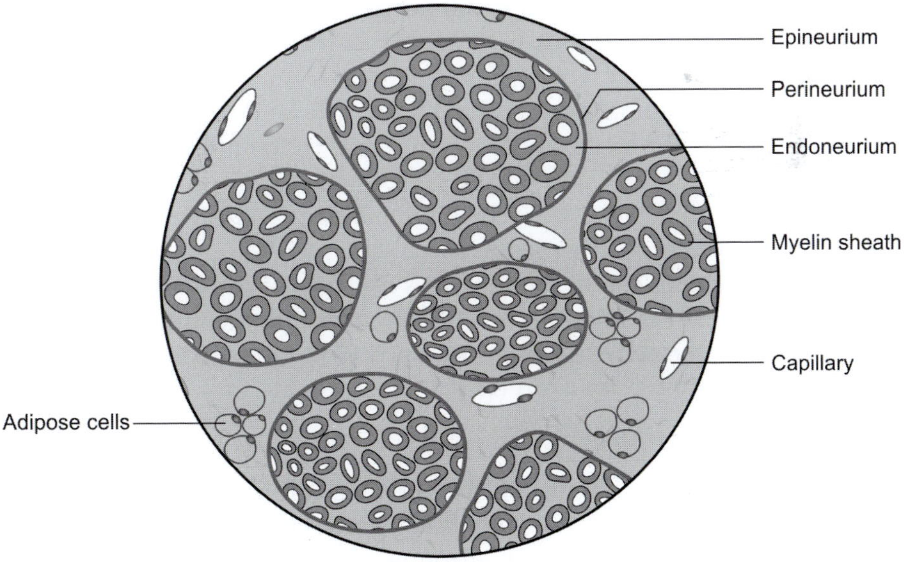

- Perineurium
- Myelin sheath
- Position of axon

FIGURE

- Epineurium
- Perineurium
- Endoneurium
- Myelin sheath
- Capillary
- Adipose cells

FACTS TO REMEMBER
1. Osmic acid preferentially stains the myelin sheath
2. Around each nerve fibre is endoneurium; around each nerve fasciculus is perineurium; and around the nerve is the epineurium
3. These support the nerve fibres

Fig. 6.5: *Transverse section of nerve trunk. Stain: Osmic acid, 100X*

- *Neuropathies* is a group of diseases of peripheral nerve. It is of two types:
  - *Polyneuropathy*: Several neurons are affected and usually long neurons like those supplying the feet and legs are affected first. This occurs mostly due to nutritional deficiencies (folic acid and vitamin B), metabolic disorders (diabetes mellitus), chronic diseases (renal and hepatic failure and carcinoma), infections (influenza, measles and typhoid fever) and toxic reactions (arsenic, lead, mercury and carbon tetrachloride)
  - *Mononeuropathy*: Usually one neuron is affected and most common cause is ischaemia due to pressure. The resultant dysfunction depends on site and degree of injury.
- *Traumatic neuroma* is a tumour like cluster formed by Schwann cells when the neurilemma of two cut ends is out of position or destroyed by the sprouted axons. It causes severe pain and mostly occurs due to some fractures or amputation of limb.

PARTS OF THE NERVOUS SYSTEM

SPINAL CORD

The spinal cord comprises a central canal surrounded by grey matter. Around this grey matter is the white matter (Fig. 6.2). Table 6.2 shows the comparison between the grey matter and white matter.

Transverse section of spinal cord stained with H & E stain (Fig. 6.2)
1. The central canal is seen as an oval cavity lined by columnar ciliated epithelium (Fig. 6.2).
2. The large cells in the anterior horn depict multiple angles/corners; the angles representing the origin of its processes.
   The grey matter reveals the neuroglial cells and lots of capillaries.
3. The peripheral white matter contains the fibres, neuroglia and fewer capillaries. In transverse sections the nerve fibres appear as hollow circles (myelin unstained) with central dots representing the axon (Fig. 6.6).

Applied Aspect
- *Herniated disc*: Intervertebral disc of the vertebral column are composed of a tough outer fibrocartilage which encases an elastic central mass called **nucleus pulposus**. During strenuous exercise or exertion in young adults and progressively due to skeletal

TABLE 6.2: Comparison of grey matter and white matter

Grey matter	White matter
1. Contains bodies of nerve cells	Bodies of nerve cells are absent
2. Has parts of dendrites and parts of the axon	Has most of the lengths of axon and dendrites
3. Contains protoplasmic astrocytes, oligodendroglia and microglia	Contains fibrous astrocytes, oligodendroglia and microglia
4. Has numerous capillaries	Has fewer capillaries

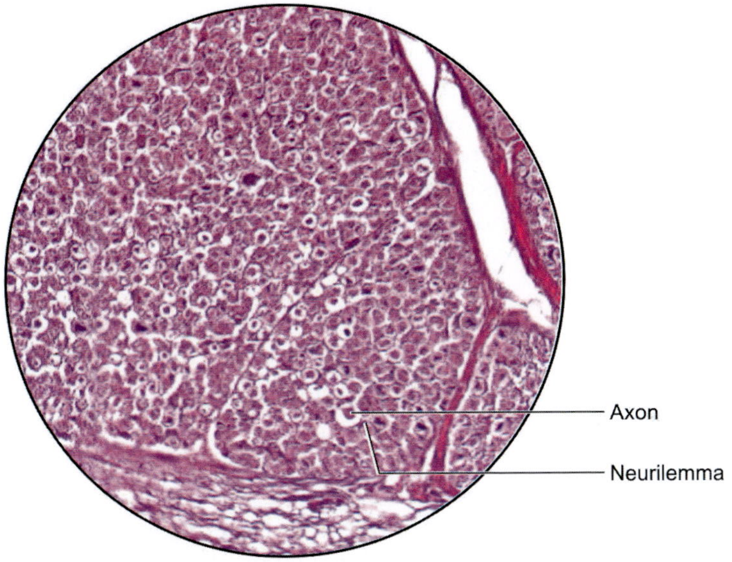

Nervous Tissue

|PHOTOMICROGRAPH|

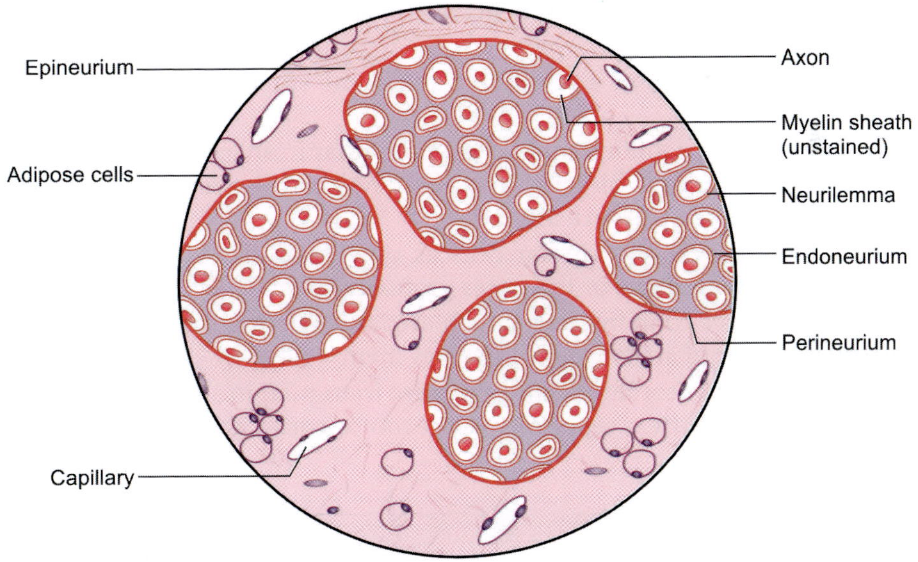

- Axon
- Neurilemma

FIGURE

- Epineurium
- Adipose cells
- Capillary
- Axon
- Myelin sheath (unstained)
- Neurilemma
- Endoneurium
- Perineurium

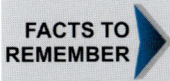

FACTS TO REMEMBER
1. The neurilemma is stained pink
2. The empty circle is the unstained myelin sheath
3. The inner structure is the stained axon

Fig. 6.6: *Transverse section of nerve trunk. Stain: Haematoxylin-eosin, 100X*

disease in older people there is herniation of nucleus pulposus into the vertebral canal. This may put pressure on the spinal nerve roots causing pain and numbness.
- *Syringomyelia* is the dilation of the central canal of the spinal cord. Dilation of central canal develops pressure which causes progressive damage to sensory and motor neurons. Early effects are insensibility to heat and pain (dissociated anaesthesia) and in long-term there is destruction of motor and sensory tracts leading to paralysis and loss of sensation and reflexes. This occurs most commonly in the cervical region and is associated with congenital abnormality of the distal end of the fourth ventricle.

GANGLIA

Collection of neurons outside the central nervous system is called ganglion. There are two types of ganglia, spinal and autonomic. These are compared in Table 6.3.

CEREBRUM

It is characterised by *heterotypical cortex*, i.e. histological structure differs in various regions of cerebral cortex. The outermost covering of the cerebral cortex is the pia mater which is the innermost meningeal layer. It carries capillaries to the grey matter. The cerebral cortex contains variety of cells. These are arranged in layers with one or more cell types predominant in each layer. The horizontal fibres are associated with each layer and give it a laminated appearance. From superficial to deep, the following six layers are seen:
1. Molecular layer consists of a few fibres and some spindle shaped or stellate cells (Fig. 6.9).
2. Outer granular layer contains small cells, triangular in shape, with an apex directed peripherally and the base directed inwards. The axons leave from the basal part of the cell. A few stellate cells are also seen.
3. Outer pyramidal layer has similar cells as outer granular layer, but the cells are distinctly larger than those of the outer granular layer.
4. Inner granular layer contains cells which are larger than outer pyramidal cells, but have large number of stellate cells between them.
5. Inner pyramidal layer contains cells which are triangular in shape and are the largest cells of the cerebral cortex, especially in the motor cortex where these are termed as the Betz cells.

TABLE 6.3: Comparison of the ganglia

Dorsal root ganglion or sensory or Spinal ganglion (Fig. 6.7)	Sympathetic ganglion or Autonomic ganglion (Fig. 6.8)
1. Consists of pseudounipolar neurons	Consists of multipolar neurons
2. Has cell bodies of afferent neurons	Has cell bodies of efferent neurons
3. The cell body is large and rounded	The cell body is smaller and irregular
4. The nucleus is central with a prominent nucleolus	The nucleus is usually eccentric and has a prominent nucleolus
5. Around each neuron is a layer of flattened cells called capsular/satellite cells	Such capsular/satellite cells are a few in number
6. The neurons lie in groups separated by nerve fibres lying in groups	The neurons and nerve fibres lie scattered

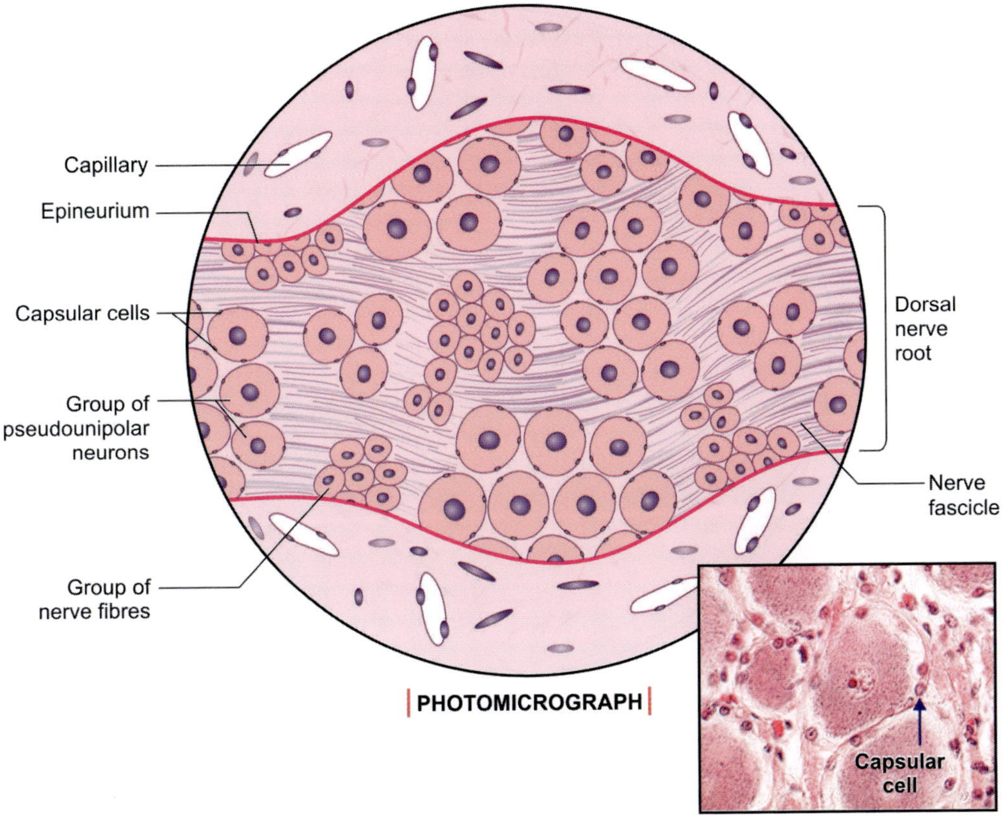

Nervous Tissue

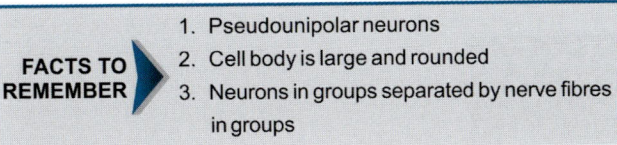

| PHOTOMICROGRAPH |

INSET — Capsular cell

FACTS TO REMEMBER
1. Pseudounipolar neurons
2. Cell body is large and rounded
3. Neurons in groups separated by nerve fibres in groups

Fig. 6.7: *Spinal/sensory/dorsal root ganglion. Stain: Haematoxylin-eosin, 400X*

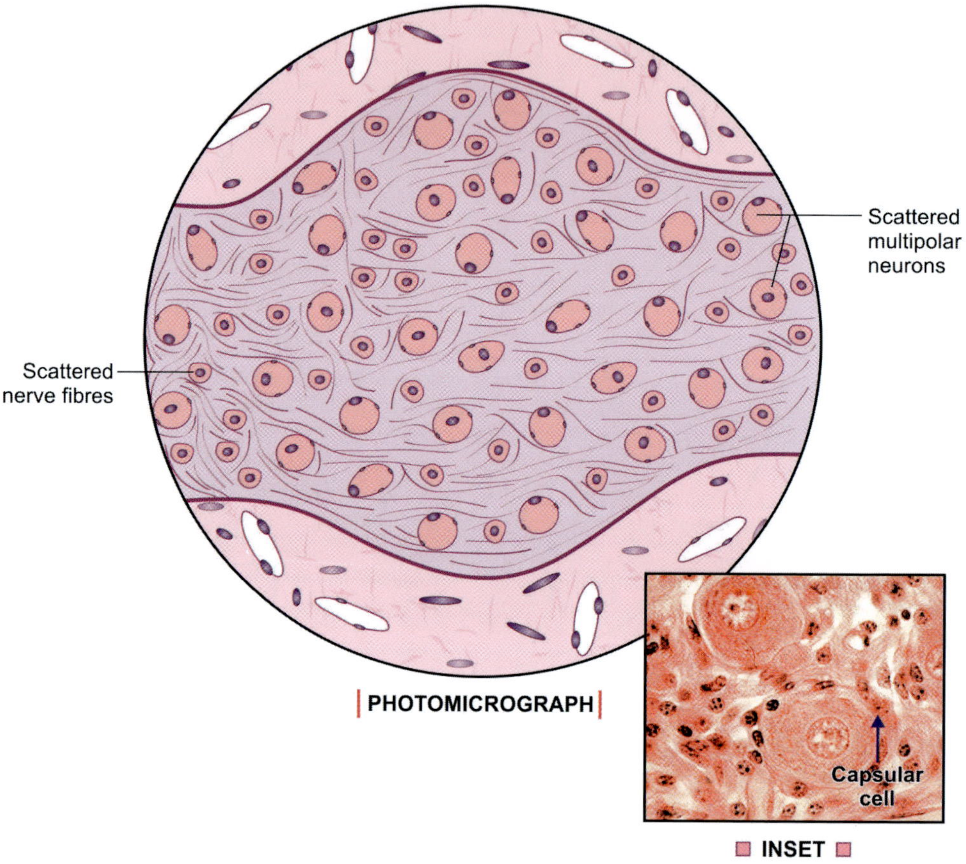

Scattered multipolar neurons

Scattered nerve fibres

| PHOTOMICROGRAPH |

Capsular cell

■ INSET ■

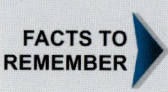

FACTS TO REMEMBER
1. Multipolar neurons
2. Cell body is small and irregular
3. Neurons and nerve fibres are scattered

Fig. 6.8: *Autonomic ganglion. Stain: Haematoxylin-eosin, 400X*

Nervous Tissue

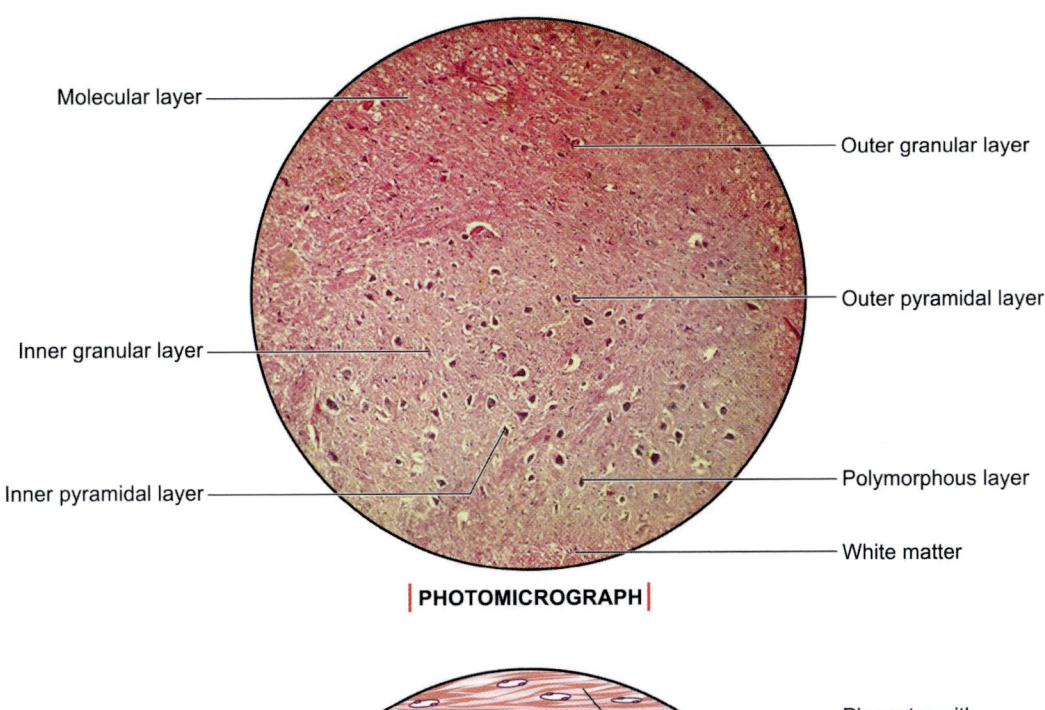

PHOTOMICROGRAPH

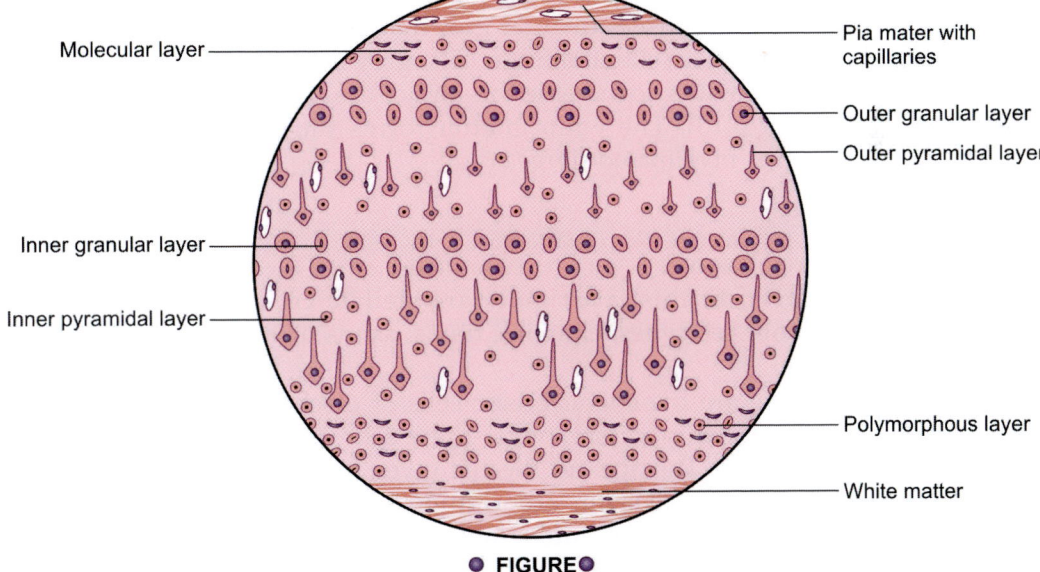

FIGURE

FACTS TO REMEMBER
1. Six layers of cells and fibres
2. Pyramidal cells more in motor cortex and granular cells more in sensory cortex
3. Numerous capillaries present

Fig. 6.9: *Grey matter of cerebrum. Stain: Haematoxylin-eosin, 400X*

6. Fusiform layer or polymorphous layer contains mainly fusiform cells with a few stellate cells. No pyramidal cells are seen in this layer.

The *granular cell* layers are *afferent* in connection and the *pyramidal* cell layers are *efferent* in nature. The pyramidal cells are more pronounced in the motor areas, whereas the granular cells are more conspicuous in the sensory areas of the brain. In between the nerve cells are the nerve fibres of these cells and capillaries. The neuroglial elements are protoplasmic astrocytes, oligodendroglia and microglia.

Applied Aspect

- *Aphasia* is a disorder of language (speech) that results from damage to that portion of the brain which are responsible for language (Wernicke's area and Broca's area). It usually occurs suddenly often as the result of a stroke or head injury. But it may develop slowly as in the case of a brain tumour.
- *Dementia* is the progressive, irreversible degeneration and atrophy of the cerebral cortex. This causes mental retardation usually over several years. It is also characterised by gradual impairment of memory, intellect and reasoning.

CEREBELLUM

The histological structure of entire cerebellum is similar and is called **homotypical cortex**. The cerebellar cortex shows many deep folds called **cerebellar folia**, separated by fissures. The cerebellum consists of outer grey matter and inner white matter. The white matter is made up of myelinated fibres. The grey matter is greatly folded over the central core of white matter to increase the surface area. The appearance is known as the *arbor vitae* (Fig. 6.10). The white matter forms the core of each folium of cerebellum. It comprises myelinated fibres.

Layers of Grey Matter

It is composed of three layers:
1. *Outer molecular layer*: In this layer there are stellate cells, basket cells, axons and dendrites of both cell types, climbing fibres, axons of granule and Golgi cells (Table 6.4).
2. *Purkinje's cells*: These are the characteristic cells of cerebellum at the junction of outer molecular and inner granular layers. These cells lie in a single row and have flask shaped cell bodies. The apex of the cell gives rise to many dendrites which branch repeatedly to form dendritic arborisations. From the base of the cell arises an axon that passes through the granular layer and becomes myelinated as it enters the white matter (Table 6.5).

TABLE 6.4: Showing types of neurons in cerebellum

Layers	Neurons	Population
Outer molecular layer	Stellate cells, Basket cells	Sparse cells in this zone
Purkinje's cell layer	Purkinje's cells are characteristic cerebellar neurons	In single layer at the junction of molecular and granular layers
Granular cell layer	Granule cell, Golgi cell	Densely populated zone

Nervous Tissue

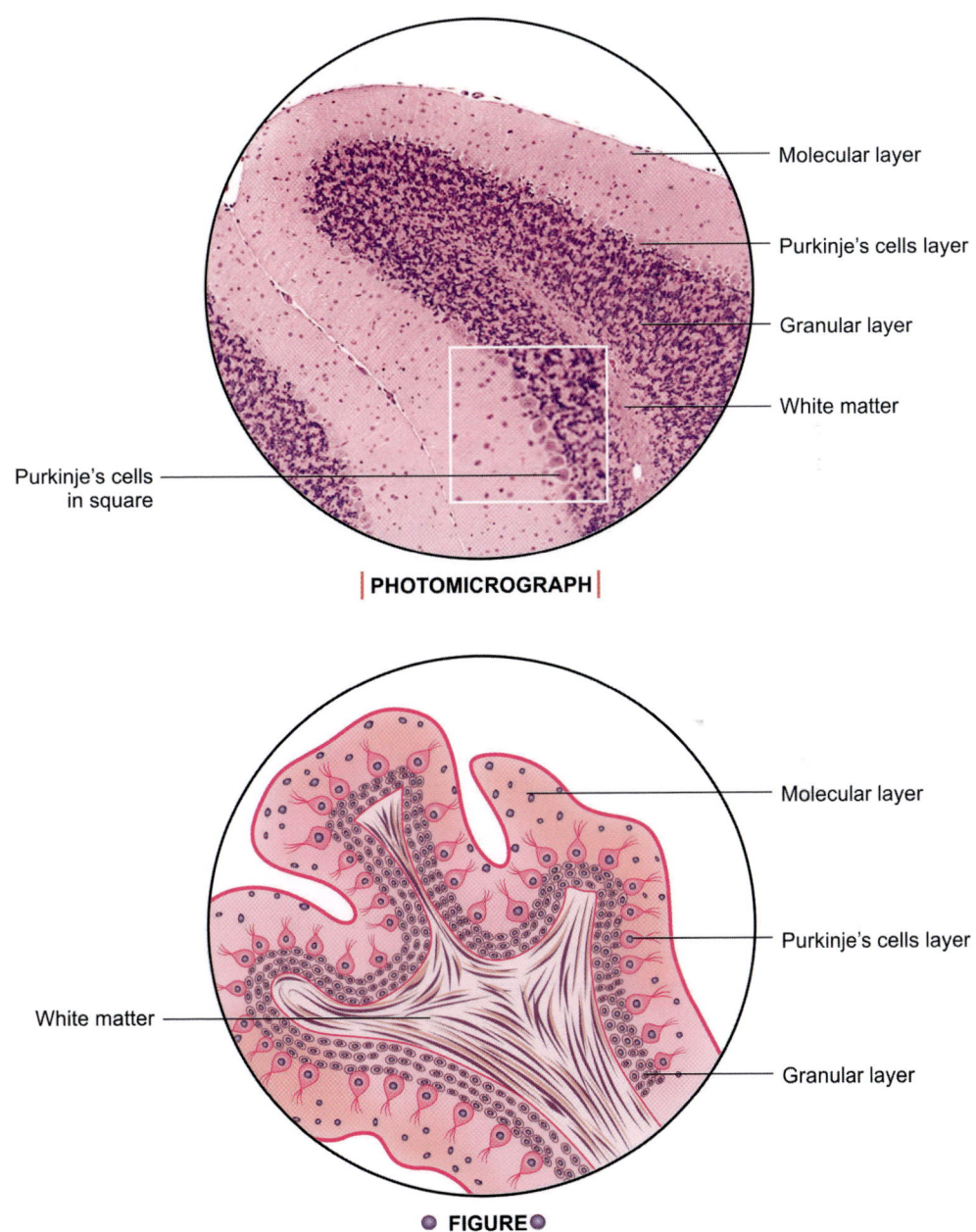

Fig. 6.10: *Structure of cerebellum cortex. Stain: Haematoxylin-eosin, 100X*

TABLE 6.5: Depicting connections of various neurons

Neuron and its placement	Course of dendrites	Course of axon
Purkinje's cells at the junction of molecular and granular layers (Fig. 6.11)	Lie in molecular layer and subdivide to form a dendritic tree. The dendrites of each Purkinje's cell lie in plane parallel to each other	Travels through the granular layer to enter the nuclei in the white matter
Granule cells in deep part of granular layer	4–6 short dendrites which synapse with **mossy** fibres in granular layer	Axon passes upwards in the molecular layer (neuron lying upside down); divides into two subdivisions which run in opposite directions (T-shaped). These subdivisions of axon are termed as parallel fibres and synapse with dendrites of Purkinje's cell
Outer stellate cell confined to the molecular layer	Synapse with parallel fibres (axons of granule cells)	Synapses with dendrites of Purkinje's cell
Basket cells in deeper part of molecular layer	Ramify in molecular layer synapsing with parallel fibres (axons of granule cells)	Form baskets around the cell bodies of Purkinje's cell
Golgi cells in superficial part of granular layer	Synapses with axons of granule cells (parallel fibres) in molecular layer	Ends in relation to dendrites of granule cells to form the glomeruli in granular layer

3. *Inner granular layer*: It contains numerous small Golgi and granule cells with dark staining nuclei and scanty cytoplasm. There are also large stellate cells which have more cytoplasm.

White Matter

The core of white matter is formed by myelinated nerve fibres or axons. The axons are afferent and efferent fibres of the cerebellar cortex.

The afferent connections of cerebellum are through **mossy** and **climbing** fibres. Mossy fibres constitute all the afferents except those of olivo-cerebellar fibres. Mossy fibres synapse with granule and Golgi cells (Table 6.5). Olivo-cerebellar fibres climb up and make synaptic connections with dendrites of Purkinje's cells and are called climbing fibres (Fig. 6.11).

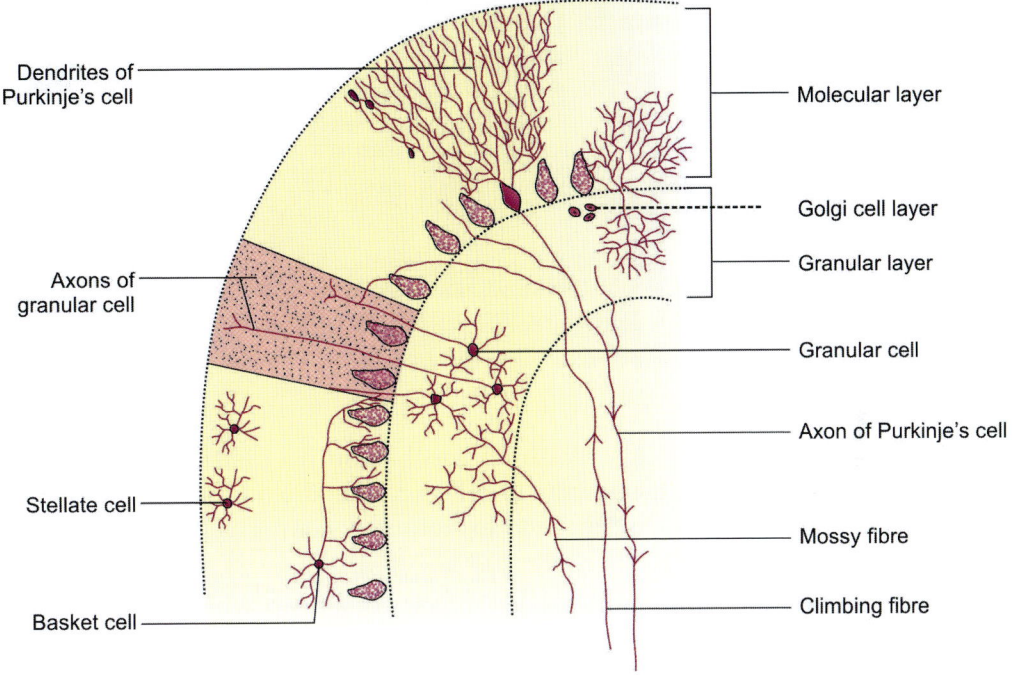

Fig. 6.11: *Schematic figure to show layers and fibres of cerebellar cortex*

MULTIPLE CHOICE QUESTIONS

1. Which cell forms myelin sheath on peripheral nerves?
   a. Astrocyte
   b. Microglia
   c. Schwann's cell
   d. Oligodendrocyte

2. Myelin sheath in CNS is laid down by:
   a. Astrocyte
   b. Oligodendrocyte
   c. Schwann's cell
   d. Ependymal cell

3. Spinal/sensory ganglion contains the following type of neuron:
   a. Multipolar neuron
   b. Bipolar neuron
   c. Unipolar neuron
   d. Pseudounipolar neuron

4. White matter contains all *except*:
   a. Astrocyte
   b. Neuronal cell body
   c. Oligodendrocyte
   d. Microglia

5. All are layers of cerebellum *except*:
   a. Molecular layer
   b. Purkinje's cell layer
   c. Granular layer
   d. Betz cell layer

ANSWERS

1. c   2. b   3. d   4. b
5. d

Blood Vessels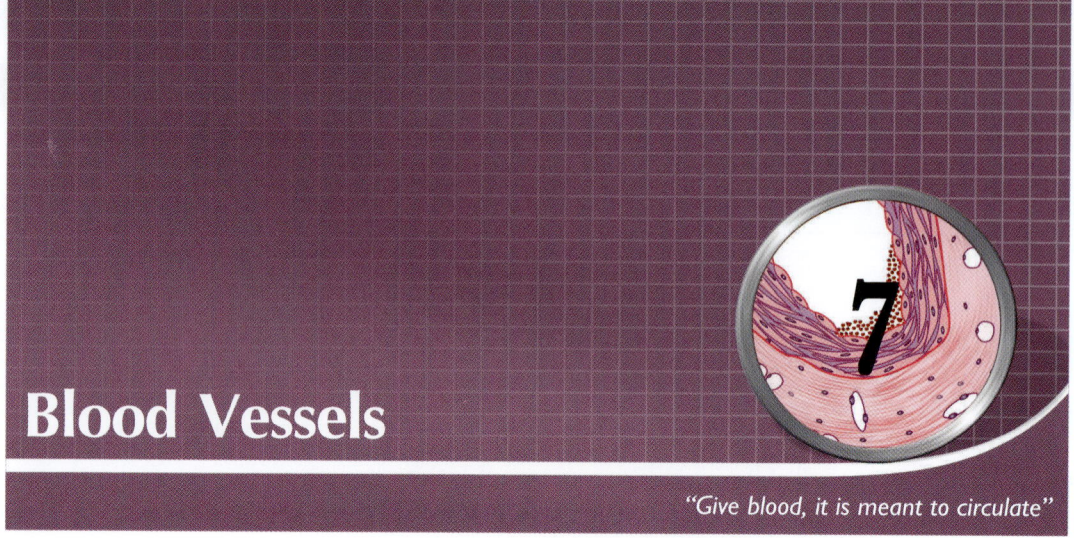

"Give blood, it is meant to circulate"

All animals and human beings require a mechanism to distribute oxygen and nutritive materials to the tissues and to collect carbon dioxide and waste products of tissue metabolism and transmit these to excretory system. This is all done by the blood vascular system.

Blood vascular system and lymph vessels consists of a heart which is the muscular pump and various types of blood vessels and lymph vessels. The latter are described in Chapter 8. The structure of heart has been described as cardiac muscle in Chapter 5.

The various types of blood vessels are (1) Arteries, (2) Capillaries, (3) Sinusoids, (4) Veins. This chapter gives histology of Arteries and Veins.

ARTERIES

Arteries are classified as:

a. Elastic or large sized arteries, e.g. aorta (Fig. 7.1)

b. Muscular or medium sized arteries, e.g. brachial, radial, popliteal.

c. Arterioles—smallest divisions of arteries with a diameter of 100 micron

A. ELASTIC ARTERIES

During systole, the elastic artery expands to accommodate increased amount of blood. During diastole of the heart, there is elastic recoil of the artery, so there is continuous blood flow to the peripheral parts of the body. Since these arteries have abundant elastic fibres in their walls, these are named elastic arteries. The lumen of the artery is surrounded by the three concentric coats (i) tunica intima, (ii) tunica media, and (iii) tunica adventitia.

i. The tunica intima consists of an endothelium, subendothelial connective tissue and an internal elastic lamina.

The **endothelium** is a thin layer, made up of flattened cells, lining the luminal surface of the artery. These cells rest on a basement membrane.

Blood Vessels

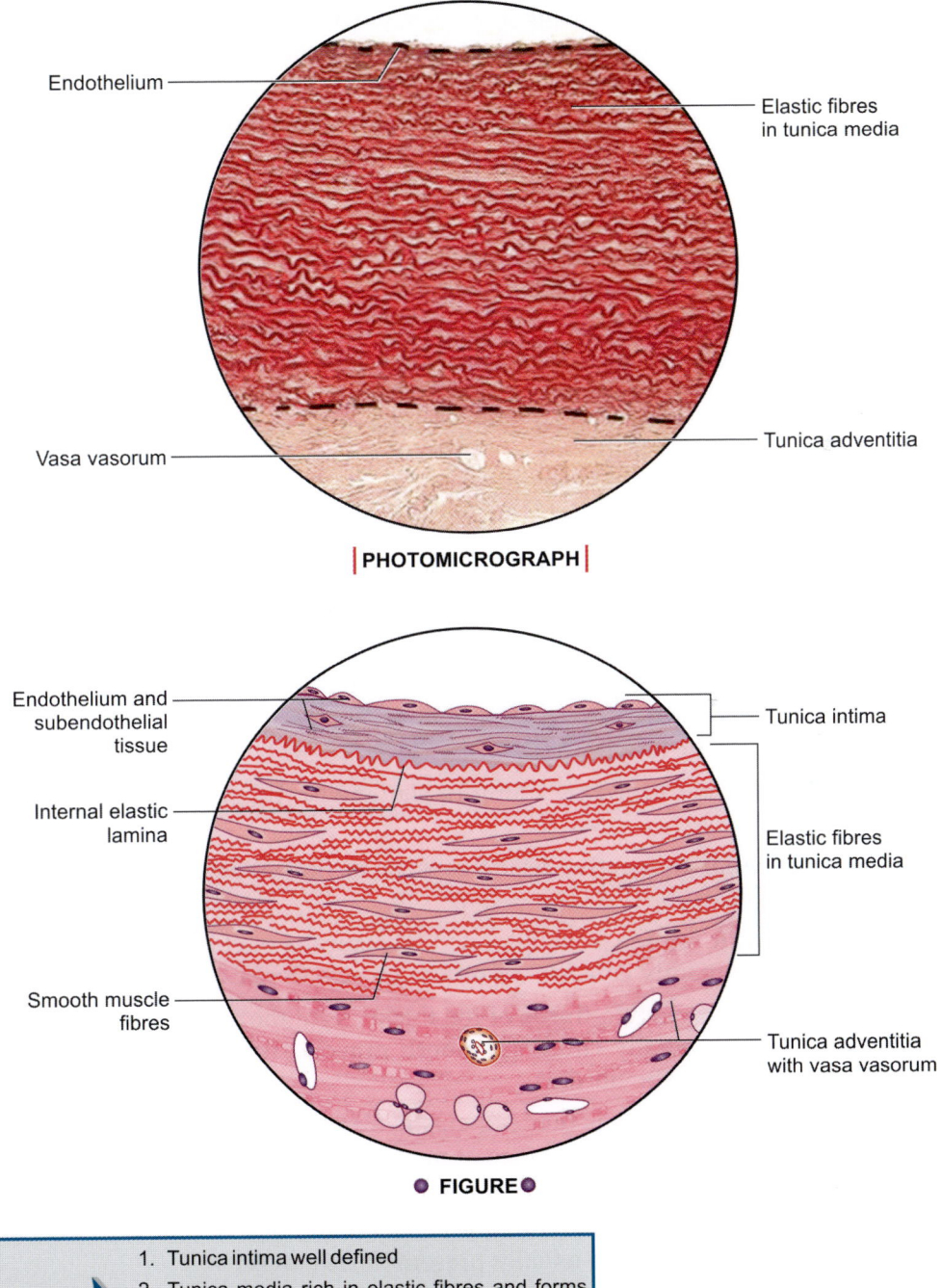

Facts to Remember
1. Tunica intima well defined
2. Tunica media rich in elastic fibres and forms 2/3rd thickness of arterial wall
3. Tunica adventitia comprises 1/3rd thickness of arterial wall

Fig. 7.1: *Layers of elastic artery. Stain: Haematoxylin-eosin, 100X*

Subendothelial connective tissue is a loose narrow layer containing elastic and collagen fibres along with nuclei of fibroblasts and macrophages.

The **internal elastic lamina** is the limiting layer of tunica intima and is made up of fenestrated elastic fibres. The internal elastic lamina is not prominent as the elastic fibres merge with the elastic laminae of the tunica media.

ii. The tunica media or middle layer is the thickest and is dominated by concentric laminae of elastic fibres with smooth muscle fibres. It comprises two-thirds of the arterial wall. The outer layer of the tunica is the **external elastic lamina,** made up of elastic fibres, which is not so conspicuous.

iii. The tunica adventitia is a layer of collagen fibres, elastic fibres and fibroblasts. It contains a few arterioles called **vasa vasorum** which nourish the tunica adventitia and outer two-thirds of tunica media, the rest being nourished by the blood flowing through the lumen of the vessels. Tunica adventitia comprises one-third of the thickness of the arterial wall.

B. MUSCULAR ARTERIES

These arteries control the amount of blood flowing through them according to the activity of the part.

It consists of a lumen surrounded by same three concentric coats (i) tunica intima, (ii) tunica media, and (iii) tunica adventitia (Fig. 7.2).

i. The **tunica intima** consists of an endothelium, subendothelial connective tissue and an internal elastic lamina.

The **endothelium** is formed by lining of flattened cells, resting on a basement membrane.

The **subendothelial connective tissue** consists of fine collagen and elastic fibres as well as fibroblasts.

The **internal elastic lamina** is well defined. The lamina of elastic fibres stands out well as the media mainly consists of smooth muscle fibres.

ii. The **tunica media** forms two-thirds of the thickness of the arterial wall. It is made up of circularly or spirally running **smooth muscle fibres**. Among the muscle fibres are scattered elastic fibres.

The **external elastic lamina** is made of elastic fibres and is better defined than in an elastic artery due to predominance of muscle fibres in the tunica media.

iii. The **tunica adventitia** is a well defined layer comprising nearly **one-third** of the thickness of the arterial wall. It contains collagen and elastic fibres. Arterioles in the form of **vasa vasorum** are usually present in this layer.

C. ARTERIOLES

These are the smallest divisions of the arteries which have a diameter of **100 micron**. These act as resistance vessels to maintain peripheral blood pressure. Three concentric coats surrounding the lumen are (i) tunica intima, (ii) tunica media, and (iii) tunica adventitia.

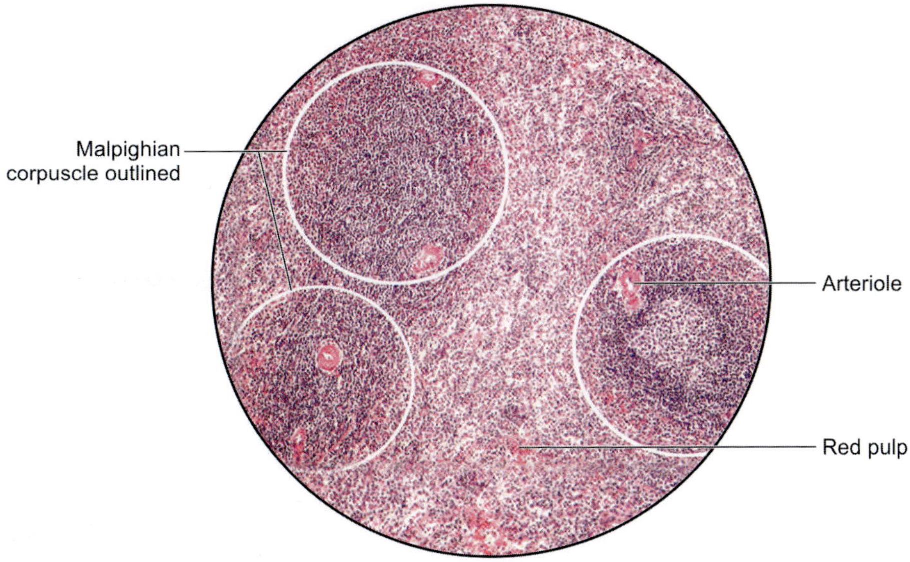

Lymphatic System

| PHOTOMICROGRAPH |

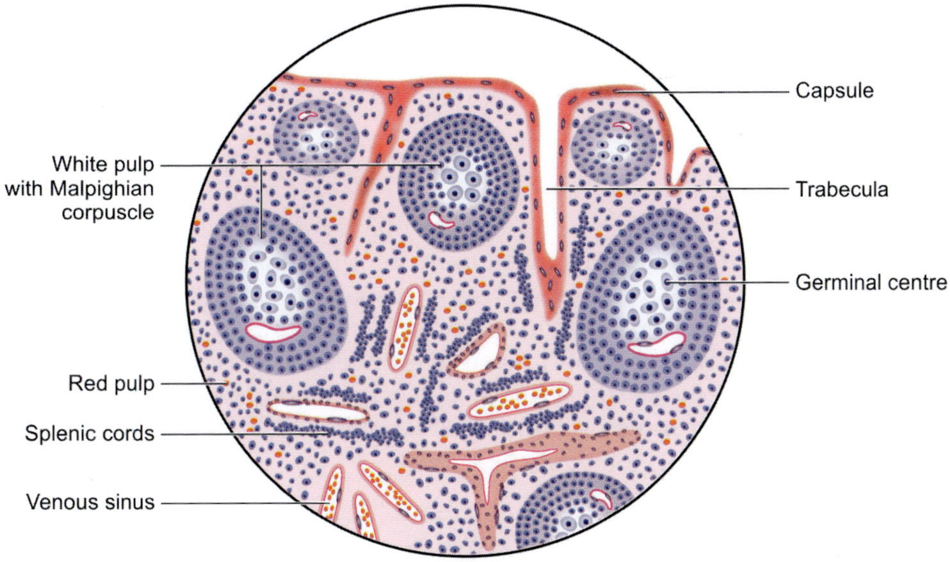

- Malpighian corpuscle outlined
- Arteriole
- Red pulp

| FIGURE |

- White pulp with Malpighian corpuscle
- Red pulp
- Splenic cords
- Venous sinus
- Capsule
- Trabecula
- Germinal centre

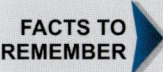
FACTS TO REMEMBER
1. Peritoneal squamous cells form outer covering
2. No differentiation into cortex and medulla
3. Red pulp and white pulp seen

Fig. 8.3: *Structure of spleen. Stain: Haematoxylin-eosin, 100X*

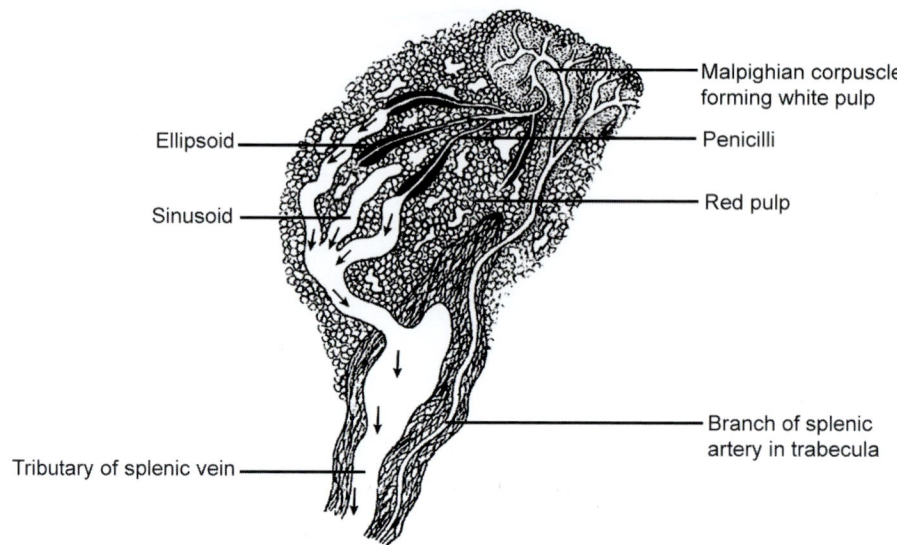

Fig. 8.4: *Splenic circulation (diagrammatic)*

2. The activated lymphocytes and antibodies produced in the spleen help in various immune/defence mechanisms of the body. It is the site of immune responses to antigens reaching it via blood.
3. Spleen produces RBC and granular series of WBC during foetal life. It is also a storehouse of blood.

Applied Aspect

- *Splenomegaly* is the enlargement of spleen mainly due to infections, circulatory disorders, blood diseases and malignant neoplasms. It causes excessive and premature haemolysis of red cells or phagocytosis of normal white cells and platelets which leads to anaemia, leukopenia and thrombocytopenia. Spleen also may enlarge due to congestion of blood in portal venous congestion in right-sided heart failure and in fibrosis caused due to cirrhosis of liver. Splenomegaly also occurs to meet the extra workload for removing damaged and abnormal blood cells.
  Commonest cause of splenomegaly is *malaria*.

THYMUS

Thymus is a lymphoepithelial lobulated organ that produces "T lymphocytes" and a lymphocyte stimulating hormone. Thymus involutes at puberty (Fig. 8.5). It is best developed in childhood. In adults it consists mainly of adipose tissue and Hassall's corpuscles. Table 8.1 shows comparison between 'T and B' lymphocytes.

STRUCTURE

It consists of a thin outer fibrous covering known as the capsule. From the capsule extend many thin connective tissue septa dividing it incompletely into various lobules. Each lobule has a peripheral darker cortex and a central lighter medulla. The

Lymphatic System

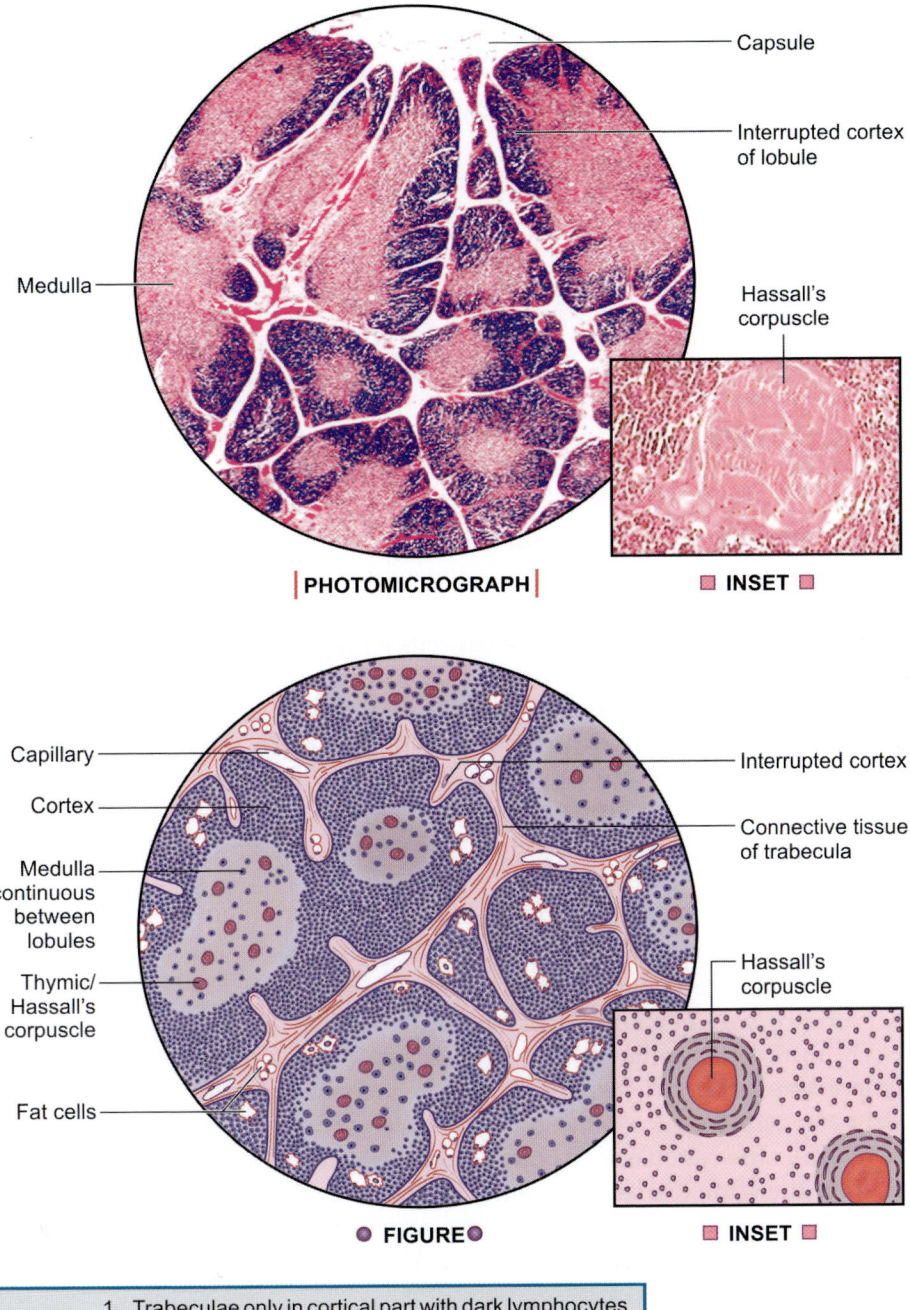

Facts to Remember
1. Trabeculae only in cortical part with dark lymphocytes
2. Medulla of adjacent lobules continuous and contains lighter reticular cells
3. Hassall's corpuscles made up of concentric lamellae of epithelial cells surrounding a hyaline mass

Fig. 8.5: *Structure of thymus of a child. Stain: Haematoxylin-eosin, 100X*

TABLE 8.1: Comparison of T and B lymphocytes

	T lymphocytes	B lymphocytes
1. Origin	Bone marrow → thymus	Bone marrow → bursa → lymphoid tissue
2. Location: lymph node	Perifollicular	Germinal centre
Spleen	Perifollicular	Germinal centre
Peyer's patches	Perifollicular	Germinal centre
3. Number in blood	80%	20%
4. Lifespan	Months to years	2–4 weeks
5. Function	Cell-mediated immunity via T cells	Humoral immunity via immunoglobulins

interlobular septa are partial and do not extend into the medulla, so that there is continuity of the medullary tissue of the various lobules.

Chief cells present in thymus are:

a. *Thymic lymphocytes*: These are situated in the interstices of the thymic reticulum. These cells develop in thymus (their precursors migrated from bone marrow to thymus) and are immunologically competent but uncommitted cells.

b. *Epithelial reticular cells*: These are flattened cells with pale nuclei. Their processes branch and lie in apposition with the processes of the adjoining cells forming thin membrane. These reticular cells develop from the endoderm of third pharyngeal pouch. These cells secrete hormones, thymosin, thymopoietin, thymulin and thymic humoral factor. These hormones are required for proliferation, differentiation, maturation of T lymphocytes. They also are necessary for expression of surface markers.

Haemothymic barrier: Between the blood capillaries of thymus and its cells there is a haemothymic barrier. This comprises:
- Endothelial lining of the capillaries
- Minimal perivascular space
- Epithelial membrane constituted by the epithelial reticular cells.

The difference between cortex and medulla is due to the varying proportion of lymphocyte to reticular cells in each. The cortex consists mainly of densely packed small lymphocytes with their dark nuclei and between them are relatively a few reticular cells with pale staining nuclei.

In the medulla the reticular cells outnumber the lymphocytes. The medulla is more vascular than the cortex. It also contains Hassall's corpuscles which are made up of concentric lamellae of epithelial cells around a central degenerated hyaline mass. These stain with acid dyes and increases with age. Thymus has only efferent lymphatics.

Functions of Thymus

It is a primary lymphoid organ actively functioning during childhood. Undifferentiated lymphocytes reach thymus from the bone marrow. It produces immunologically competent "T lymphocytes", helper T lymphocytes, cytotoxic T lymphocytes which settle in other lymphatic tissues.

Thymus controls lymphopoiesis and thus maintains the lymphocytic population in various lymphoid organs. It produces a hormone, i.e. *competence inducing factor* which imparts responsiveness to antigens in the newly formed lymphocytes. Thymus is essential till puberty, i.e. the time when the lymphatic tissues are fully developed. After puberty thymus involutes and production of T cells gets diminished. Since T lymphocyte progeny is established, immunity continues without the requirement of new 'T' cells.

Applied Aspect

- Enlargement of thymus may cause **myasthenia gravis**, which produces extreme weakness of the skeletal muscles. It may be treated by removal of enlarged thymus, or by drug treatment.
- It thymus gland is removed in a newborn, lymphoid organs will not receive T lymphocytes, which are immunocompetent. The infant may die during early years as he/she lacks the competence to kill the pathogens.

PALATINE TONSIL

It is a collection of paired lymphoid tissue at the oropharyngeal isthmus. Its oral aspect is covered by stratified squamous non-keratinised epithelium which dips into the underlying tissue to form crypts (Fig. 8.6). The lymphocytes lie beneath the epithelium and on the sides of the crypts. These are collected to form nodules. The germinal centre/secondary nodule may or may not be present. If present, these contain B lymphocytes, large lymphocytes and plasma cells. "T lymphocytes" are present in the perifollicular area. The serous and mucous acini are seen on the deeper aspect of tonsil. Their ducts open on the sides of crypts. The outer aspect is covered by a capsule (hemicapsule). The deep aspect of tonsil contains serous and mucous acini and sections of skeletal muscle fibres. Table 8.2 shows the comparison of lymph node, spleen, thymus and palatine tonsil.

Functional Aspect

- Palatine tonsils are one of the components of Waldeyer's ring of lymphoid tissue at the oropharyngeal isthmus. Others components are lingual, tubal and nasopharyngeal tonsils. All these try to prevent the entry of antigens and even attempt to destroy the antigens entering via nose and mouth.

Applied Aspect

- *Tonsillitis* is the inflammation of palatine tonsils, palatine arches and walls of pharynx caused by the viruses and *Streptococcus haemolyticus*. Severe infection may lead to suppuration and abscess formation which spreads into the neck causing cellulitis. Endotoxins released due to tonsillitis may cause rheumatic fever and glomerulonephritis.
- Repeated infection of palatine tonsils causes chronic inflammation, fibrosis and permanent enlargement. Thus the palatine tonsils themselves become a source of infection and may have to be removed.

TABLE 8.2: Comparison of the lymphatic organs

Features	Lymph node	Spleen	Thymus	Palatine tonsil
1. Outer covering	Connective tissue capsule with fat cells. Subcapsular sinus present	Connective tissue capsule covered with squamous epithelium of peritoneum	Thin connective tissue capsule	Connective tissue capsule on pharyngeal aspect is covered with stratified squamous non-keratinised epithelium, invaginating to form crypts
2. Lymph vessels	Both afferent and efferent lymph vessels	Only efferent lymph vessels	Only efferent lymph vessels	Only efferent lymph vessels
3. Trabeculae	Thin trabeculae all over	Abundant thick trabeculae with blood vessels	Trabeculae only in peripheral or cortical part	Occasional thin trabeculae from the capsule
4. Cortex	Contains well defined lymph nodules with central germinal centre	Not differentiated into cortex and medulla. Instead there is white pulp with lymphatic nodules and red pulp	Contains collections of dark staining lymphocytes, and a few endodermal epithelial cells	Not differentiated into cortex and medulla Lymphocytes aggregated as small follicles along the sides of crypts. Germinal centre seen in a few follicles
5. Medulla	Lymphocytes are arranged in cords around lymph sinuses. These cords are known as medullary cords	Absent instead there is white pulp and red pulp	Medulla of one lobule is continuous with that of the adjoining lobules. Epithelial cells are arranged concentrically to form Hassall's corpuscles	Absent

Lymphatic System

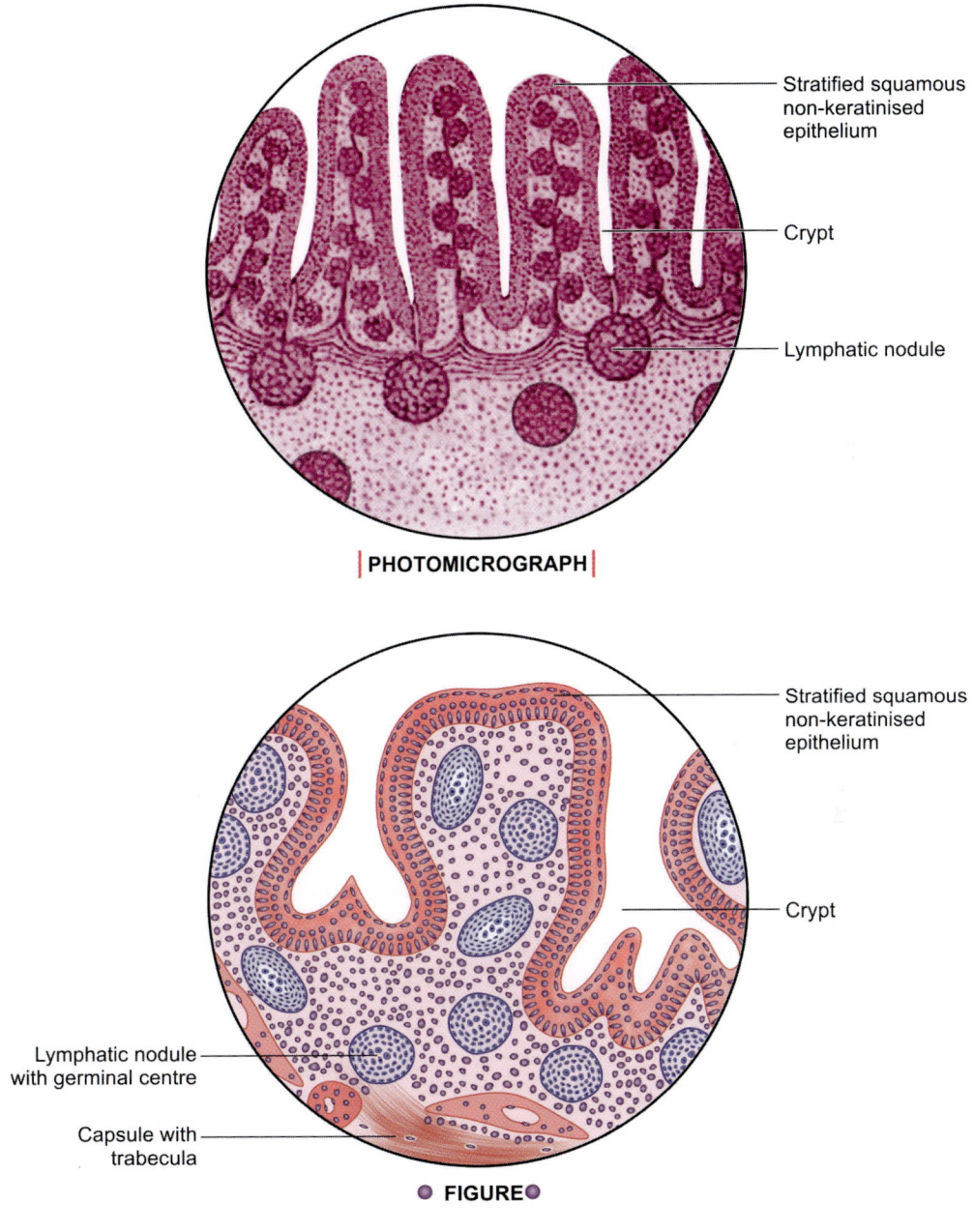

Fig. 8.6: *Structure of palatine tonsil. Stain: Haematoxylin-eosin, 100X*

FACTS TO REMEMBER
1. Capsule shows stratified squamous non-keratinised epithelium on its oral aspect
2. The epithelium forms crypts
3. No differentiation into cortex and medulla

MULTIPLE CHOICE QUESTIONS

1. **Name the thymus dependent zone of lymph node:**
   a. Cortex
   b. Medulla
   c. Paracortex
   d. Medullary cords

2. **Which lymphoid tissue contains Hassalls's corpuscle?**
   a. Lymph node
   b. Thymus
   c. Spleen
   d. Palatine tonsil

3. **Lymphatic nodules are present in all of the following *except*:**
   a. Lymph node   b. Thymus
   c. Spleen   d. Palatine tonsil

4. **Afferent and efferent lymphatics are present in one of the following lymphoid organs:**
   a. Thymus   b. Palatine tonsil
   c. Spleen   d. Lymph node

5. **Which of the following lymphoid organ is lobulated?**
   a. Lymph node
   b. Thymus
   c. Palatine tonsil
   d. Spleen

6. **Which of the following lymphoid organ has abundant blood supply?**
   a. Thymus   b. Spleen
   c. Lymph node   d. Palatine tonsil

ANSWERS

| 1. c | 2. b | 3. b | 4. d |
| 5. b | 6. b | | |

9
The Glands

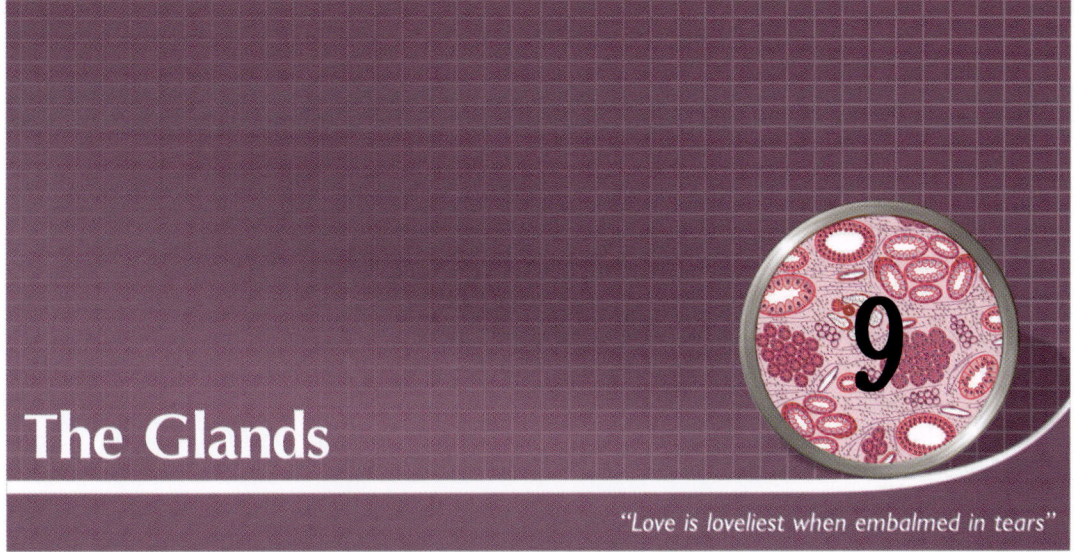

"Love is loveliest when embalmed in tears"

The glands are epithelial invaginations of the surface epithelium, which are modified for the purpose of elaboration of secretion. These are classified as endocrine and exocrine glands.

Endocrine glands discharge their secretion directly into the blood or lymphatics and are called ductless glands, e.g. thyroid, suprarenal, hypophysis cerebri, etc.

Exocrine glands discharge their secretions onto a surface directly or by means of ducts and can be classified in five different ways as follows:

1. According to the branching of ducts: Simple and compound glands.

   Simple: For example, gastric glands, pyloric glands, sweat glands. The secretion of these glands is conveyed to the surface by a single or unbranched duct (Fig. 9.1).

   Compound: For example, pancreas, parotid, Brunner's glands. The ducts of these glands divide into many branches.

2. According to the shape of the secretory unit:

   Tubular racemose: For example, gastric glands, Brunner's glands of duodenum where the secretory unit is tubular in shape.

   Acinar: For example, salivary glands, where the secretory unit is rounded or oval in shape.

3. According to the mode of elaboration of secretion: Holocrine, apocrine or merocrine also called epicrine.

   Holocrine: For example, sebaceous glands. The secretory products first collect in the cytoplasm of the cell and then the cell disintegrates to form part of secretion.

   Apocrine: For example, mammary glands. Only the apical part of the cell forms part of secretion. Some authorities believe it to be merocrine in type.

   Merocrine or epicrine: For example, lacrimal and salivary glands. The secretion passes through the free surface of the cells into the lumen of the acinus. The wall of the secretory unit remains intact.

4. According to the type of secretion: Serous, mucous and mixed glands.

Serous: For example, parotid, exocrine part of pancreas. The secretion of these glands is a watery clear fluid. The cells have rounded nuclei close to the base of the cell with basal basophilia. Zymogen granules are in apical part of the cell.

Mucous: For example, sublingual gland. It is predominantly mucus in nature. The gland secretes mucin, which when mixed with water gets converted into mucous. These cells have flattened peripheral nuclei, lying against the bases of the cells. The cytoplasm is eosinophilic and vacuolated.

Mixed gland: For example, tracheal gland, submandibular gland. These have both serous and mucous type of acini.

5. According to number of cells: Unicellular and multicellular.

   Unicellular: For example, goblet cells. These are unicellular glands situated in the epithelium of the trachea and intestines (Fig. 9.1).

   Multicellular: For example, lacrimal, parotid gland. Most of the glands in the body are multicellular.

SALIVARY GLANDS

Three pairs of salivary glands secrete saliva which is poured into the oral cavity. These are:
  i. Parotid gland is chiefly serous.
 ii. Submandibular gland is mixed, predominantly serous.
iii. Sublingual gland is mixed, predominantly mucous.

These glands are of the compound tubulo-alveolar variety. The connective tissue capsule and septa divide the gland into many lobes and lobules, carrying blood vessels, nerves and ducts. Various types of ducts are *intralobular, interlobar* and the *main duct*. These ducts are lined by cuboidal, columnar and stratified columnar epithelia respectively.

SEROUS GLAND

PAROTID GLAND

The acini of the gland secrete enzymes. The acinus is rounded and is lined by pyramidal cells surrounding a very small lumen. The cells show basal basophilia and lighter apical portion. The nuclei are rounded and basal in position. With higher magnification, the active cells show basal striations and apical eosinophilic zymogen granules (Fig. 9.2).

MIXED GLAND

SUBMANDIBULAR GLAND AND TRACHEAL GLAND

These glands consist of both serous and mucous acini (Table 9.1). The mucous acinus is lined by truncated columnar cells. The size of the acinus is larger than the serous one and shows a bigger lumen. The nucleus is flattened against the basement

The Glands

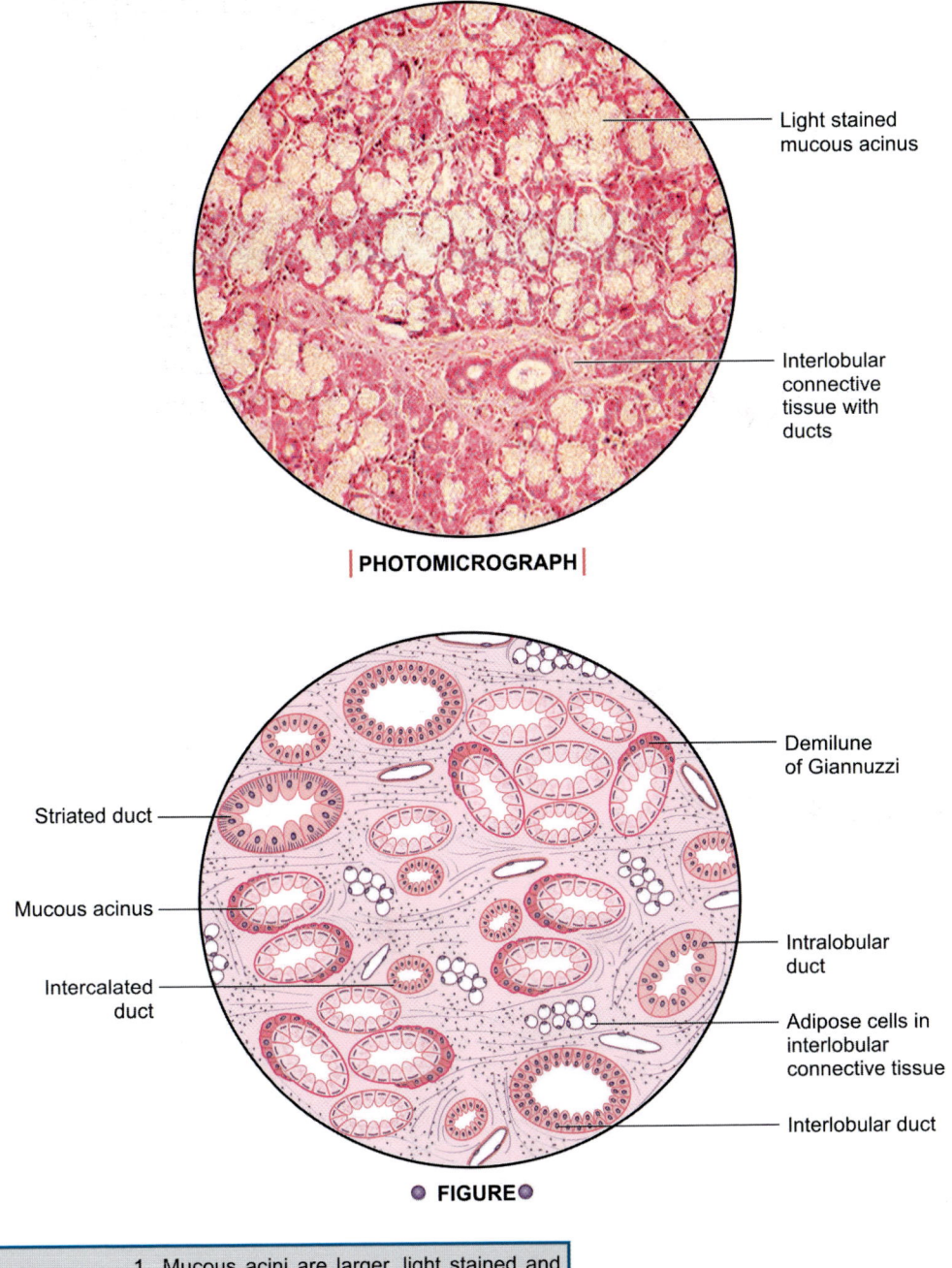

Fig. 9.4: *Structure of sublingual gland. Stain: Haematoxylin-eosin, 100X*

- *Calculi* in duct of submandibular gland are formed due to crystallisation of the secretion. Blockage leads to swelling of the gland, after food. Later it leads to atrophy of the gland.
- *Tumours* arising in parotid gland are usually benign, while those arising in submandibular or sublingual glands may be malignant.

MULTIPLE CHOICE QUESTIONS

1. Which one of the following glands is holocrine in nature?
   a. Sweat
   b. Sebaceous
   c. Duodenal
   d. Gastric
2. Goblet cells are present in all the following organs *except*:
   a. Ileum
   b. Stomach
   c. Colon
   d. Vermiform appendix
3. Apocrine sweat glands are not found in one of the following areas:
   a. Axilla
   b. Areola of mammary gland
   c. Palm
   d. Anus
4. Sweat gland belongs to which following variety of glands:
   a. Simple acinar
   b. Compound acinar
   c. Simple coiled tubular
   d. Compound tubular
5. Which types of acini are present in submandibular gland?
   a. Serous
   b. Mucous
   c. Seromucous
   d. All of the above

ANSWERS

1. b   2. b   3. c   4. c
5. d

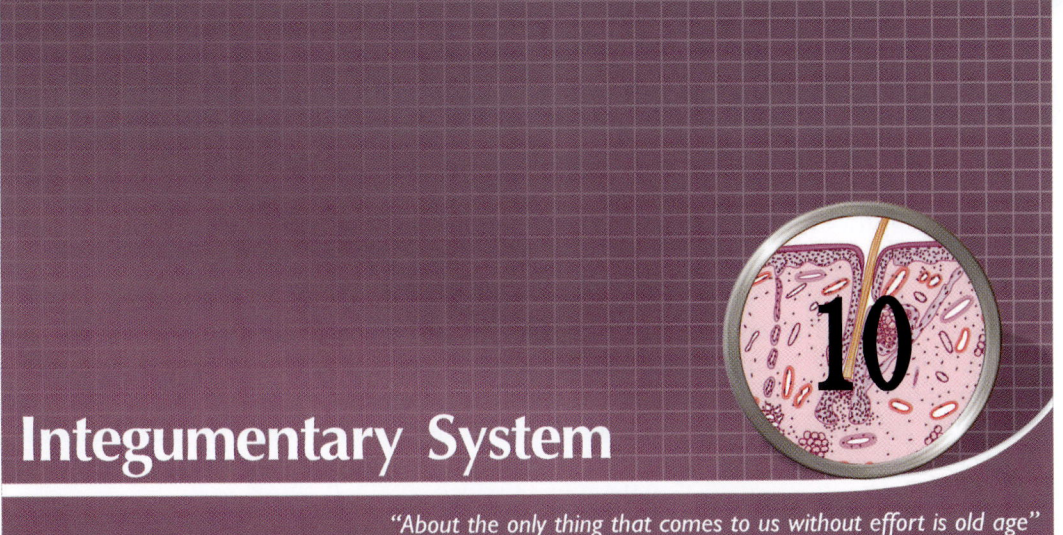

Integumentary System

"About the only thing that comes to us without effort is old age"

Integumentary system consists of skin and its various appendages. Skin covers the surface of the body and consists of two main layers:
a. The surface epithelium or epidermis derived from ectoderm,
b. Subjacent deeper connective tissue layer or the dermis derived from mesoderm.

Thickness of skin varies from less than one millimeter to few millimeters. The skin rests on a loose connective tissue layer called the superficial fascia.

EPIDERMIS

Consists of stratified squamous keratinised epithelium nourished by diffusion from the capillaries of the dermis. It is primarily protective in nature. The epithelium is made up of the following.

i. *Stratum basale*: It is the deepest single layer of columnar cells resting on the basement membrane with a few melanocytes in between, which produce melanin pigment. This pigment prevents the skin against ultraviolet rays of sun. In albinism (genetic disorder) the melanocytes are absent.

ii. *Stratum spinosum*: It is made up of 3–7 layers of polygonal cells which are attached to each other by unstable desmosomes, giving it a prickly appearance (Fig. 10.1).

iii. *Stratum granulosum*: Consists of 2–3 layers of diamond shaped cells containing granules which stain deeply with basic dyes. These are keratohyalin granules.

iv. *Stratum lucidum*: These cells lose their nuclei and form a zone of flattened ill-defined cells. These cells contain refractile eleidin granules.

v. *Stratum corneum*: The cells in this stratum are flat and cornified. The nucleus and cytoplasm are replaced by a protein called keratin. This zone is waterproof and protective in nature. The most superficial cells are constantly being desquamated.

A few Langhans' or clear cells may be seen in the stratum basale or stratum spinosum. These cells act as antigen—presenting cells to T lymphocytes. Langhans' cells recognise, phagocytose and process the antigens before presenting to T lymphocytes. A small number of Merkel's cells is seen in basal layer of epidermis. These act as mechanoreceptors to detect pressure in the finger tips.

Functional Aspect
- *Stratum basale*: This layer is a region of cell division. This layer also contains Merkel cells in addition to melanocytes. Merkel cells are closely associated with non-myelinated axons. These function as mechanoreceptor.
- *Stratum spinosum*: This layer also contains Langerhans' cells or clear cells and processes of melanocytes. Langerhans' cells help in fighting with the antigens. These cells recognize the antigenic cells.
- *Stratum granulosum*: This layer is absent in thin skin.
- *Stratum lucidum*: This layer is absent in thin skin.
- *Stratum corneum*: The cells in this stratum are flat and cornified. The nucleus and cytoplasm are replaced by a protein called keratin. This zone is waterproof and protective in nature. The most superficial cells are constantly being desquamated. This layer is thickest in the palm and sole.

DERMIS

Consists of an outer papillary and a deeper reticular layer. The outer **papillary layer**, in contact with the epidermis, is usually uneven and projects into papillae between the ridges on the deep surface of epidermis. These papillae, primary and secondary, bring about close contact between the capillaries of the dermis and cells of the epidermis. The papillary layer is thin and is made of fine collagen and elastic fibres with lymphocytes and plasma cells. It is very rich in capillaries and nerve endings. The deeper portion of the dermis is named the **reticular layer** and consists of dense irregular connective tissue with lymphocytes, fat cells, capillaries, lymphatics and nerve fibres.

APPENDAGES OF SKIN

HAIR FOLLICLES
Hair follicles are follicular invaginations of the epidermal epithelium. The hair follicle thus produced dips down from the epidermis into the dermis and is surrounded by connective tissue. The active follicle has a bulbous terminal expansion with a concavity at its bottom occupied by a connective tissue papilla. The papilla is covered by the epithelial matrix cells of hair and is called "**germinal matrix**" which germinates the hair. The cells on the dome of convexity of the papilla form a hair root which develops into a *hair shaft*. Thus, the hair root is the part of hair inside the skin and hair shaft is protruding beyond the level of epidermis. The hair root is comprised of *medulla, cortex* and *cuticle* from within outwards. The hair root is covered by *inner root sheath* derived from stratum corneum. The inner root sheath consists of a cuticle, lying adjacent to cuticle of hair root, Huxley's layer of 2–3 layers of flattened nucleated cells and Henle's layer of single layer of cuboidal cells, from inside out. The *outer root sheath* is comprised of nucleated cells from stratum spinosum and stratum basale. Still outside is the connective tissue sheath (Figs 10.2 and 10.3).

Integumentary System

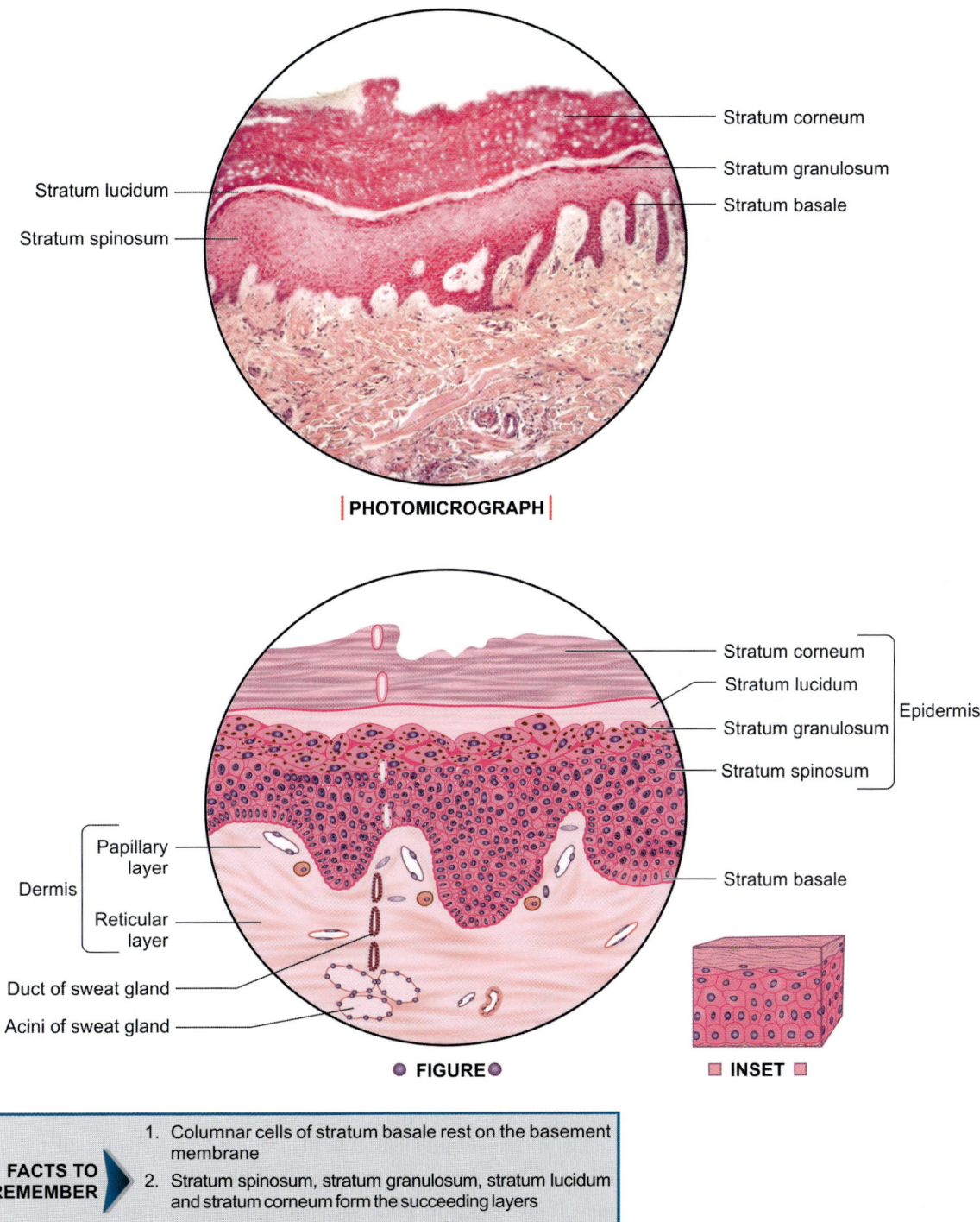

Fig. 10.1: *Layers of epidermis of thick skin. Stain: Haematoxylin-eosin, 400X*

HAIR

The hair projects obliquely outside the skin and consists of a central medulla, outer cortex and outermost cuticle. The cells of medulla are vacuolated and keratinising. The cells of cortex are keratinised. The cells of cuticle are heavily keratinised.

Arrector pilorum muscle arises from connective tissue sheath of hair follicle and gets inserted into papillary layer of dermis. Its contraction causes depression in the skin where the muscle is attached to the dermis. It is called gooseflesh.

SEBACEOUS GLAND

Sebaceous glands are *holocrine* glands and are scattered in the superficial layer of the dermis. These are absent in the palm and sole. The glands secrete sebum and open by ducts into upper one-third of hair follicle. The secretory portions of these glands comprises rounded acini lined by a single layer of epithelial cells with round nuclei. Towards the centre of the acini, cells become polyhedral and occupied by fat droplets. Their nuclei shrink; the cells break down and are called holocrine glands. Their oily secretion or sebum is conducted by short ducts into the hair follicle. Sebum acts as a lubricant for the hair shaft (Fig. 10.4). Sebum keeps the skin smooth and prevents it from drying. It also acts as a waterproof layer on the skin.

ARRECTOR PILI MUSCLE

Arrector pili is a band of smooth muscle fibres, attached at one end to the papillary layer of dermis and at the other to the connective tissue sheath of the hair follicle. The muscle is supplied by sympathetic nerves and on contraction moves the hair into a more vertical position. Thus, the hair becomes straight and the skin in the region of its exit gets elevated and neighbouring region which gives attachment to arrector pili muscle is depressed to give rise to gooseskin. The muscle contracts and the hair stands erect in response to cold, fear and danger. Erect hair entrap air between them. Air being a bad conductor of heat prevents loss of body heat.

Nails of the fingers and toes, hair, feathers and horns are made up of hard keratin.

SWEAT GLANDS

Sweat glands are distributed all along in the dermis, except at the margins of the lips and the glans penis; being more numerous in thick skin, i.e. palm and sole. These produce sweat which regulates the temperature of the body.

The glands are of simple coiled tubular type, which have secretory and conducting parts. The secretory part is a simple tube convoluted in several unequal twists into a ball, the conducting part of duct is a narrow unbranched tube (*see* Fig. 9.1).

The cells lining the secretory part or acini are columnar and rest on a basement membrane. Between the basement membrane and the lining acinar cells are a few **myoepithelial cells,** which help in the expulsion of secretion. The duct or conducting portion of the gland passes through the dermis into the epidermis to open on its surface. The duct is lined by stratified cuboidal cells. The secretory cells are larger and lighter stained as compared to the cells lining the ducts (Fig. 10.4).

Integumentary System

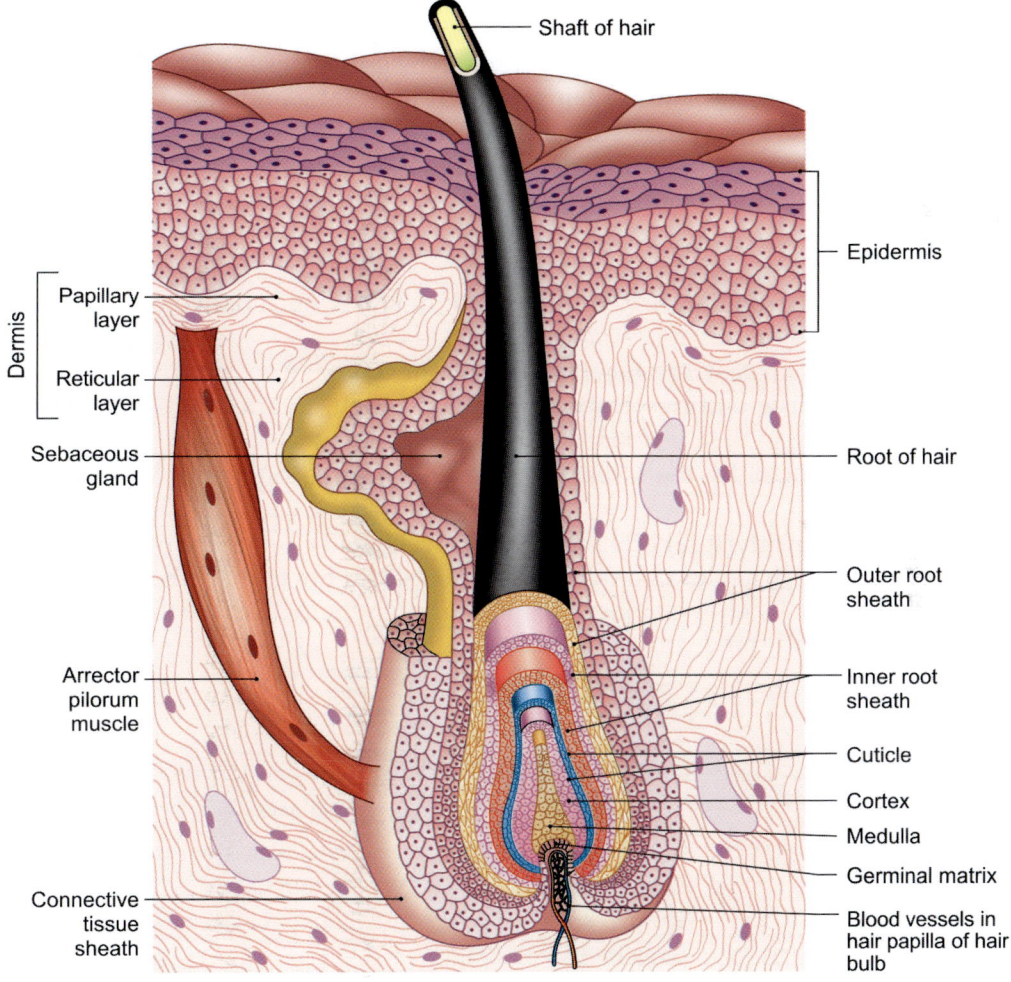

Fig. 10.2: *Structure of the hair follicle*

There are two types of sweat glands; eccrine and apocrine. Eccrine glands are simple tubular coiled glands. The gland consists of clear cells and dark cells. Dark cells secrete mucus whereas clear cells secrete watery fluid. The secretory acinus is surrounded by myoepithelial cells which help to expel the secretion. These glands help in temperature regulation.

Apocrine glands are located chiefly in the axilla. These are large glands. Their ducts open into the hair follicle. They produce a viscous secretion.

TYPES OF SKIN—THICK AND THIN

Thick skin (Fig. 10.1), e.g. skin of palm and sole. The epidermis is very thick especially the stratum corneum. This skin contains numerous sweat glands.

Thin skin (Figs 10.1 and 10.4), e.g. skin over the rest of the body. Its characteristic features are the presence of hair follicles, sebaceous glands and arrector pili muscles. Table 10.1 shows the differences between thick skin and thin skin.

Functional Aspect

- The keratinised epithelium is the first line of defense. The skin is impermeable to water.
- The skin is the largest sensory organs of the body. Free nerve endings and encapsulated nerve endings respond to pain, touch, temperature and pressure sensations.
- The sweat produced by the sweat gland excretes some salts and water from the body.
- The skin maintains the temperature of the body. In cold climate the blood vessels to the skin get constricted and blood flow is also less. In hot climate the blood vessels get dilated and have enough blood flowing through them, to expel the heat out and keep the body and mind cool.

TABLE 10.1: Shows comparison between thick skin and thin skin

Features	Thick skin	Thin skin
Epidermal layers	Comprises 5 layers: Stratum basale Stratum spinosum Stratum granulosum Stratum lucidum Stratum corneum	Comprises 3 layers Stratum basale Strtum spinosum – – Thin stratum corneum
Epidermal ridges	Present	Absent
Sebaceous gland hair follicle and arrector pili muscle	Absent	Present
Sweat gland	Many	Few
Sensory receptors	Many	Few
Location	Palm and sole and palmar aspects of digits	All parts of body except palm, sole and palmar aspects of digits

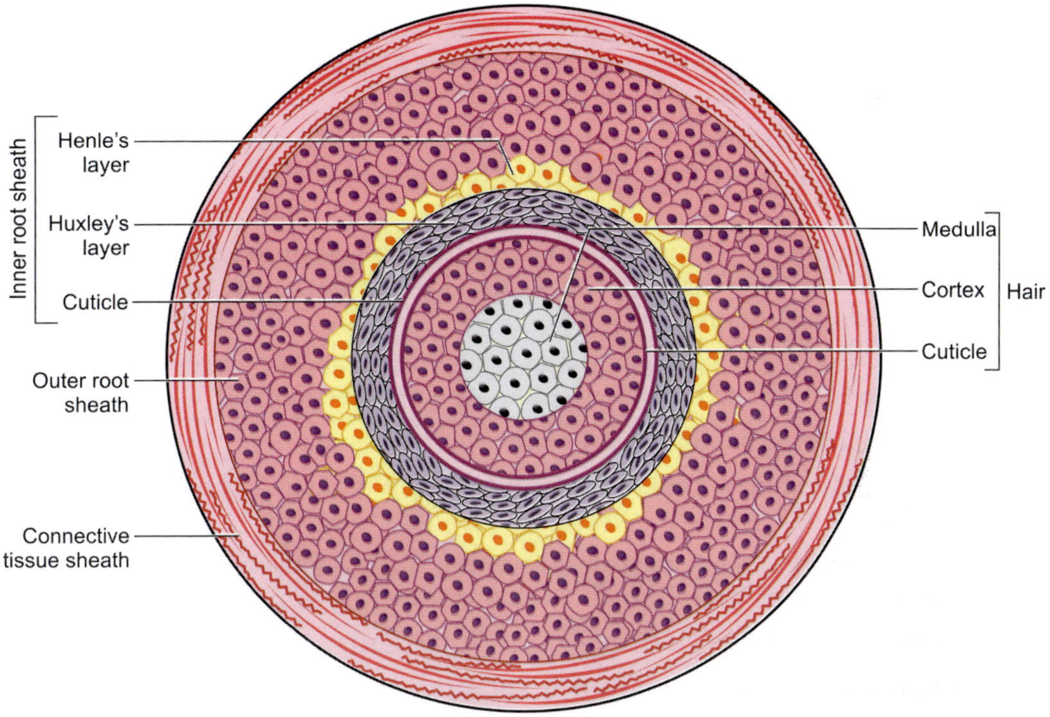

Integumentary System

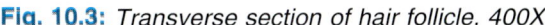

Fig. 10.3: *Transverse section of hair follicle, 400X*

FACTS TO REMEMBER
1. Consists of shaft of hair comprising medulla, cortex and cuticle
2. Next is inner root sheath, comprising cuticle, Huxley's layer and Henle's layer
3. Outermost is outer root sheath and connective tissue sheath

- Vitamin D is synthesised by epidermal cells with the help of ultraviolet rays of the sun.
- Optimum amount of vitamin D may also decrease incidence of cancer in the body.

Applied Aspect
- *Dermatitis* is the acute or chronic inflammation of skin. Acute dermatitis is characterised by redness, swelling, itching and exudation of serous fluid. This is often followed by crusting (formation of hard coating) and scaling (scale formation). In chronic dermatitis, the skin becomes thick and leathery due to long-term scratching.
- *Psoriasis* is a disease of skin with proliferation of the basal layer cells of the epidermis. This leads to incomplete maturation of upper layer and skin appears shiny, silver coloured and scaly. Bleeding may occur when scales are scratched or rubbed off. Mostly affected parts are elbows, knees and scalp.
- *Squamous cell carcinoma*: Mostly found on the exposed surfaces of the skin. The epithelial cells invade the deeper dermis. Irregular ulcer with everted edges is seen on the surface.
- *Malignant melanoma* is due to malignant multiplication of melanocytes of the epidermis. It mostly occurs in white people. The tumour causes metastases in liver, lung, intestine and brain.
- *Basal cell carcinoma:* It is most common type of skin cancer occurring in face, head, and neck. It is associated with long-term exposure to sunlight.
- Skin is the outer garment and is subjected to many maladies:
  - *Albinism:* The child is born without any melanin pigment in the skin. It is usually inherited.
  - *Eczema/dermatitis:* There is redness, swelling, itching and exudation in acute cases. It may become chronic. Dermatitis may be due to allergy to soap or cosmetics.
  - *Herpes virus:* It causes chickenpox and herpes zoster.
  - *Fungal infections:* Ringworm is a superficial fungal infection with rings of inflammation. It most commonly affects the scalp.

    In 'athlete's foot' there is fungal infection between the toes. If toes and area between toes is kept dry, it improves.
  - *Pressure sores:* The skin slowly dies over pressure sites, e.g. pressure sores on the lower back when patient is too sick to get up.
  - *Acne:* It usually occurs at puberty due to blockage of sebaceous glands in the hair follicle. Acne mostly appears on face and chest.
  - *Burns:* It is common condition and occurs due to heat, too much cold, strong alkalis or acids, electricity, etc. It only epidermis is involved, the burn is superficial. But if both epidermis and dermis are affected by burns, the burn is deep. Severe burns result in shock, dehydration, renal failure and contratures.
  - *Impetigo:* It is bacterial infection of skin caused by *Staphylococcus aureus* or *Streptococcus pyogenes*. Superficial pustules develop around the nose and mouth.

Integumentary System

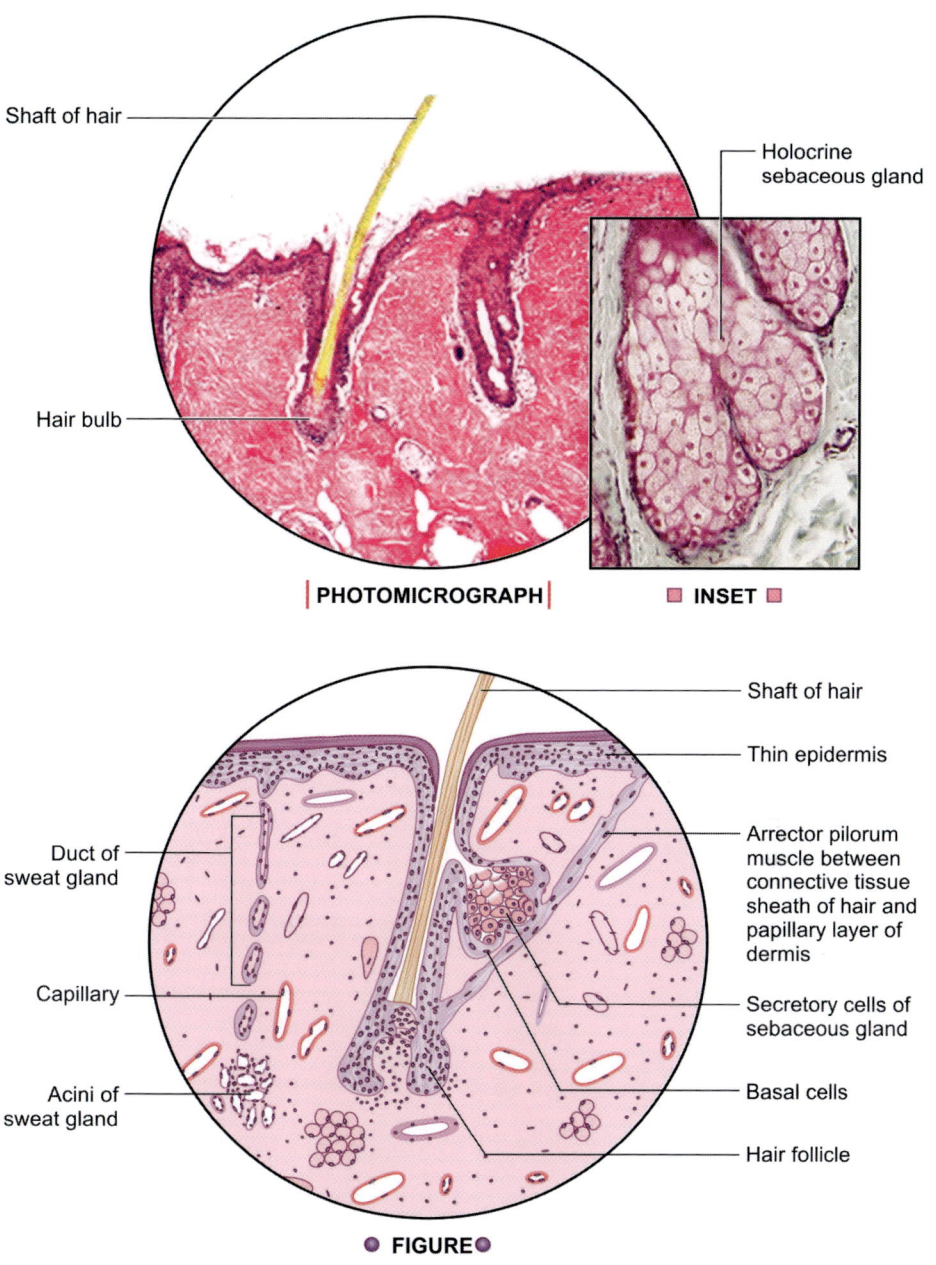

FACTS TO REMEMBER
1. Epidermis is thin
2. Hair follicle, sebaceous gland with arrector pilorum muscle
3. Sweat gland with its duct

Fig. 10.4: *Structure of thin skin. Inset shows the sebaceous gland. Stain: Haematoxylin-eosin, 100X*

MULTIPLE CHOICE QUESTIONS

1. Which one of the following is *not* an antigen presenting cell?
   a. Merkel
   b. Kupffer
   c. Macrophage
   d. Langerhans'

2. Which layer/stratum of epidermis contains melanocytes?
   a. Spinosum   b. Basal
   c. Lucidum   d. Corneum

3. What type of muscle is arrector pilorum?
   a. Skeletal   b. Smooth
   c. Cardiac   d. None of the above

4. What is the nerve supply of arrector pilorum muscle?
   a. Somatic
   b. Sympathetic
   c. Parasympathetic
   d. Cranial nerve

5. Free nerve endings are present in which of the following layer of skin?
   a. Epidermis
   b. Papillary layer of dermis
   c. Reticular layer of dermis
   d. All of the above

ANSWERS

1. b 2. a 3. b 4. b
5. a

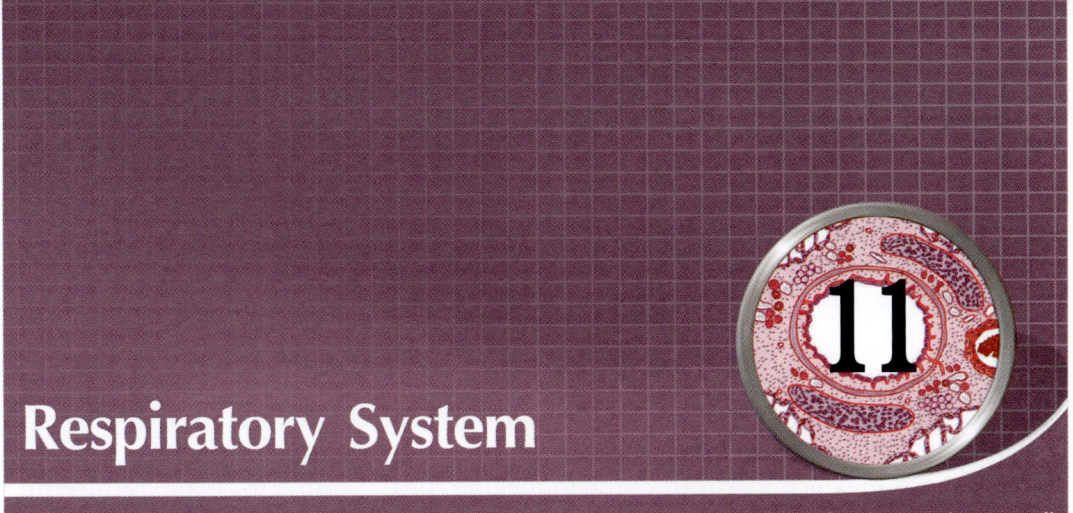

Respiratory System

"Pattern of right and left bronchial tree are mirror images, but the heart on left side gives less room"

The respiratory system provides for the intake of oxygen and elimination of carbon dioxide, which are transported to and from the tissues of the body by the circulatory system.

Organs of respiration are nose comprising external nares, nasal cavity, posterior nares including the paranasal air sinuses.

Nasopharynx

Larynx

Trachea

Pleura, lungs including the bronchial tree.

Functionally the respiratory system is divided into:

i. Conducting part which comprises nose, nasopharynx, larynx, trachea and bronchial tree till the level of terminal bronchioles. These are always patent for respiration.

ii. Respiratory part comprising of respiratory bronchioles, alveolar duct, atria alveolar sac and alveoli. These are present in the spongy part of lung for exchange of gases.

HISTOLOGY OF NOSE, NASOPHARYNX AND LARYNX

NOSE

Comprises two nasal cavities separated by a nasal septum. Its functions are:

i. Filtering, warming and moistening the inspired air

ii. Conducting air to and from the lungs

iii. As an organ for smell. The receptors for smell are placed in the upper one-third of nasal cavity and is lined by olfactory mucosa with special olfactory neurons. It is described in Chapter 19. The lower two-thirds of nasal cavity is lined by respiratory mucosa, which is pseudostratified ciliated columnar epithelium with goblet cells. The lamina propria contains mucous and serous secreting glands, lymphocytes, plasma cells and large venous plexus.

Functions

The cilia of the columnar cells carry foreign particles towards oropharynx to be swallowed. Goblet cells produce mucus to trap foreign particles. The cells in lamina propria provide necessary immunity.

Clinical Features

The nose, nasopharynx get attacked by various bacteria, pollutants and allergans causing sinusitis, and tonsillitis.

The venous plexus may rupture due to picking/heat, leading to epistaxis (bleeding from nose).

NASOPHARYNX

It is situated between the posterior nares of nose and nasopharynx. It is lined by pseudo-stratified ciliated columnar epithelium with goblet cells.

LARYNX/VOICE BOX

It is made up of number of cartilages. It begins at root of tongue and ends at the trachea. Most of the larynx is lined by pseudostratified ciliated columnar epithelium interspersed with goblet cells.

Epiglottis is a very important elastic cartilage of larynx. There is lamina propria on both sides of the elastic cartilage. The anterior surface of epiglottis facing the tongue and upper part of posterior surface are lined with stratified squamous non-keratinised epithelium. The rest of the posterior surface is lined with respiratory epithelium, i.e. pseudostratified ciliated columnar epithelium.

TRACHEA AND CONDUCTING PART

Trachea is a thin walled flexible tube. Its lumen is kept permanently patent by means of C-shaped hyaline cartilages. The trachea is lined by *pseudostratified ciliated columnar epithelium* with interspersed goblet cells resting on a basement membrane. The *lamina propria* consists of elastic fibres, lymphocytes both segregated and aggregated and short ducts of the glands (Fig. 11.1).

These ducts open on the free surface of the epithelium.

The deeper part of lamina propria is the *submucosa* which contains both mucous and serous acini that keep the epithelium moist. The mucus provided by mucous acini entangle the dust particles. Cilia move the mucous towards pharynx. Coughing also moves the mucus towards larynx and pharynx to be expelled from the respiratory system.

The most characteristic feature of trachea is its supporting framework of 16–20 C-shaped hyaline cartilages that encircle it on its ventral and lateral aspects. The posterior wall of the trachea adjacent to the oesophagus is devoid of cartilage. Its place is taken by transverse smooth muscle fibres, the *trachealis* muscle. The cartilage is covered by perichondrium on all sides which separates it from the neighbouring structures. The outermost layer is the adventitia which contains blood vessels and nerves.

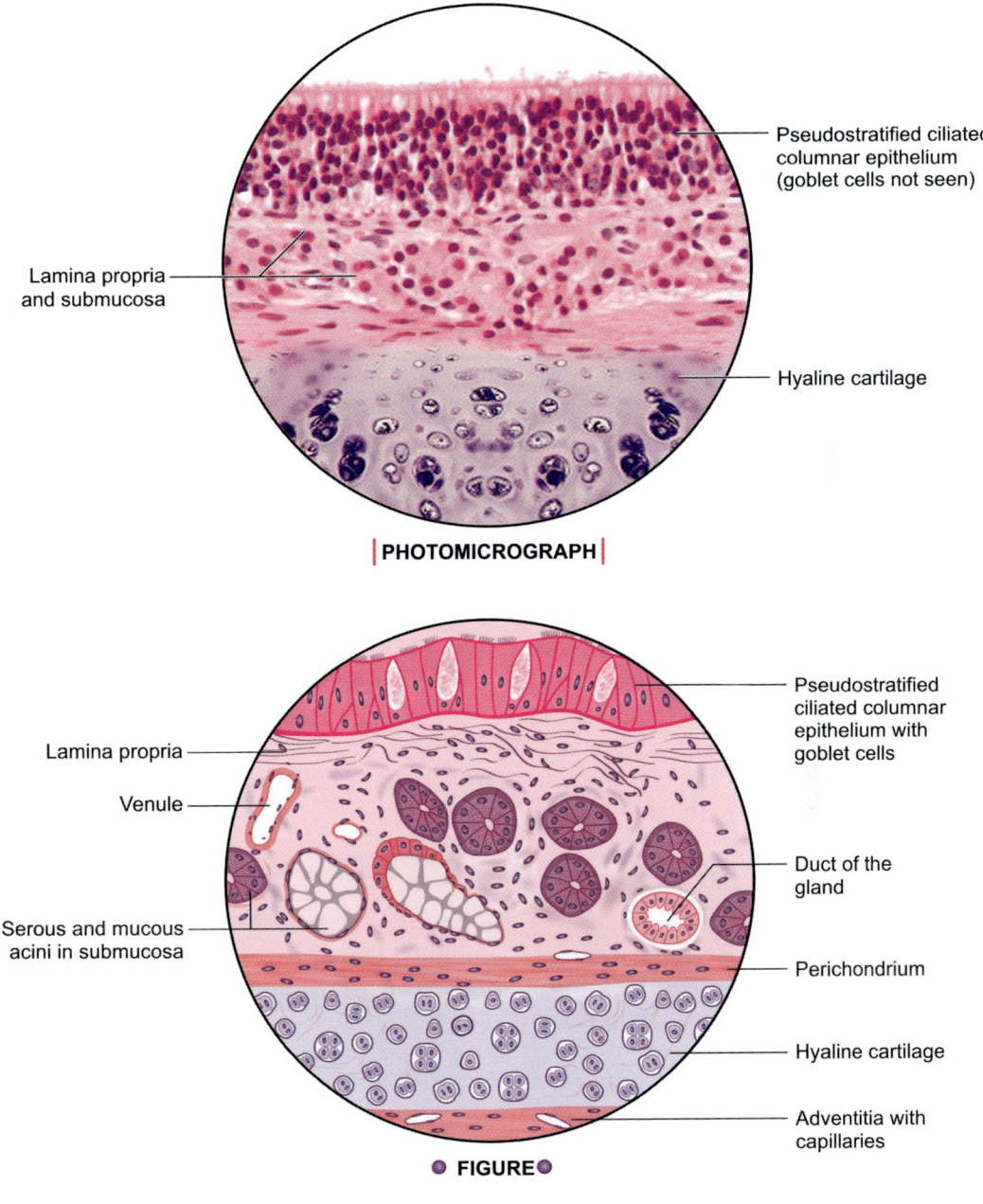

Fig. 11.1: *Various layers of wall of trachea. Stain: Haematoxylin-eosin, 100X*

Applied Aspect

- *Tracheitis* is the viral or bacterial infection of trachea. This is characterized by acute inflammation of mucous membrane causing tissue congestion and profuse secretion of watery fluid. The infection may become chronic in tobacco smokers and people who live or work in polluted atmosphere.
- *Diphtheria* is the infection of the pharynx caused by *Corynebacterium diphtheriae*, which may extend to the nasopharynx and trachea. A thick fibrous membrane forms over the area which obstruct the airway. Immunization is used as a remedy of diphtheria.

BRONCHIAL TUBES

The trachea divides into two divisions called *primary bronchi* which traverse for a short distance before entering the lungs at their hila. These primary bronchi run downwards and outwards and divide into two *secondary bronchi* on the left side and three secondary bronchi on the right side. Each secondary bronchus divides into 2–5 *tertiary* or *segmental bronchi*. Each aerates a *bronchopulmonary segment*. The tertiary bronchi continue to divide dichotomously till the diameter of the tube reaches 1 mm and is known as the *terminal bronchiole*. Up to this stage is the conducting part of respiratory system. Hereafter, the respiratory part starts where exchange of gases takes place.

Each terminal bronchiole continues to divide into 2–4 *respiratory bronchioles*. These break up into 2–10 *alveolar ducts* which give rise to *atria, alveolar sacs* and *alveoli*.

In a section of the lung, the mesothelial covering of visceral pleura may be visible. The structure of the lung is a lacework of alveoli separated by thin walled septa. This is traversed by system of intrapulmonary bronchi (Fig. 11.2), bronchioles and alveolar ducts, into which atria, alveolar sacs and alveoli open.

INTRAPULMONARY BRONCHUS

Intrapulmonary bronchus is lined by *pseudostratified ciliated columnar epithelium* with **goblet cells** resting on a thin basement membrane. **Cilia** prevent the accumulation of mucus in the bronchial tree. The **lamina propria** consists of reticular and elastic fibres. The **submucous coat** contains both mucous and serous acini. A complete layer of smooth muscle fibres is present which is responsible for infoldings of the mucous membrane. Outermost is the hyaline cartilage which is visible as small cartilaginous plates of varying sizes and shapes (Fig. 11.2) with tunica adventitia.

TERMINAL BRONCHIOLE

Terminal bronchiole is part of the conducting system of respiratory pathway which is less than 1 mm in diameter. It is lined by simple columnar epithelium. The lamina propria contains elastic and smooth muscle fibres. Both the glands and cartilage plates are absent (Fig. 11.3). There are following distinct epithelial cell types in the conducting airways. These are:

- *Ciliated columnar cells:* These cells form the force of mucociliary current in the bronchial tree. The 300 cilia project from the apical part of the cell. The rate of ciliary beating is 12–16/second.

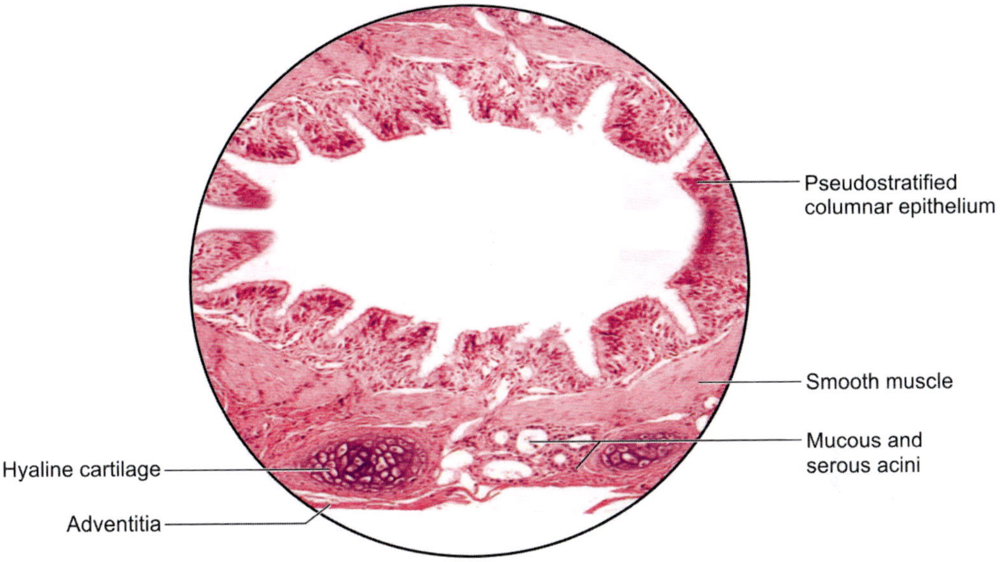

Respiratory System

Photomicrograph labels:
- Pseudostratified columnar epithelium
- Smooth muscle
- Mucous and serous acini
- Hyaline cartilage
- Adventitia

| PHOTOMICROGRAPH |

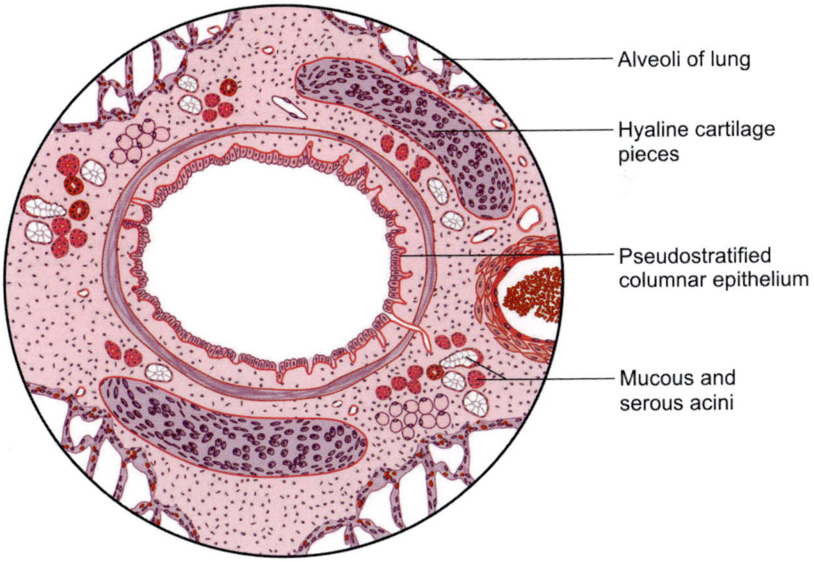

Figure labels:
- Alveoli of lung
- Hyaline cartilage pieces
- Pseudostratified columnar epithelium
- Mucous and serous acini

● FIGURE ●

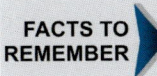

FACTS TO REMEMBER
1. Epithelium is pseudostratified columnar in nature
2. Cartilage in pieces seen all around
3. Mucous and serous acini also seen

Fig. 11.2: *Intrapulmonary bronchus. Stain: Haematoxylin-eosin, 100X*

- *Goblet cells:* These cells are present from trachea to the smallest bronchi, excluding the bronchioles. In the smokers, the goblet cells increase in number and extend into the bronchioles as well.
- *Clara cells:* These are non-ciliated cuboidal cells, bulging into the lumen. These contain secretory granules and lysosomes. These cells may regulate the surface tension.
- *Basal cells:* These cells are seen in the airways lined by pseudostratified epithelium. These are mitotic stem cells.
- *Brush cells:* These are delicate non-ciliated cells with long apical microvilli, which are stiff in nature. These have sensory receptor function.
- *Neuroendocrine cells:* These are rounded cells and form part of neuroendocrine system of amine precursor uptake and decarboxylation (APUD) cells. These cells are maximum in fetal lungs and their number decreases after birth.
- *Lymphocytes:* Lymphocytes derived from thymus (T lymphocytes) are present. These are concerned with immune mechanism of the respiratory system.
- *Mast cells:* These are present in the basal region of the epithelium. Their secretory granules release histamine in response to irritants.
- *Columnar cells:* These line the terminal bronchiole (Fig. 11.3).

RESPIRATORY PART

RESPIRATORY BRONCHIOLE

Respiratory bronchiole is lined by cuboidal epithelium. The walls consist of collagenous connective tissue containing bundles of interlacing smooth muscle fibres and elastic fibres. At number of places, the alveolar sacs and alveoli arise from the respiratory bronchiole and its cuboidal epithelium is continuous with the squamous epithelium of alveolar sacs and alveoli.

ATRIA, ALVEOLAR DUCTS AND ALVEOLAR SACS

The alveolar ducts have a long tortuous course and give off several branches. These are closely beset with thin-walled outpouchings, the atria, the alveolar sacs and alveoli. The atria, alveolar ducts and alveoli are lined with squamous epithelium.

ALVEOLI

Alveoli are thin walled polyhedral sacs. The alveoli are lined by two types of cells, which rest on a basement membrane. The main support of the alveoli is provided by elastic fibres. Majority of cells lining the alveoli are the *squamous cells* or *type I pneumocytes*. A few are larger cells or *type II pneumocytes*. Type II cells secrete the *surfactant* which lowers surface tension and prevents alveoli from collapsing.

Between the adjacent alveoli is the interalveolar septum containing numerous capillaries lined by continuous non-fenestrated endothelial cells (Fig. 11.4). Alveolar pores of 10–15 micron are present along the interalveolar wall to equalise pressure in alveoli. These pores also permit collateral air circulation.

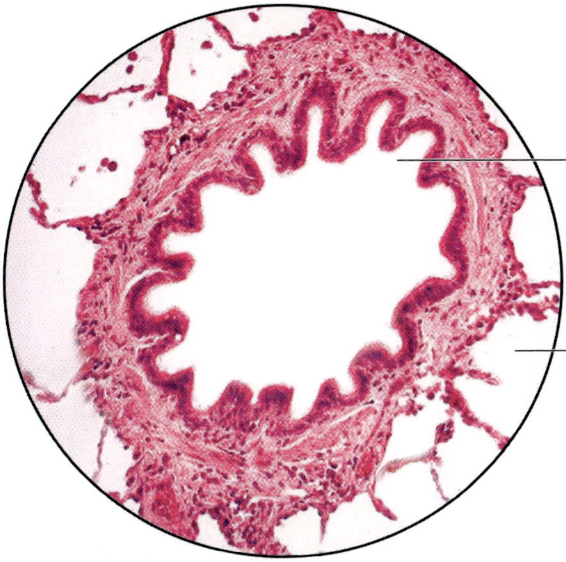

Respiratory System

PHOTOMICROGRAPH

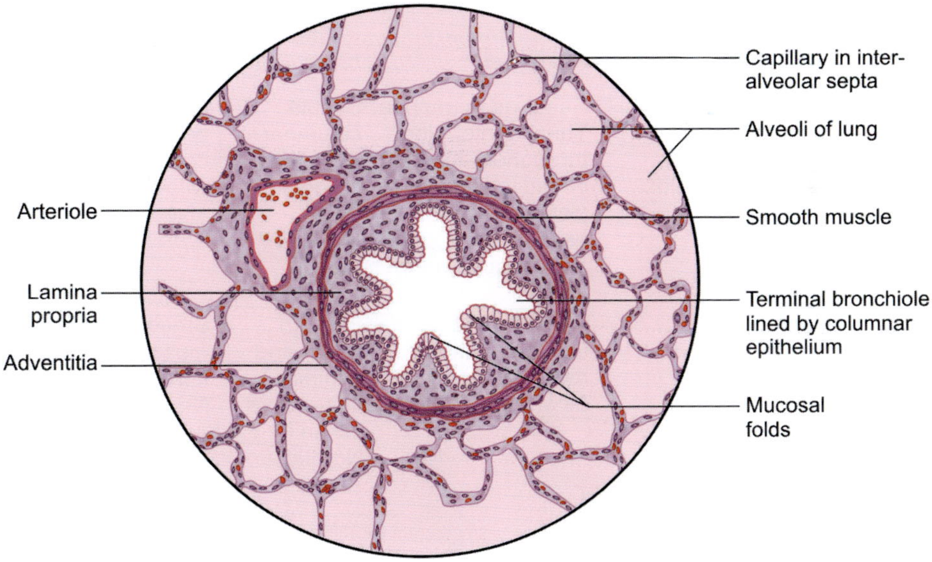

- Terminal bronchiole
- Alveoli of lung

FIGURE

- Capillary in inter-alveolar septa
- Alveoli of lung
- Smooth muscle
- Terminal bronchiole lined by columnar epithelium
- Mucosal folds
- Arteriole
- Lamina propria
- Adventitia

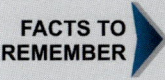

FACTS TO REMEMBER
1. Continuous squamous epithelium of alveoli with capillaries in interalveolar septa
2. Bronchioles do not have glands or cartilages
3. Arteriole seen adjacent to bronchiole

Fig. 11.3: *Structure of terminal bronchiole. Stain: Haematoxylin-eosin, 400X*

Various cell types present in the interalveolar septum are the goblet cells, basal cells, lymphocytes, serous cells, leucocytes and macrophages (Fig. 11.5). In congestive cardiac failure, heart failure cells are present in the sputum. These cells are the alveolar macrophages, containing hemosiderin of the red blood cells from the ruptured capillaries.

The exchange between the blood in the capillaries and air in the alveoli takes place through the following.
i. Cytoplasm of endothelial cell of a capillary (Fig. 11.4 Inset)
ii. Basement membrane of the capillary
iii. Basement membrane of the alveolus
iv. Cytoplasm of the epithelial cells of the alveolus.

Table 11.1 shows the differentiating features of various parts of the respiratory passages.

Functional Aspect

- The epithelium of the respiratory tract gradually thins downwards. It is squamous in the alveoli to permit exchange of gases efficiently. The conducting part is kept patent due to presence of hyaline cartilage.

TABLE 11.1: Provides differentiating features of various parts of the respiratory passages

Features	Trachea and extra-pulmonary bronchus	Intrapulmonary bronchus	Terminal bronchiole	Respiratory bronchiole	Alveoli
1. Epithelium	Pseudostratified ciliated columnar with goblet cells. Thrown into folds posteriorly	Same as in trachea. Thrown into folds throughout lumen because of a complete layer of muscle between cartilage and mucous membrane	Simple columnar cells. No cilia, no goblet cells	Cuboidal cells, continuous with that of alveoli	Continuous epithelium squamous cells
2. Lamina propria	Comprises connective tissue, elastic fibres, lymphatics and ducts of glands. Smooth muscle fibres are seen only between ends of cartilage	Same as in trachea Contains smooth muscle fibres, all around	Smooth fibres and minimal connective tissue No ducts	Smooth muscle fibres No ducts	Interalveolar septa contains capillaries and various types of cells
3. Glands	Both mucous and serous acini present between mucous membrane and cartilage	Both mucous and serous acini lie between muscle and cartilage	No glands	No glands	No glands
4. Hyaline cartilage	C-shaped single cartilage	Seen as many irregular plates	No cartilage	No cartilage	No cartilage
5. Muscle layer	Only present posteriorly outside the submucosa	Forms a complete layer outside submucosa with elastic fibres	Well-defined muscle with elastic fibres	Muscle layer with only elastic fibres	No muscle

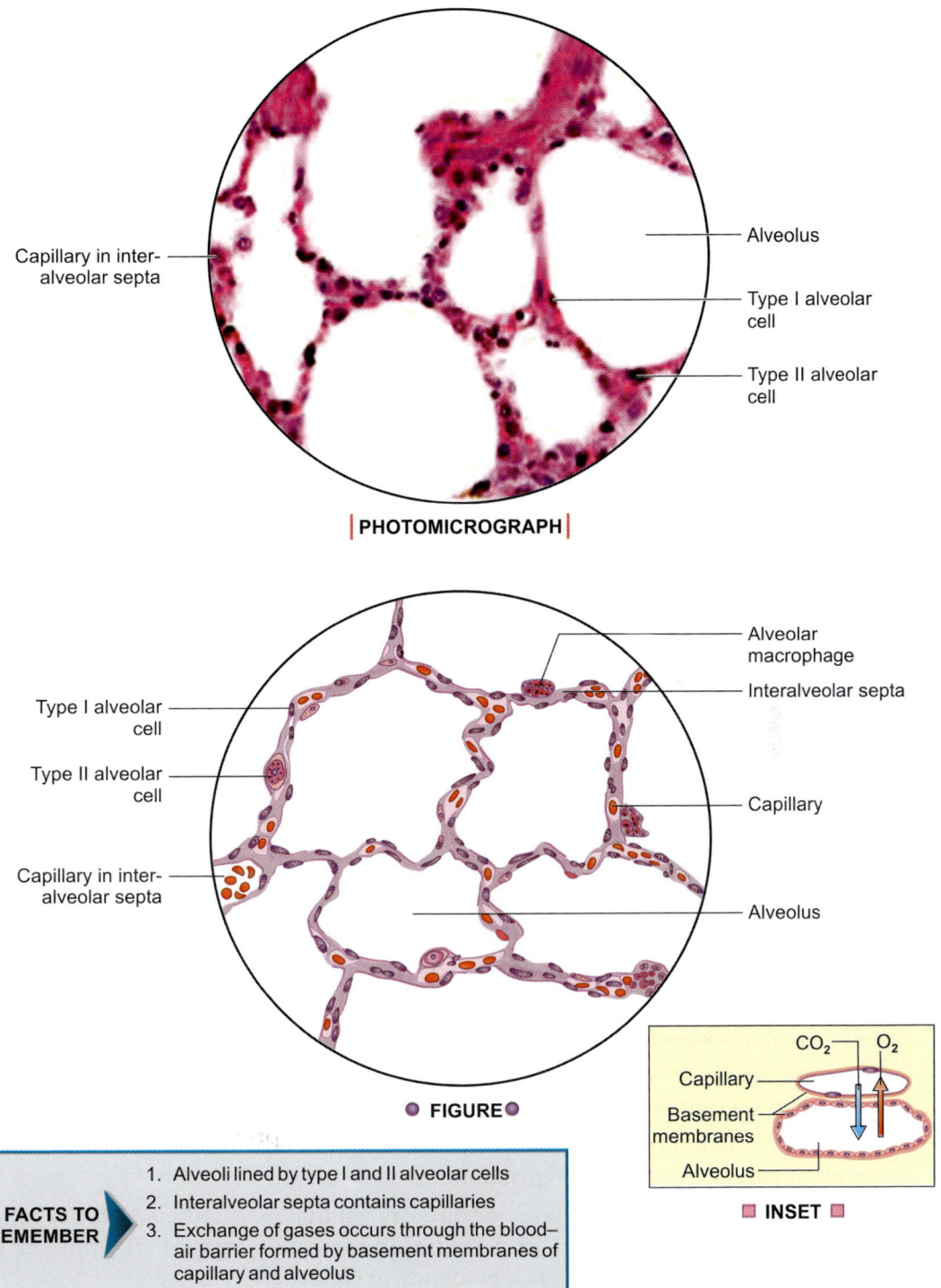

Fig. 11.4: Alveoli and interalveolar septa. Haematoxylin-eosin, 400X

- The alveoli are lined by squamous cells. A few surfactant producing cells lower the surface tension and prevent alveoli from collapsing.

Applied Aspect
- *Asthma* is an inflammatory disease of respiratory system. Mucous membrane and muscle layers of bronchi are thickened and the mucous glands enlarged causing reduced airflow in the lower respiratory tract.
- *Atelectasis* is the collapse of alveoli due to the obstruction in bronchus or bronchiole. The gas in the alveoli beyond the obstruction is absorbed and leads to collapse.
- *Emphysema* is a potentially fatal pulmonary disease characterized by decreased elasticity of the lungs due to the disruption of elastic tissue. Alveoli are replaced by large air sacs due to breakdown of the walls between the alveoli. Heavy cigarette smoking is the most common cause of emphysema.
- *Pneumonia* is the disease of lungs caused by inhaled or blood borne microbes. It is of two types—lobar pneumonia and bronchopneumonia. In lobar pneumonia, watery inflammatory exudates accumulate and fill up many alveoli in a lobule and then overflow into adjacent lobule. This drastically reduces or cuts off the air entry into it. In bronchopneumonia, there is an influx of leucocytes and accumulation of fibrous exudates.
- *Tuberculosis (TB)*: It affects the lung most commonly especially in developing countries like India. Cough is the usual symptom. If it is persists for about one month investigations must be done for diagnosis of TB. Treatment must be taken for full period as advised by the physician.

Reflexes associated with Respiratory System
1. *Hering-Breuer reflex:* Hering-Breuer reflex is a respiratory reflex which regulates the depth of inspiration. The receptors for this reflex are the stretch receptors present in the walls of the bronchi and bronchioles which respond to stretch of the lung tissue.
2. *Cough reflex:* A reflex apnoea takes place during swallowing to prevent aspiration of food or water into tracheobranchial tree.
3. *Speech:* An inspiratory effect precedes the slow expiratory process.
4. *Swallowing reflex:* A reflex apnoea takes place during swallowing to prevent aspiration of food or water into tracheobronchial tree.
5. *Sneezing reflex:* Irritation of the nasal mucosa triggers this protective reflex. Deep inspiration precedes exposive expiration.
6. *Yawning reflex:* A peculiar infectious respiratory act that is usually initiated when a person spends a long period in a monotonous environment. It appears in underventilated alveoli which has a tendency to collapse.
It may be a response to slight increase in arterial pCO_2.

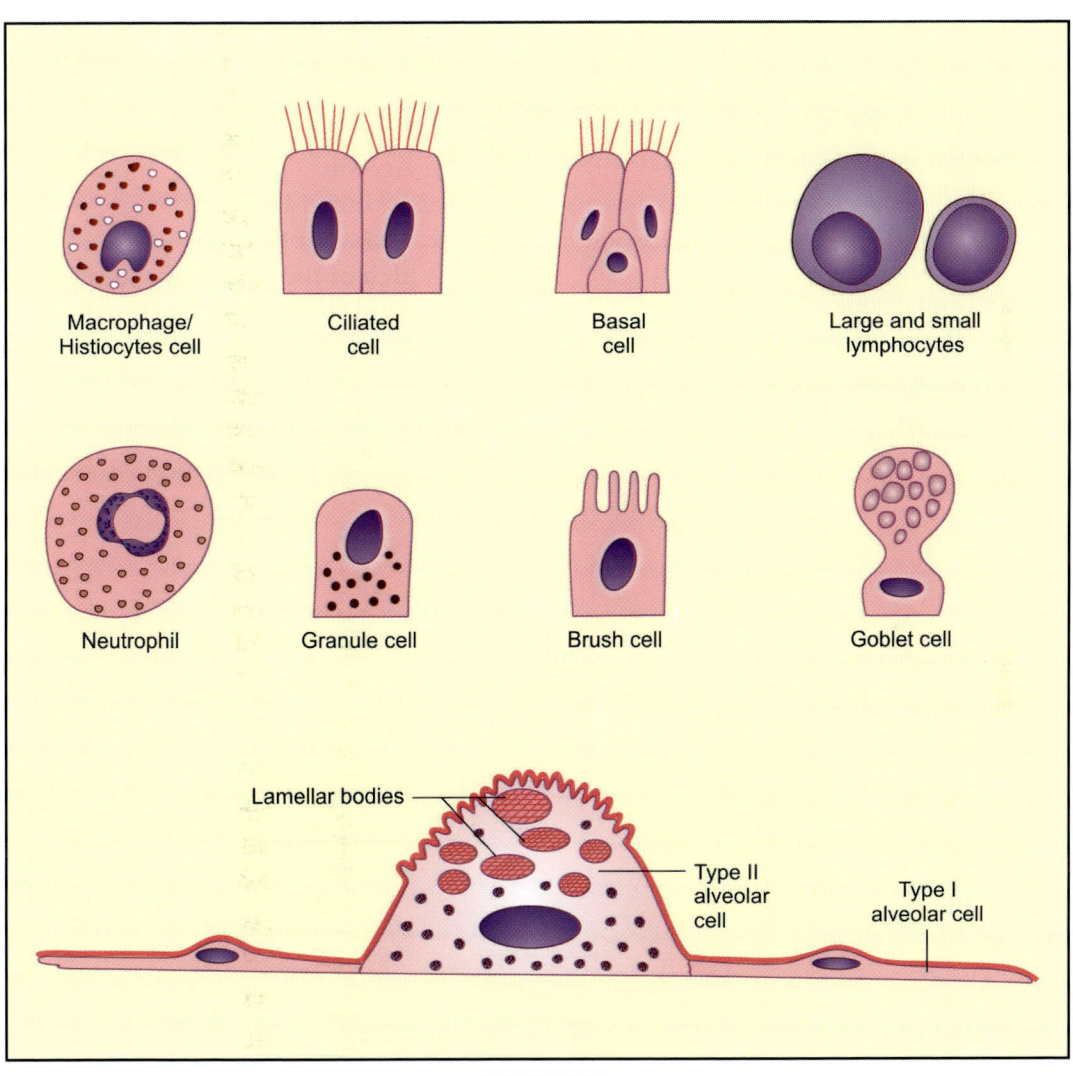

Fig. 11.5: *Cells in interalveolar septa and cells lining the alveoli*

MULTIPLE CHOICE QUESTIONS

1. **What is the epithelium of conducting part of the respiratory system?**
   a. Columnar
   b. Cuboidal
   c. Pseudostratified columnar
   d. Stratified columnar

2. **What is the main epithelial lining of the alveoli?**
   a. Columnar
   b. Cuboidal
   c. Squamous
   d. Pseudostratified columnar

3. **Which cartilage is present in the bronchial tree:**
   a. Fibrocartilage
   b. Hyaline
   c. Elastic
   d. All of the above

4. **Surfactant producing cells are present in one of the following areas:**
   a. Respiratory bronchiole
   b. Alveoli
   c. Terminal bronchiole
   d. Tertiary bronchus

5. **Which of the following connective tissue fibres is predominantly present in the respiratory system?**
   a. Collagent fibrres
   b. Elastic fibres
   c. Reticular fibres
   d. All of the above

ANSWERS

| 1. c | 2. c | 3. b | 4. b |
| 5. b | | | |

Digestive System: Oesophagus and Stomach

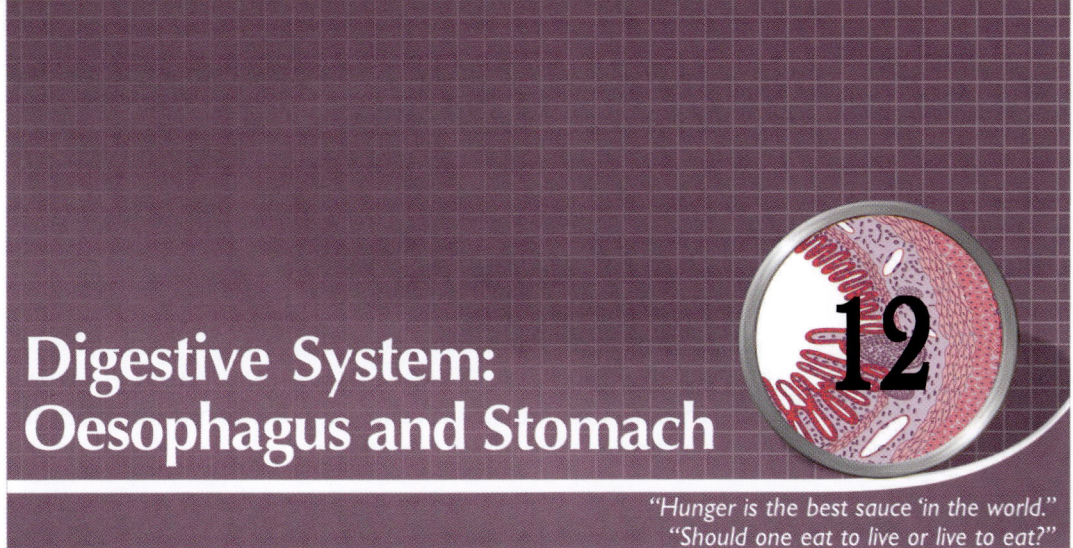

"Hunger is the best sauce 'in the world."
"Should one eat to live or live to eat?"

The **digestive system** consists of digestive tract: (i) oral/mouth cavity, oesophagus, stomach, small and large intestines, rectum and anal canal, and its associated glands (ii) salivary glands, liver, gall bladder and pancreas.

Function
- Ingestion of food necessary for maintenance, development and growth.
- Absorption of broken down small molecules from lining of digestive tract.
- Its mucous membrane acts as a protective barrier to harmful substances.
- Expulsion of solid waste.

Accessory organs and glands: These are teeth, tongue, salivary glands, liver, gall bladder and pancreas.

DIGESTIVE SYSTEM

ORAL CAVITY

Digestive system comprises: Long gastrointestinal tract/alimentary canal.

Canal: It starts at oral cavity, and continues as pharynx, oesophagus, small and large intestines to end at anus.

The oral cavity is divided into an outer smaller portion, the vestibule and an inner larger part the oral cavity proper. Vestibule of the mouth is narrow, bounded externally by the lips and cheeks and internally by the teeth and gums. The parotid duct opens into the vestibule. The vestibule communicates with the oral cavity when the mouth is open. The lining of vestibule is stratified squamous non-keratinised epithelium. The oral/mouth cavity proper contains teeth, openings of submandibular and sublingual salivary glands. Most of it is occupied by the tongue, described in Chapter 19. The opening of mouth cavity is guarded by the lips.

Lips: The lips are fleshy folds lined externally by skin and internally by mucous membrane. The mucocutaneous junction lines the edge or red margin of the lip, part of the mucosal surface is also normally seen. Each lip is composed of:
- Skin lined by stratified squamous keratinised epithelium with hair follicles, sweat and sebaceous glands in the dermis

- Superficial fascia
- Orbicularis oris muscle
- Submucosa, containing mucous labial glands and blood vessels
- Mucous membrane is lined by stratified squamous non-keratinised epithelium. The labial mucous glands are present in the lamina propria
- Mucocutaneous junction/red margin shows the transition from keratinised to non-keratinised epithelium, i.e. thick epithelium of skin changing to thin pink epithelium of mucous membrane, due to underlying blood vessels.

TEETH

Teeth form part of the masticatory apparatus and are fixed in the jaws. In man, the teeth are replaced only once (*diphyodont*) in contrast with non-mammalian vertebrates where teeth are constantly replaced throughout life (*polyphyodont*). The teeth of the first set (dentition) are known as *milk*, or *deciduous teeth*, and the second set, as *permanent teeth*.

The deciduous teeth are 20 in number. In each half of each jaw, there are two incisors, one canine, and two molars.

The permanent teeth are 32 in number, and consist of two incisors (Latin *to cut*) one canine (Latin *dog*) two premolars (Latin *millstone*) and three molars in each half of each jaw.

Parts of a Tooth

Each tooth has three parts:
1. A *crown*, projecting above the gum
2. A *root*, embedded in the jaw beneath the gum
3. A *neck*, between the crown and root and surrounded by the gum

Structure

Structurally, each tooth is composed of:
1. The pulp in the centre
2. The dentine surrounding the pulp
3. The enamel covering the projecting part of dentine, or crown
4. The cementum surrounding the embedded part of the dentine
5. The periodontal membrane.

The *pulp* is loose fibrous tissue containing vessels, nerves and lymphatics, all of which enter the pulp cavity through the apical foramen. The pulp is covered by a layer of tall columnar cells, known as *odontoblasts* which are capable of replacing dentine any time in life.

The *dentine* is a calcified material containing spiral tubules radiating from the pulp cavity. Each tubule is occupied by a protoplasmic process from one of the odontoblasts. The calcium and organic matter are in the same proportion as in bone.

The *enamel* is the hardest substance in the body. It is made up of crystalline prisms lying roughly at right angles to the surface of the tooth.

Digestive System: Oesophagus and Stomach

The *cementum* resembles bone in structure, but like enamel and dentine it has no blood supply, nor any nerve supply. Over the neck, the cementum commonly overlaps the cervical end of enamel; or, less commonly, it may just meet the enamel.

The *periodontal membrane (ligament)* holds the root in its socket. This membrane acts as a periosteum to both the cementum as well as the bony socket.

The pharynx contains the palatine tonsil, described in Chapter 8.

The gastrointestinal tract from oesophagus to rectum follows a general plan.

General plan of gastrointestinal tract: The wall of the gastrointestinal tract (GIT) (Fig. 12.1) from oesophagus to anal canal is made up of the following four layers.

1. Mucous membrane consists of three layers:
    a. Epithelium resting on a basement membrane
    b. Lamina propria
    c. Muscularis mucosae
2. Submucosa
3. Muscularis externa
4. Serosa or adventitia

MUCOUS MEMBRANE

a. *Epithelium*: It varies in different parts of GIT and is protective, absorptive and secretory. Its protective function against thermal, mechanical and chemical injury is clearly evident in oesophagus. This function is also seen in the distal part of the anal canal. Besides oesophagus and anal canal, the epithelium is single layered with various types of secretory cells. Its secretions are supplemented by the secretions of the glands which are present in different layers. The short ones are in the lamina propria, slightly longer ones in the submucosa and the other glands like liver, gall bladder and pancreas lie outside the gut.

b. *Lamina propria*: It consists of compact connective tissue with collagen, elastic and reticular fibres. It supports the epithelium. It contains capillaries, glands, fibroblasts, lymphocytes and sensory nerves which carry sensation of stretch and distension. This layer also contains extensions of muscularis mucosae. Lymphoid follicles are present in many regions like Peyer's patches in ileum. Cells in the lamina propria are also the source of growth factors which regulate the differentiation, turnover and repair of the epithelial cells.

c. *Muscularis mucosae*: It is made of an inner circular and an outer longitudinal layer of smooth muscle fibres. It is developed from oesophagus till distal part of rectum.

- It causes localised movements of the mucous membrane helping in digestion and absorption.
- The extensions of muscularis mucosae into the villus exert a milking effect on the lacteals of the villi of small intestine and promotes vascular exchange.
- Its circular layer helps in emptying of the glands of lamina propria.

By its contraction, it modifies the shape of the local mucous membrane, permitting it to adapt to the altered shape due to its contents.

SUBMUCOSA

Submucosa consists of dense connective tissue, blood vessels and *Meissner's* or *submucous plexus* of nerves, ganglion cells, lymphatics and glands. It is a strong layer of the gut. It contains largest arterial network for supply of mucous membrane and muscularies externa. Submucosa enters into folds of oesophagus, stomach and intestine. Does not enter into the villus.

MUSCULARIS EXTERNA

Muscularis externa is comprised of an inner circular and an outer longitudinal layer of smooth muscle. The antagonistic activities of these two layers result in peristalsis. Circular layer is mostly thicker than the longitudinal layer. Only in colon the longitudinal layer is thicker, forming taenia. The contraction of this layer results in peristaltic movements along the intestines. Between the two layers of muscle fibres is the *Auerbach's* or *myenteric plexus* of autonomic nerves with a few ganglion cells. Parasympathetic system is (i) secreto-motor to the glands, (ii) motor to the smooth muscle of the gut, and (iii) inhibitory to the sphincters of gut. Sympathetic system has the opposite effect.

SEROSA OR ADVENTITIA

Serosa is the outermost protective layer which carries some blood vessels, nerves and lymphatics. A double layer of serosa forms the mesentery by which various organs are suspended from the abdominal wall.

NERVE SUPPLY

The gastrointestinal tract is richly supplied by both the components of autonomic nervous system and an additional enteric nervous system. The neurons of enteric nervous system lie between the outer longitudinal and inner circular layers of muscularis externa and also in the submucosa. These connect with extrinsic motor, sensory and sensorimotor nerves of cranial and spinal nerves and provide intrinsic motor and sensory nerve supply to the gut wall.

Extrinsic Innervation

The extrinsic innervations comes from sympathetic and parasympathetic nervous system. The sensory endings respond to ischaemia, distension and stretching of the gut wall. The cell bodies of parasympathetic system are present in nodose ganglion of vagus while that of sympathetic arise from thoracic and upper lumbar segments of the spinal cord and relay in coeliac and mesenteric plexuses.

Intrinsic Innervation

The intrinsic innervations of the gut wall comes from neurons in intramural ganglionated plexuses. The myenteric plexus is situated between the outer longitudinal and inner circular layers. There are two submucosal plexuses, the most superficial being the Meissner's plexus.

Digestive System: Oesophagus and Stomach

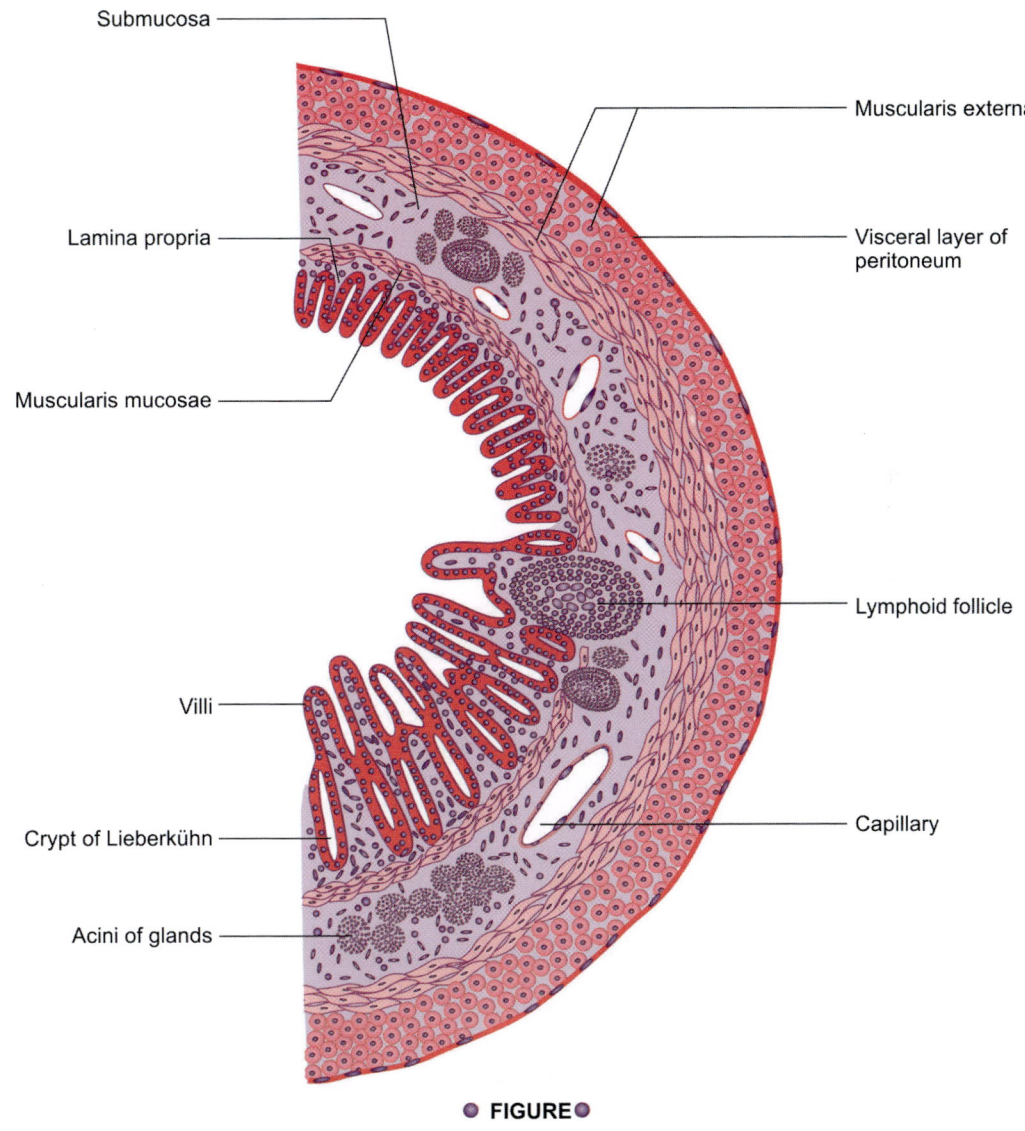

● FIGURE ●

FACTS TO REMEMBER
1. Mucous membrane comprises epithelium, lamina propria and muscularis mucosae
2. Submucosa contains glands, nerve plexus and capillaries
3. Muscularis externa mostly comprises two layers with an outer covering of peritoneum

Fig. 12.1: *General plan of gastrointestinal tract (diagrammatic)*

Nerve plexuses without ganglia are present at various levels in the gut wall. These are:
i. In lamina propria
ii. At the junction of submucosa and muscularis externa
iii. Between circular and longitudinal layers of muscularis externa
iv. Between internal and external parts of the circular muscle coat

All these muscle plexuses are connected with each other. These are also connected with extrinsic nerve fibres.

OESOPHAGUS

The oesophagus is a muscular tube that rapidly propels the food from pharynx into the stomach. It is about 25 cm long. Its wall includes all the layers included in the general plan of GIT.

The **mucous membrane** is thrown into longitudinal folds when empty. These folds become smooth as the bolus of food passes through the oesophagus. The epithelium is *stratified squamous non-keratinised* in character and protective in function. The lamina propria sends papillae into the epithelium. The muscularis mucosae is indistinct at the beginning of oesophagus, but becomes distinct lower down. It is made up of longitudinal layer of smooth muscle fibres (Fig. 12.2).

The **submucosa** contains *oesophageal glands*. These are mucus secreting glands with acini which are round or oval in shape. The lining cells are truncated columnar with flattened peripheral nuclei. The cytoplasm is lightly stained and contains mucigen droplets.

The **muscularis externa** has striated muscle fibres in upper third, mixed, i.e. both striated and smooth muscle fibres in the middle third and smooth muscle fibres in the lower third of oesophagus.

The outermost layer is the **adventitia** which is made up of loose connective tissue with capillaries and nerves.

Functional Aspect

- The oesophagus only conducts the bolus from its upper end to the stomach, with no digestive activity.
- The thick epithelium prevents injury to its wall from too hot or too cold food or fluid. The mucus helps in easy passage of the food.
- The functional sphincter at the gastro-oesophageal junction prevents the regurgitation of gastric contents into the oesophagus.

Applied Aspect

- *Hiatal hernia* is a condition in which the upper portion of the stomach protrudes into the chest cavity through oesophageal hiatus (an opening of the diaphragm).
- *Achalasia* is a problem of oesophagus which mostly occurs in young adults. It is due to constriction of cardiac sphincter, which obstructs or blocks the passage of ingested food materials into the stomach. This causes dilation of oesophagus and hypertrophy of muscle layer.

Digestive System: Oesophagus and Stomach

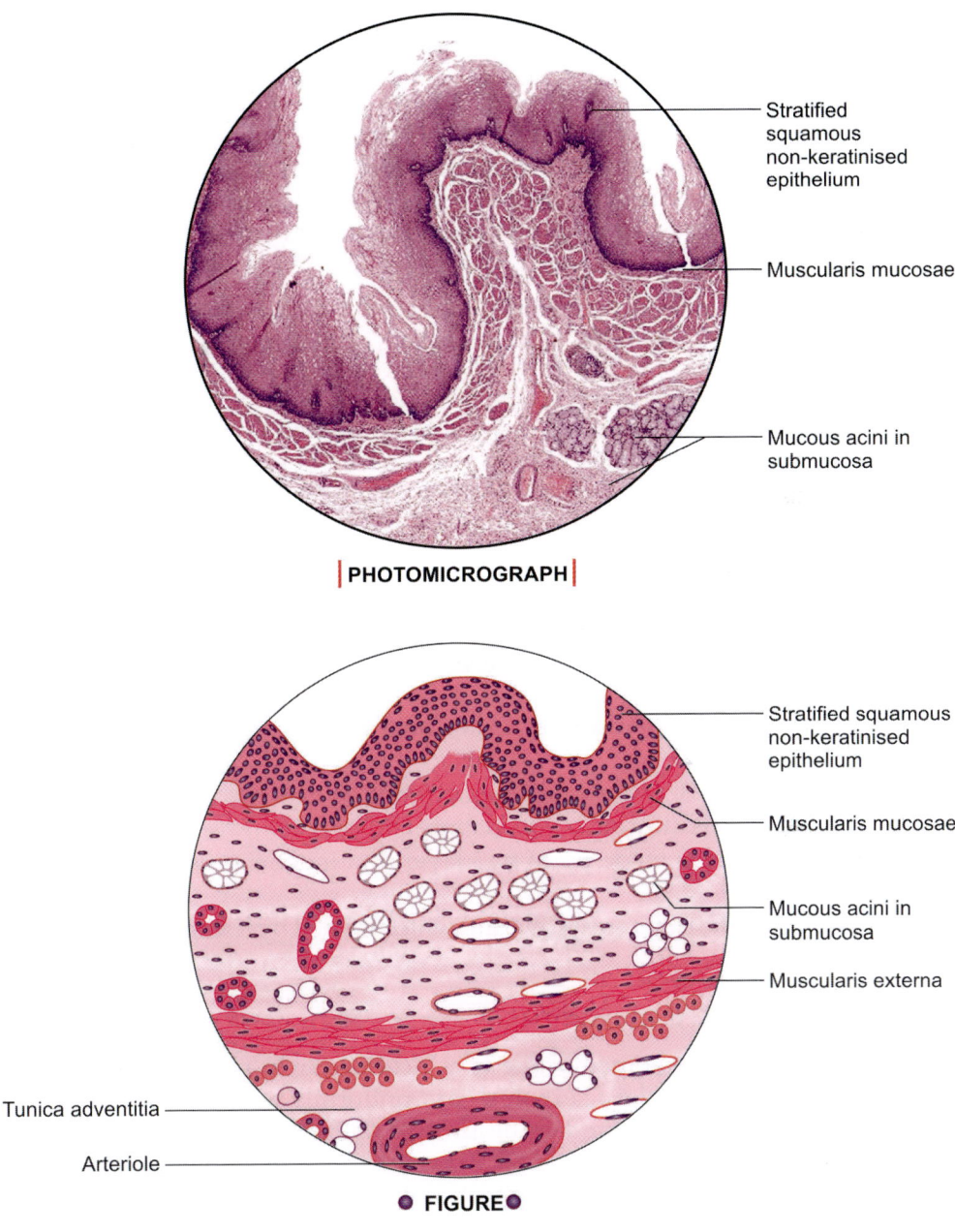

Fig. 12.2: *Oesophagus. Stain: Haematoxylin-eosin, 100X*

STOMACH

The stomach is the most distensible part of the gastrointestinal tract. It is a mechanical mixer, chemical digester and a temporary storage receptacle of food. The entire thickness of the mucous membrane is occupied by glands, which open into the gastric pits. The first part which includes a narrow ring-shaped area around the beginning of stomach is called the *cardiac end*. The succeeding largest part is the fundus and the *body*. Fundus and body are similar histologically. The terminal part of the stomach is called the *pyloric part*.

CARDIO-OESOPHAGEAL OR GASTRO-OESOPHAGEAL JUNCTION

At the cardio-oesophageal junction, the *stratified squamous epithelium* of the **mucous membrane** changes *abruptly* into simple columnar epithelium. The columnar cells *all look alike* with basal oval nuclei. The supra-nuclear portion is filled with mucigen granules, the precursors of mucus. *No goblet cells* are present in this epithelium. The columnar cells line the surface epithelium as well as the gastric-pits indenting the surface epithelium.

The lamina propria contains small tubular glands, oriented perpendicular to the surface. **Basal half** of the gland is lined by secretory columnar cells with a few parietal and zymogenic cells. The **apical half** is lined by short columnar cells and is conducting in nature.

The muscularis mucosae consists of an inner circular and an outer longitudinal layer of smooth fibres.

The **submucosa** may show few mucous secreting acini of oesophageal glands besides the loose connective tissue, fine blood vessels and nerves.

Muscularis externa is made up of two layers; an inner circular layer and an outer longitudinal layer.

The **serosa** forms the outermost covering which is lined by a single layer of squamous cells (Fig. 12.3).

FUNDUS AND BODY OF STOMACH

The epithelium of **mucous membrane** is tall columnar in nature. *All cells look alike*. These cells have basal oval nuclei which are uniformly stained. The free surface of epithelium invaginates into the lamina propria to form *gastric pits*. Three to seven gastric glands open into each gastric pit. Thus the whole of lamina propria is studded with tall **gastric glands**. These glands are straight, except near the muscularis mucosae where they may be bent. Thus the *deeper two-thirds* of each gland is secretory, while the *upper one-third*, the common pit for 3–7 glands is for conducting the secretions.

Parts of gastric glands and cell types:

The deepest portion close to muscularis mucosae is called the *base*, major middle portion is the *body* and upper part is the *neck* which is continuous with the *pit*. The base and body are lined by:

1. Chief or zymogenic or peptic cells. These are pyramidal in shape with rounded central nuclei and basophilic granular cytoplasm. These cells secrete enzymes like pepsin and lipase. These are strongly basophilic.

Digestive System: Oesophagus and Stomach

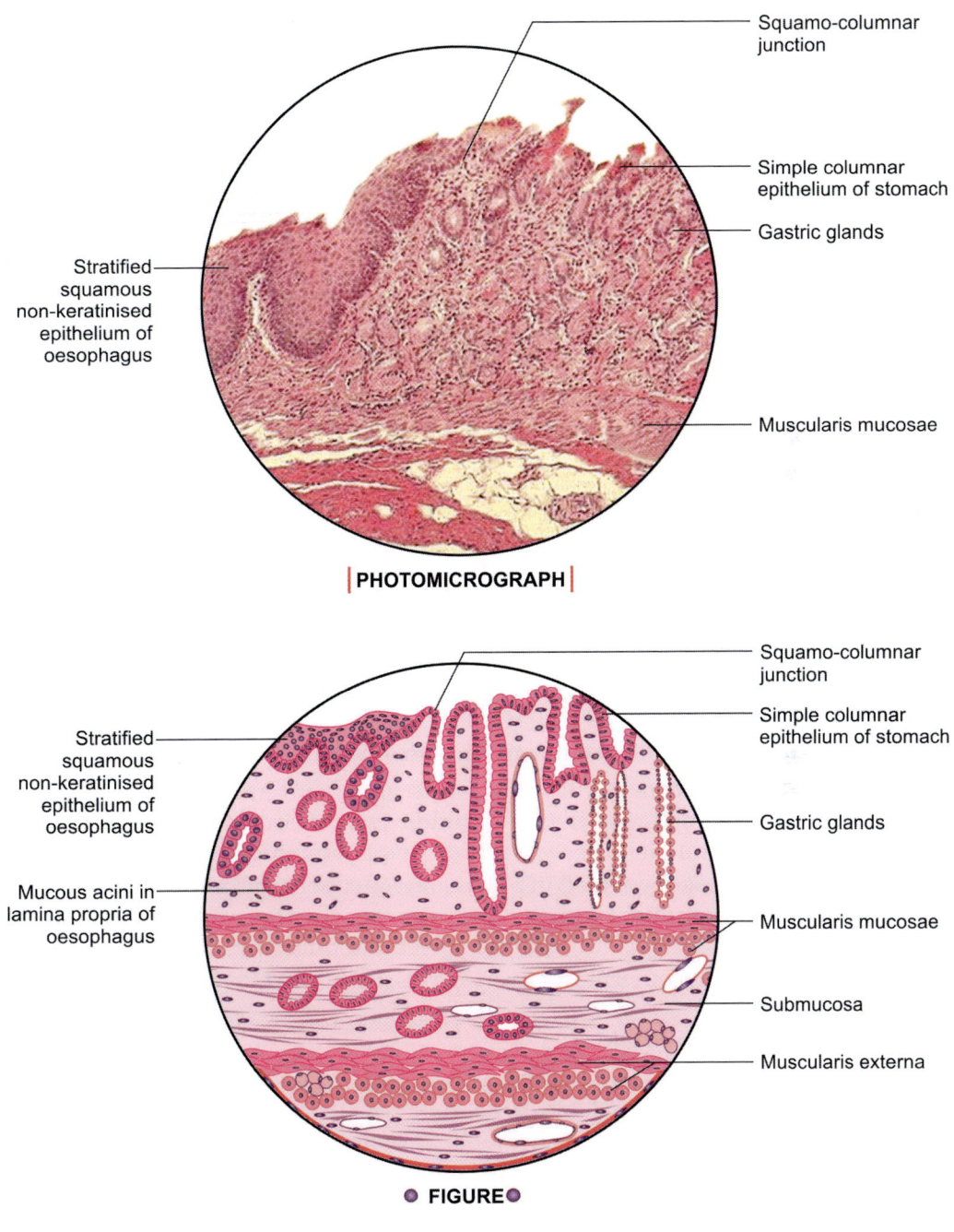

Fig. 12.3: *Cardio-oesophageal junction. Stain: Haematoxylin-eosin, 100X*

2. **Oxyntic or parietal cells** mainly in the apical half of the gland are scattered between the zymogenic or chief cells. These are large oval cells with central nuclei. The cytoplasm is bright acidophilic. These cells lie between the zymogenic cells and the basement membrane causing a bulge on the outer aspect of the gland into the lamina propria, giving a *beaded appearance* to the gland. The cells pour their secretion of hydrogen and chloride ions through canaliculi which pass between the adjacent chief cells. They also secrete *intrinsic factor* required for the absorption of vitamin B_{12}.
3. **Argentaffin cells** are seen as few triangular cells at the base of the gland. These cells are stained by silver salts and form part of gastro-enteropancreatic endocrine amine precussor uptake and decarboxylation (APUD) system. Argentaffin cells secrete *serotonin* into the capillaries of lamina propria which exerts a regulatory action on the gut.
4. *Mucous neck cells* line the neck of the gastric gland. These are short columnar cells, full of mucus with round nuclei. This mucus is different histochemically from that of the surface mucous cells. A few parietal cells are also seen in the region of the neck of the gland. The pit is lined by columnar cells which is continuous with those of surface epithelial cells. The mucous neck cells and surface epithelial cells secrete mucus which protects gastric lining against its own secretion of acid and enzymes.
5. **Undifferentiated cells** are small number of stem cells replacing surface mucous cells every third day and mucous neck cells every seventh day (Fig. 12.4).
6. **Surface mucous cells** line the surface epithelium.

Muscularis mucosae is made of three thin layers, inner circular, middle longitudinal layer and a discontinuous external circular layer of smooth muscle fibres.

Submucosa only has loose connective tissue, fine blood vessels and nerve fibres.

Muscularis externa consists of three layers of smooth muscle fibres. There is an innermost coat of oblique muscle fibres, middle coat of circular muscle and an outer coat of longitudinal muscle fibres and Meissner's autonomic plexus.

Circular layer is best developed in pyloric region, poorly developed in oesophageal region. The outer longitudinal layer is most prominent in upper two-thirds of stomach, the inner oblique is well developed in the lower half only (Fig. 12.5).

The **serosa** forms the outermost covering of squamous cells.

PYLORIC PART OF THE STOMACH

In pyloric region the pits or ducts are deeper than elsewhere in the stomach. The epithelium of the mucous membrane consists of tall columnar cells which all look alike. The epithelium dips down to line the *deep pit* into which open the *short pyloric glands*. The deeper **one-third is secretory** while superficial **two-thirds is conducting** (Fig. 12.6). The lumen of pyloric glands is larger than that of gastric glands. Their terminal parts are coiled. The acini are lined chiefly by columnar light staining cells with flattened peripheral nuclei, including some oxyntic cells. A few argentaffin cells may also be present. The glands open into the bases of the pits. **Mucus** and the **hormone gastrin** is secreted by the cells of pyloric glands. The acini of pyloric glands and their ducts are all situated in the lamina propria. In between the glands the lamina propria also contains gastric lymphatic follicles, especially in young age. Muscularis mucosae is made up of two layers of smooth muscle fibres, an inner circular coat and an outer

Digestive System: Oesophagus and Stomach

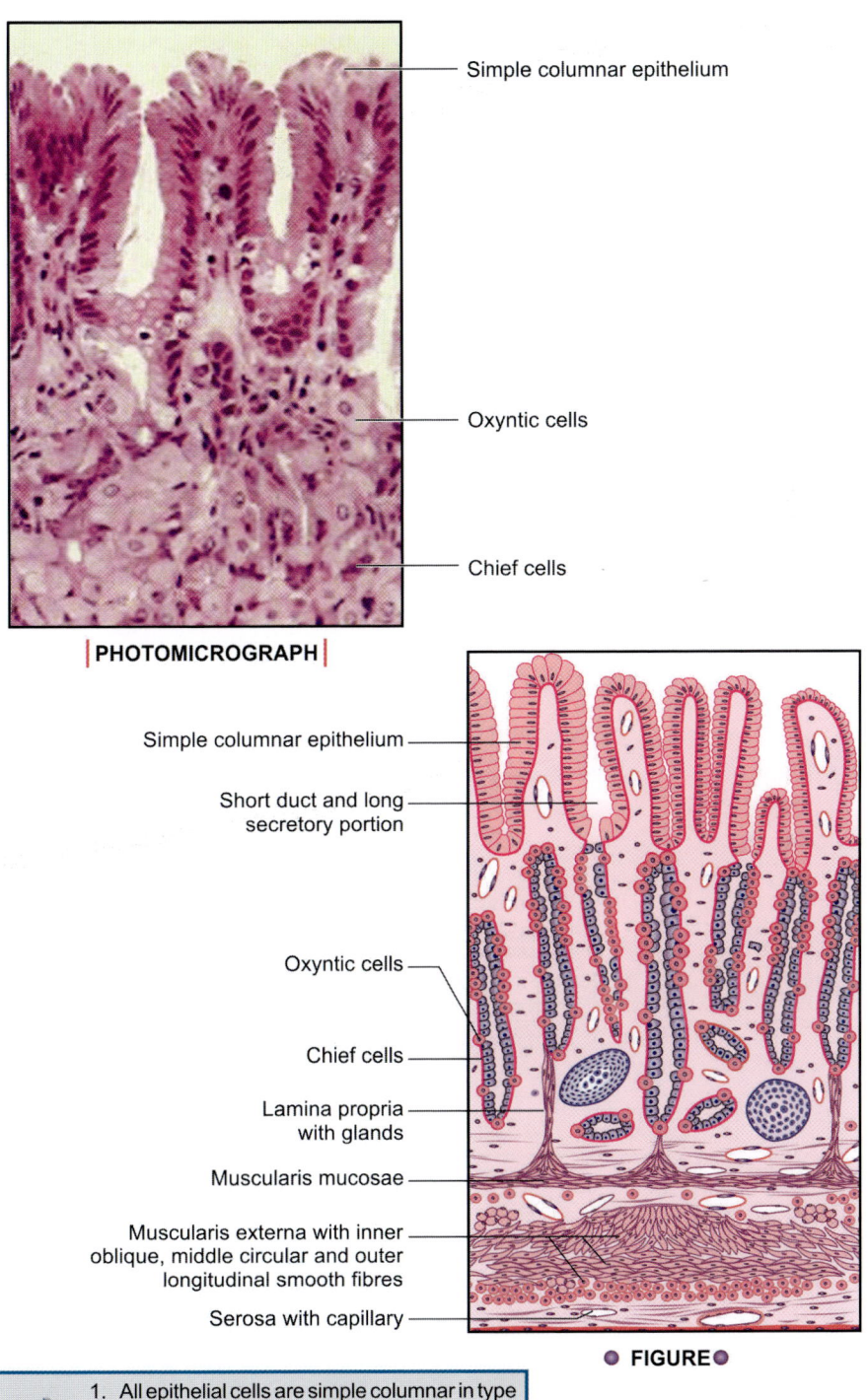

FACTS TO REMEMBER
1. All epithelial cells are simple columnar in type
2. Parietal cells are large and pink, chief cells are small and blue
3. Duct is 1/3rd and secretory part is 2/3rd

Fig. 12.4: *Stomach fundus/body of stain: Haematoxylin-eosin, 100X*

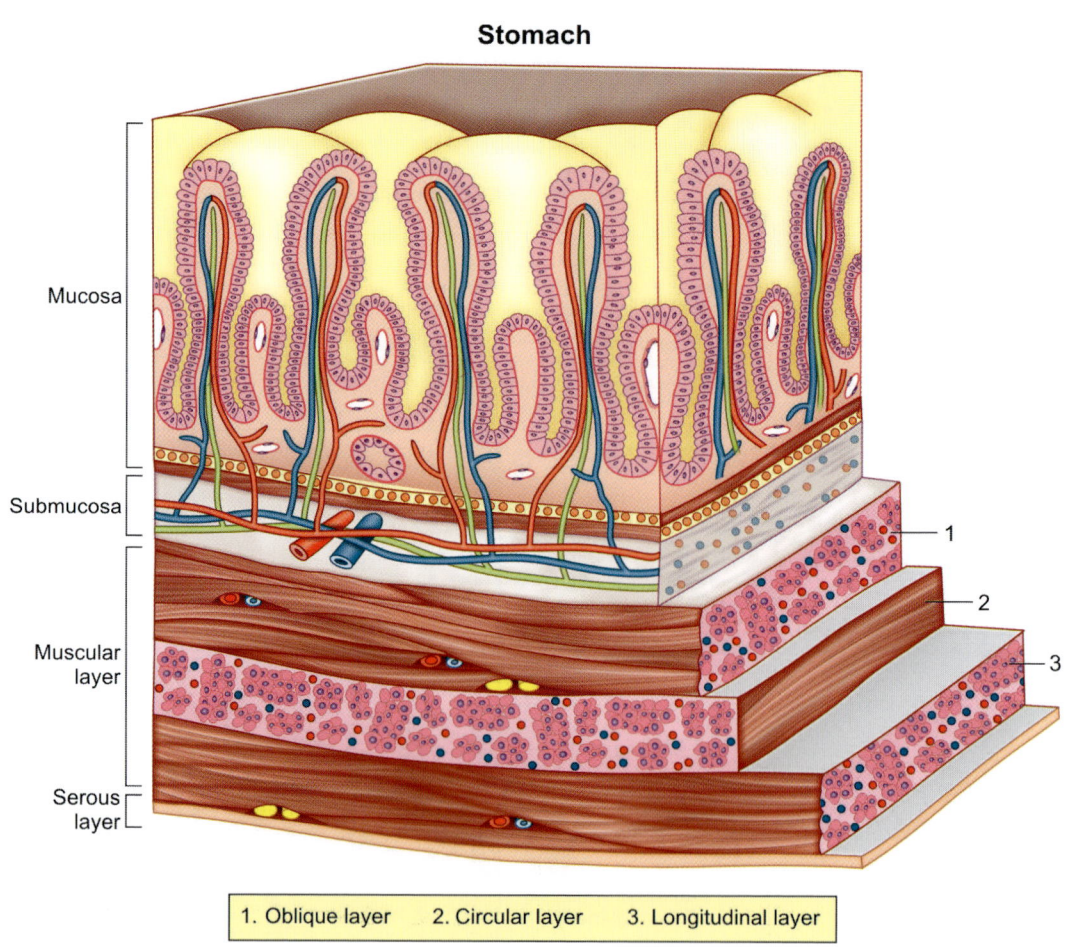

Fig. 12.5: *Various layers of wall of stomach (diagrammatic)*

Digestive System: Oesophagus and Stomach

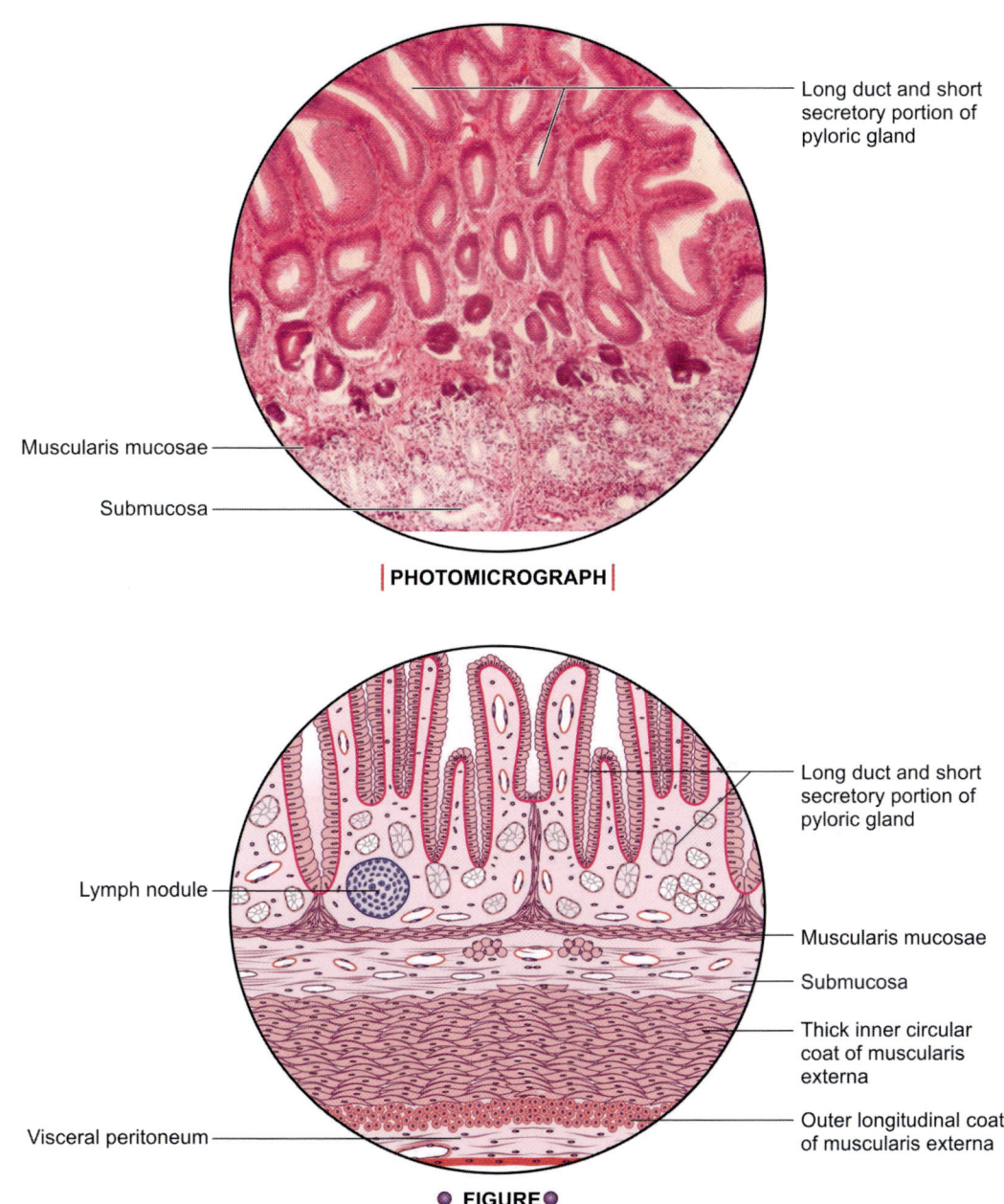

Fig. 12.6: *Pylorus of stomach. Stain: Haematoxylin-eosin, 100X*

FACTS TO REMEMBER
1. The epithelium is simple columnar in type
2. Duct is 2/3rds and secretory part is 1/3rd
3. Muscularis externa has thick circular coat which forms pyloric sphincter

longitudinal coat. The inner circular coat sends a few fibres between the glands which help in contraction of gland.

The **submucosa** is comprised of loose connective tissue, nerve fibres and smaller blood vessels.

The **muscularis externa** is chiefly made up of thickened inner circular layer which forms pyloric sphincter (*pylorus* = gate keeper) to control the timely emptying of the stomach.

The **serosa** is constituted by a single layer of squamous cells.

Table 12.1 shows the features of various parts of stomach.

Functional Aspect

- Stomach mixes and partially digests the food by mechanical and chemical actions. It only absorbs alcohol, water and a few drugs.
- Mucus produced by columnar cells lines and lubricates the mucosa.
- The parietal cells secrete hydrochloric acid and gastric intrinsic factor, for the absorption of B_{12} from the small intestine.
- The zymogenic cells contain pepsinogen. The released pepsinogen gets converted into pepsin in acidic pH. Pepsin breaks down the proteins. A few argentaffin cells are also seen.

Applied Aspect

- *Gastritis* is a condition which occurs due to disruption of normal balance between the protective effect of mucus on the gastric mucosa and the corrosive action of gastric juice. There is insufficient amount of mucus in the stomach to protect the surface epithelium from the destructive effects of hydrochloric acid.
- *Peptic ulcer* is the ulceration of the gastrointestinal mucosa. This is due to break down of the protective mucus barrier of the gastric mucosa, exposing it to irritation

TABLE 12.1: The features of various parts of stomach

Features	Cardiac end	Fundus and body	Pyloric part
1. Epithelium	Tall columnar cells which are all alike. No goblet cells	Same	Same
2. Gland	Very short gland 1/2 is body and 1/2 is duct	Tubular J-shaped gland. Lower 2/3rd is secretory and upper 1/3rd is conducting	Coiled pyloric gland. Lower 1/3rd is secretory and upper 2/3rd is conducting
3. Cells of the glands	Mucous cells and a few parietal cells	Chief or zymogenic, parietal or oxyntic, mucous neck cells and a few argentaffin cells	Mucous cells and a few argentaffin cells
4. Muscularis externa	Inner circular and outer longitudinal muscle fibres	Innermost oblique layer, middle circular layer and outer longitudinal muscle fibres	Circular muscle fibres are thickened to form pyloric sphincter and outer longitudinal layer

by food and autodigestion from its own secretory product. Stomach and first few centimeters of duodenum are the most common sites for ulcer. Hurry, worry and hot spicy curry are the predisposing factors.

- *Ulcer/cancer of oesophagus*: The oesophagus has to bear the brunt of too hot fluids or food from the mouth. Due to "hard to leave habits", it gets ulcerated.
  The lower end of the oesophagus has to bear the insult of acid from the stomach, leading to reflux oesophagitis and even cancer.
- *Ulcer/cancer of stomach*: Due to erratic eating habits and spicy food one is likely to get gastritis, followed by gastric or duodenal ulcer.
  The chronic ulcer more commonly along the lesser curvature of stomach may become cancerous in nature.

MULTIPLE CHOICE QUESTIONS

1. In which organ are the oxyntic cells present?
   a. Oesophagus
   b. Stomach
   c. Duodenum
   d. Colon
2. Which of the following layers is not a part of mucous membrane?
   a. Epithelium
   b. Lamina propria
   c. Submucosa
   d. Muscularis mucosae
3. Which of the following epithelium lines the oesophagus in human?
   a. Columnar
   b. Stratified columnar
   c. Stratified squamous non-keratinised
   d. Stratified squamous keratinised
4. Goblet cells are absent in which of the following parts of the alimentary canal?
   a. Stomach
   b. Duodenum
   c. Colon
   d. Vermiform appendix
5. Myenteric plexus is present in which layer of the alimentary/digestive canal?
   a. Mucous membrane
   b. Submucosa
   c. Muscularis externa
   d. Serosa

ANSWERS

1. b   2. c   3. c   4. a
5. c

Small and Large Intestines

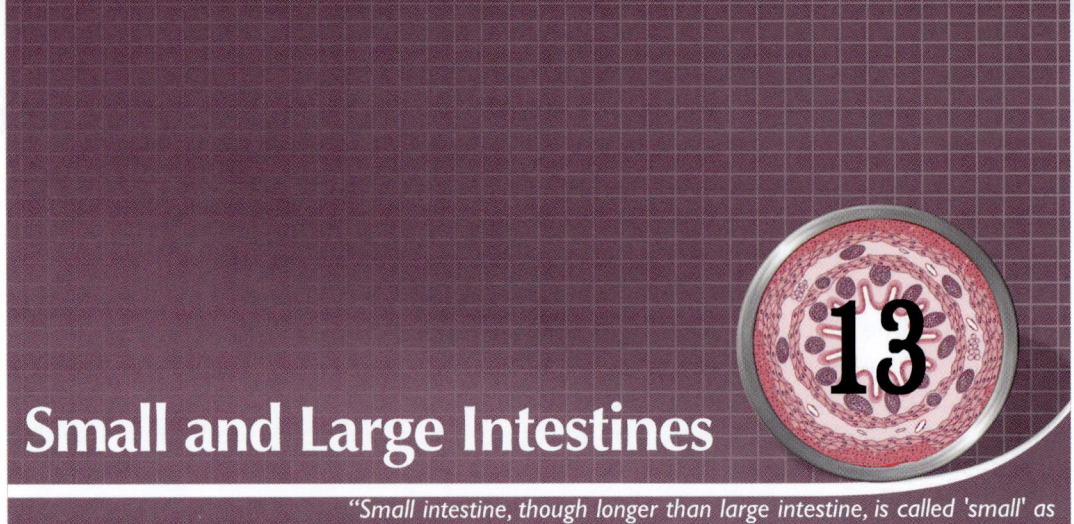

"Small intestine, though longer than large intestine, is called 'small' as it is less distensible than large intestine"

SMALL INTESTINE

GENERAL PLAN

The small intestine is the portion of the gastrointestinal tract between the stomach and the caecum which is the beginning of large intestine. It is divisible into three parts—duodenum, jejunum and ileum. The luminal surface of small intestine is modified for the purpose of increasing the surface area for absorption of digested food by the following mechanisms.

  i. The surface area of the small intestine is increased by the formation of circular folds. These are permanent folds, involving both mucosa and submucosa. These begin to appear 5 cm beyond pylorus. In second part of duodenum these become large and close together and continue to be large till proximal half of jejunum. From here onwards these start to diminish and almost disappear in distal ileum. The circular folds slow the passage of intestinal contents and also increase the surface area for absorption. These can be seen in X-rays after a barium meal.

  ii. The epithelium of the mucous membrane is evaginated to form finger like processes, *the villi* (Fig. 13.1). They evaginate to varying heights and increase the surface area for absorption by eight times. Villi give intestine a velvety appearance.

  iii. The columnar epithelial cells have striated border or *brush border* which is made up of numerous parallel cylindrical processes called *microvilli*. These further aid in increasing the surface area for absorption. These columnar cells are replaced by thin membrane cells over the lymphatic follicle. These are specialised cells for transport of antigens. The lamina propria contains invaginations of the epithelium forming crypts of Lieberkühn. The openings of these crypts lie between the bases of the villi. The crypts secrete intestinal juices.

Lamina propria contains fibroblasts, connective tissue fibres, lymphocytes, eosinophils, macrophages, mast cells, non-myelinated nerve fibres, lymph vessels and capillaries. Lymphocytes may be clustered to form follicles.

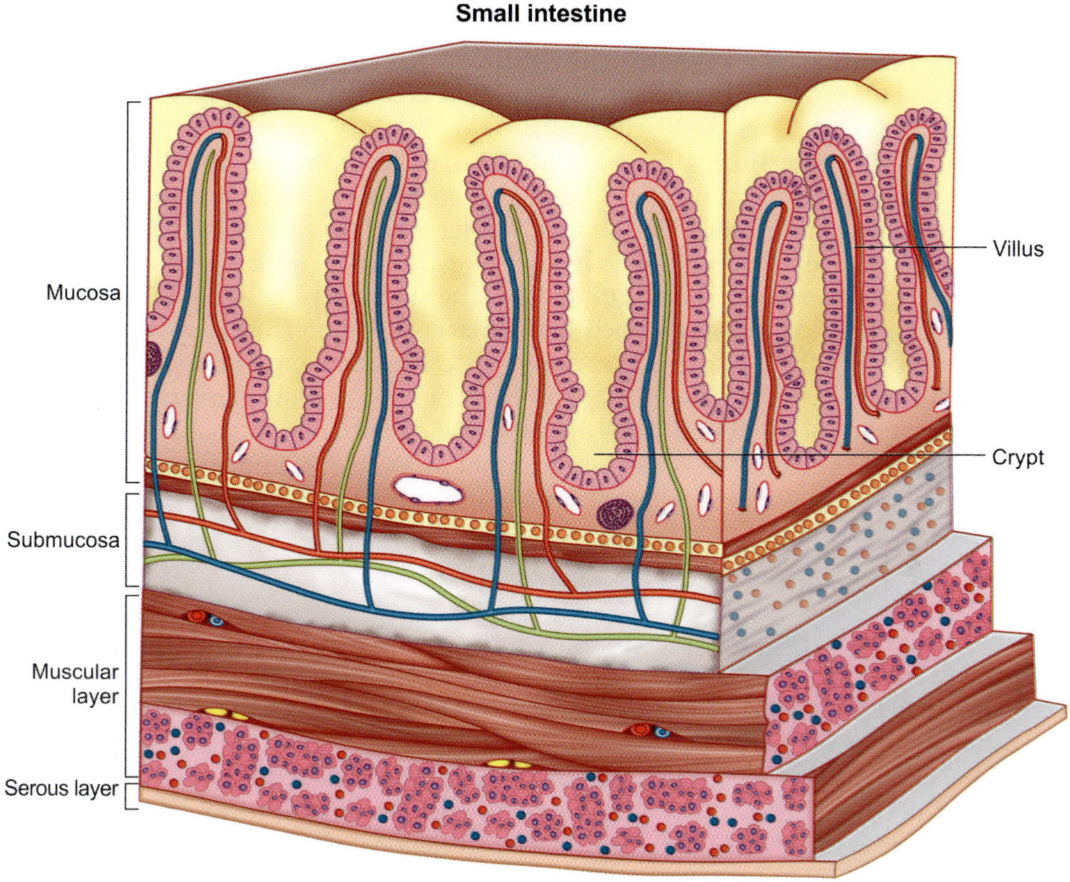

Small and Large Intestines

Fig. 13.1: *Various layers of wall of small intestine (diagrammatic)*

STRUCTURE OF A VILLUS

i. The centre of the villus contains a lymphatic vessel, the *lacteal*, which ends blindly at the top of the villus. It is lined by a single layer of endothelial cells. This lacteal is responsible for absorption of fatty acids and glycerol.
ii. There are capillaries which are radicles of portal vein in its core, for the absorption of amino acids and glucose. These are lined by **fenestrated endothelium** (Fig. 13.2).
iii. Core of connective tissue contains fibres and cells, e.g. lymphocytes, fibroblasts including autonomic nerve fibres.
iv. There are extensions of muscularis mucosae around the lacteal from base to the apex of the villus. Since some of these myocytes are attached to the basement membrane of epithelium and the lacteal, their contraction causes milking of the lacteals.
v. The surface epithelial cells covering a villus are most numerous tall columnar/ enterocytes with striated border. Their life span is 5 days. Tight junctions between the enterocytes are present. The striated border is rich in *alkaline phosphatase* and is associated with absorption. Enzymes such as *disaccharides* are bound to the striated borders. These help in intestinal digestion. The surface epithelial cells do not look alike, in contrast to those of stomach. Columnar cells are interrupted by the presence of goblet cells. Mucin of the goblet cells is discharged in a merocrine manner.

Microfold cells (M cells) are present in the dome epithelium covering localised collection of lymphoid tissue. M cells are cuboidal or flattened in shape with widely spaced microfolds. These cells sample luminal antigens by endocytosis and then transport antigens to lymphocytes which occupy spaces between M cells. All these cells are derived from the stem cells of the crypt of Lieberkühn.

STRUCTURE OF CRYPT OF LIEBERKÜHN

The epithelium covering the villi continue into the crypt of Lieberkühn. The wall of the crypt is lined by:
i. Columnar epithelial cells or enterocytes, which secrete ions and alkaline fluid to dilute chyme and aid absorption.
ii. Stem cells which are the undifferentiated cells. These cells divide mitotically and ascend along the side walls of villi, where these differentiate into goblet or columnar cells. These lie on a zone just above the basal regions of the crypts.
iii. Paneth cells are numerous in the deeper part of the crypt. These cells are rich in zinc and have eosinophilic granules, secreting lysozyme and antibacterial substance.
iv. Enterochromaffin/Argentaffin cells are present in the crypt amongst other cells. These are columnar/pyramidal in shape. Their granules stain black with silver salts and brown with chromium salts and have been classified as a type of APUD (amine precursor uptake and decarboxylation) cells. Such cells may be seen in the stomach, small intestine and are abundant in vermiform appendix. These cells secrete a hormone called serotonin or 5-hydroxytryptamine.
v. Mucous cells: The mucous cells in the crypts are similar to the goblet cells of the villi.

Lamina propria: This is composed of connective tissue. If provides support to the epithelium. It forms the core of the villi. It contains smooth muscle cells, macrophages, mast cells, capillaries, nerve fibres, solitary and aggregated lymphatic follicles.

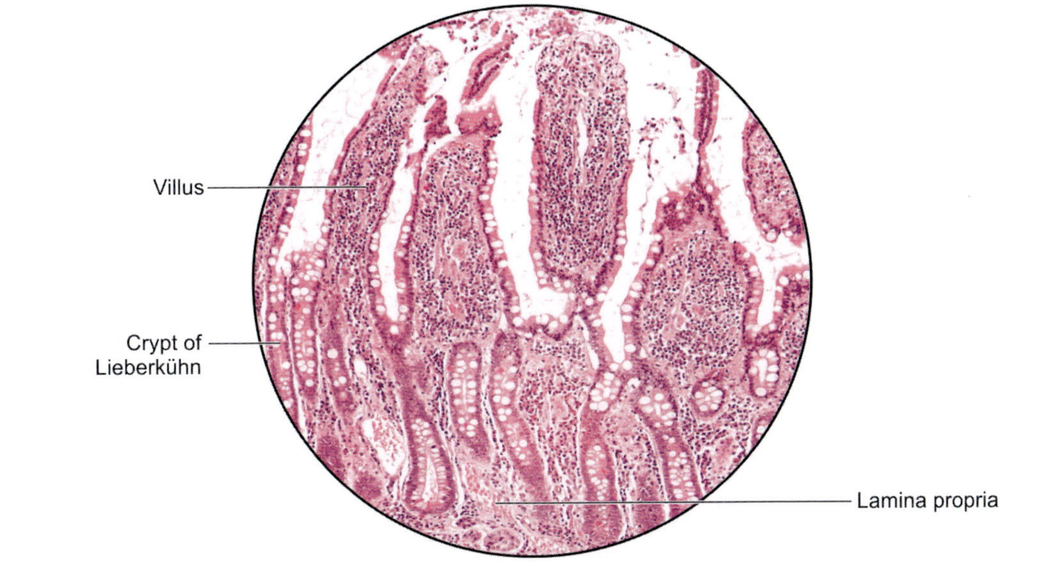

Small and Large Intestines

PHOTOMICROGRAPH

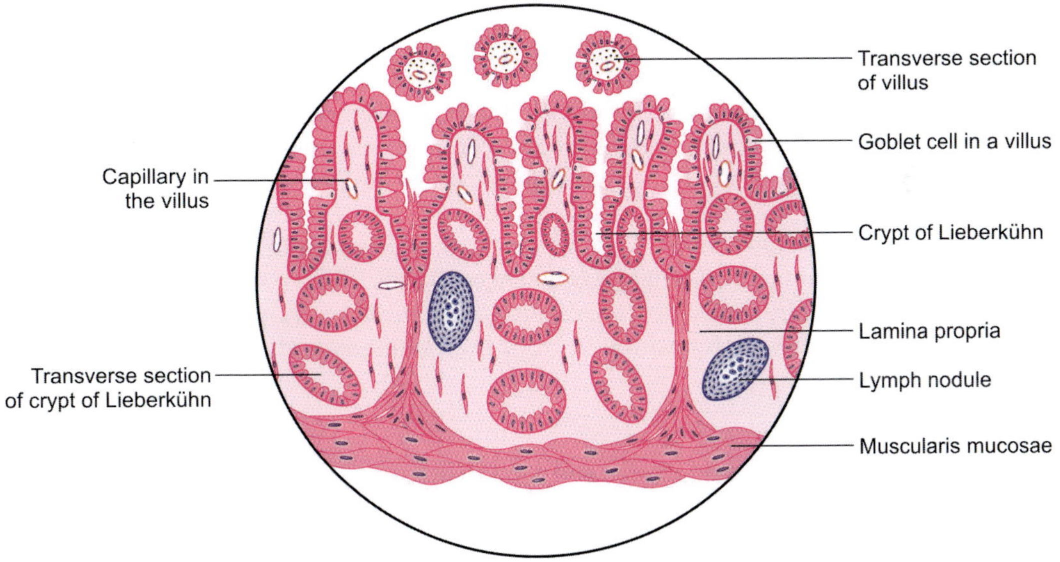

- Villus
- Crypt of Lieberkühn
- Lamina propria

FIGURE

- Transverse section of villus
- Goblet cell in a villus
- Capillary in the villus
- Crypt of Lieberkühn
- Lamina propria
- Transverse section of crypt of Lieberkühn
- Lymph nodule
- Muscularis mucosae

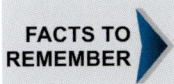

FACTS TO REMEMBER
1. Villi are evaginations
2. Crypts are invaginations
3. Villi contain capillaries and lacteals

Fig. 13.2: *Villi of small intestine. Stain: Haematoxylin-eosin, 100X*

Muscularis mucosae consists of an inner circular and outer longitudinal coats of smooth muscle fibres and extends into the circular folds to follow its profile.

Submucosa: Comprises loose connective tissue, capillaries and submucous plexus. In duodenum there are Brunner's glands while in ileum there are Peyer's patches.

MUSCULARIS EXTERNA

Muscularis externa comprised of inner circular and outer longitudinal coats of smooth muscle fibres. Myenteric plexus of nerves and ganglia are present between these two layers. This coat is responsible for the peristaltic waves.

SEROSA

Whole of jejunum and ileum have a single layer of squamous cells resting on a basement membrane. Parts of the duodenal walls have either serosa or adventitial covering.

Functional Aspect

Small intestine completes the digestion of various components of food. It absorbs the final products of digestion via the capillaries and lacteals and pushes the remainder components to the large intestine.

Table 13.1 depicts the differences between pylorus and duodenum.

PARTS OF THE SMALL INTESTINE

Duodenum

The **epithelium** shows numerous broad villi lined by columnar cells with brush border and goblet cells. Lamina propria contains crypts, connective tissue and diffuse lymphocytes.

Muscularis mucosae is made of two thin layers of muscle fibres. The inner layer sends extensions into the villi (Fig. 13.3).

The **submucosa** is characterised by the presence of compound racemose mucous glands called Brunner's or duodenal glands. These glands fill up most of the submucosa. Their secretions contain mucosubstances, small amounts of enzyme and bicarbonate ions which help to activate trypsinogen from the pancreas and also to neutralise the acidity of the chyme.

TABLE 13.1: Differences between pylorus and duodenum

Pylorus	Duodenum
1. All the cells of surface epithelium look alike. It dips in to form deep pits	Cells of surface epithelium do not look alike. It evaginates to form "villi" of varying heights. Also invaginates to form "crypts"
2. Columnar cells do not exhibit striated (brush) border	Columnar epithelial cells exhibit striated border
3. No goblet cells	Goblet cells present
4. Mucous acini are present in the lamina propria	Crypts of Lieberkühn are present in lamina propria.
Submucosa only contains connective tissue, nerve fibres, fine blood vessels	Submucosa contains mucus secreting Brunner's glands
5. Thickened circular muscle fibres form pyloric sphincter	Outer longitudinal and inner circular layer of smooth muscle fibres are seen without thickening of circular muscle fibres.

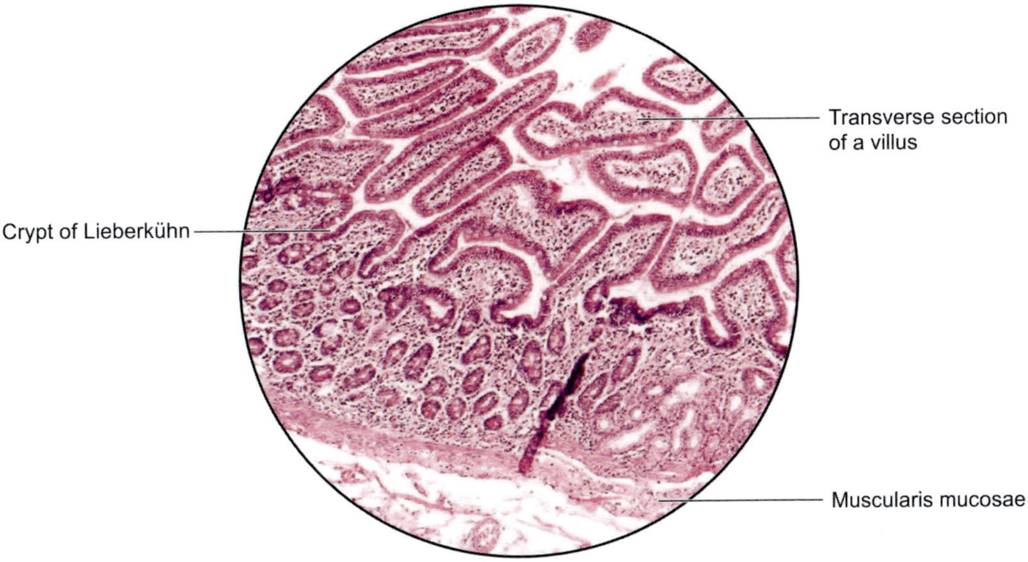

Small and Large Intestines

PHOTOMICROGRAPH

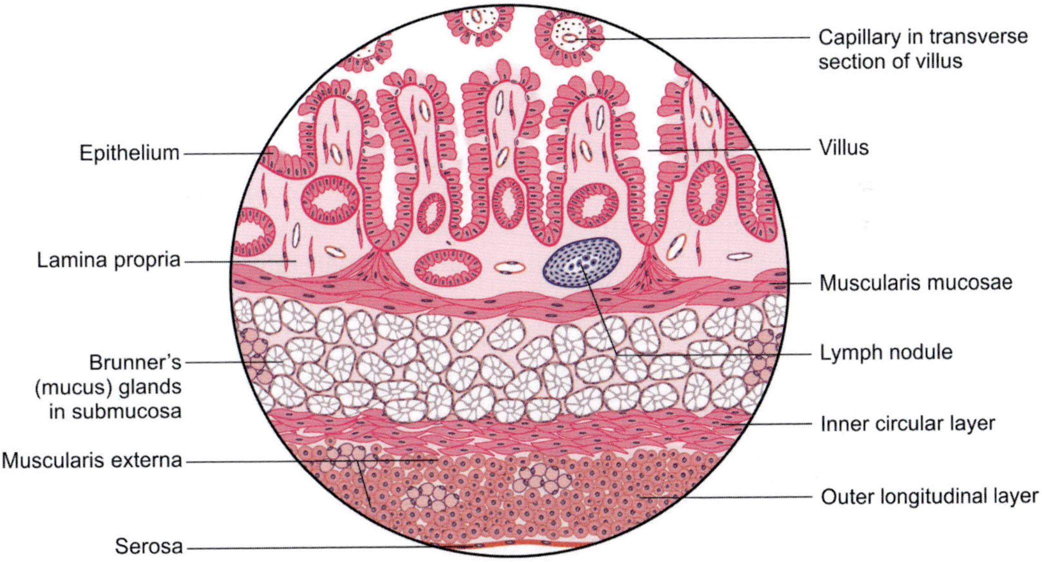

- Crypt of Lieberkühn
- Transverse section of a villus
- Muscularis mucosae

FIGURE

- Epithelium
- Lamina propria
- Brunner's (mucus) glands in submucosa
- Muscularis externa
- Serosa
- Capillary in transverse section of villus
- Villus
- Muscularis mucosae
- Lymph nodule
- Inner circular layer
- Outer longitudinal layer

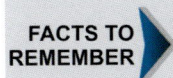

FACTS TO REMEMBER
1. Spatulate broad closely packed villi
2. Crypts of Lieberkühn in lamina propria
3. Mucus-secreting Brunner's glands in submucosa

Fig. 13.3: *Duodenum. Stain: Haematoxylin-eosin, 100X*

Muscularis externa comprises two layers of smooth muscle fibres.
The outermost layer is **serosa/adventitia**.

Functional Aspect

Besides villi, the presence of duodenal glands is a characteristic feature. These glands secrete alkaline mucus and bicarbonate ions to neutralize the acidic chyme from the stomach. These glands also secrete a hormone urogastrone which inhibits the secretion of hydrochloric acid by the oxyntic/parietal cells of the stomach. It also stimulates epithelial proliferation in small intestine.

Jejunum

The **mucous membrane** contains numerous tall tongue shaped villi.

Lamina propria reveals cut sections of **crypts of Lieberkühn**, diffuse lymphocytes and connective tissue.

Muscularis mucosae is in two usual layers (Fig. 13.4).

Submucosa has only connective tissue, nerve plexus, ganglion cells and blood vessels. No Brunner's glands or Peyer's patches are seen.

Muscularis externa is comprised of two layers of smooth muscle fibres.

The entire jejunum is covered with a single layer of squamous cells forming the **serosa** (Fig. 13.4).

Ileum

The **villi** are few smaller, finger like and narrow. The **lamina propria**, besides cut sections of crypts of Lieberkuhn, shows solitary lymphoid follicles and aggregated lymphoid follicles known as *Peyer's patches*. Solitary lymphoid follicles, most numerous in distal ileum, are covered with rudimentary villi (Fig. 13.5).

Table 13.2 shows differences among three parts of small intestine.

TABLE 13.2: Differences among three parts of small intestine

	Duodenum	Jejunum	Ileum
1. Epithelium	Columnar epithelium with striated border. A few goblet cells seen	Columnar epithelium with goblet cells. Striated border seen in columnar cells	Same epithelium, goblet cells are more
2. Villi	Spatulate, broad, closely packed villi reaching up to varying heights	Tongue-shaped villi of different heights	A few thin finger-shaped villi. Their upper level is variable
3. Lamina propria	Contains sections of crypts of Lieberkühn, segregated lymphocytes and loose connective tissue	Sections of crypts of Lieberkühn, diffuse infiltration of lymphocytes	Cut sections of crypts. Lymphocytes aggregated to form nodules of Peyer's patches which break through the muscularis mucosae into submucosa
4. Submucosa	Mucus secreting Brunner's glands are typical feature	Only connective tissue, blood vessels and nerves	Peyer's patches form a characteristic feature

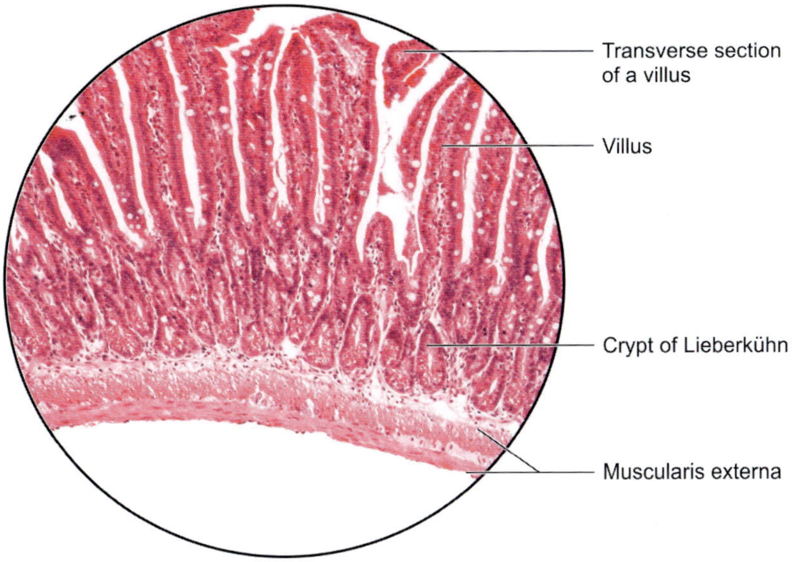

Small and Large Intestines

PHOTOMICROGRAPH

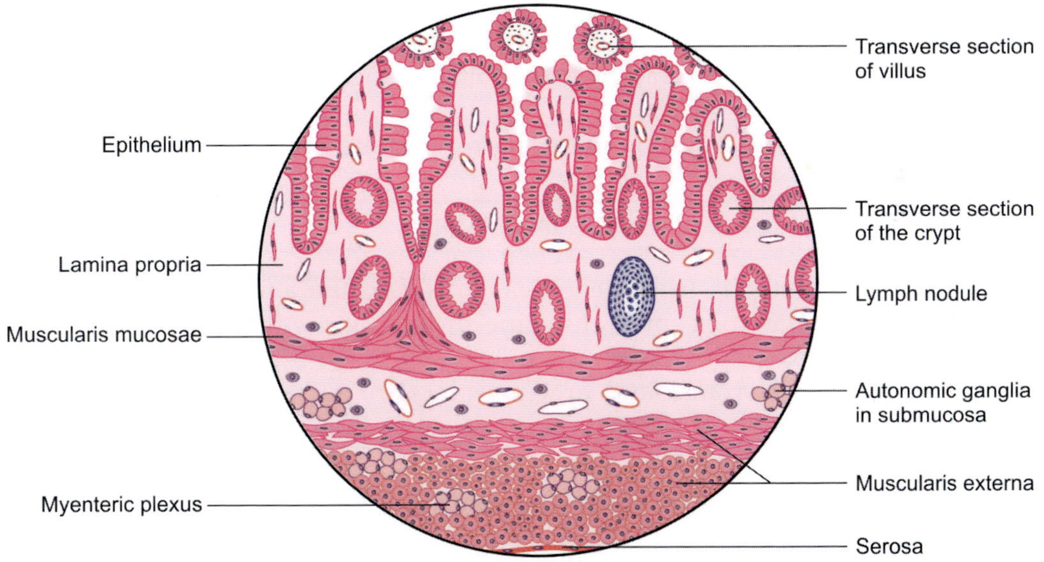

- Transverse section of a villus
- Villus
- Crypt of Lieberkühn
- Muscularis externa

FIGURE

- Transverse section of villus
- Epithelium
- Transverse section of the crypt
- Lamina propria
- Lymph nodule
- Muscularis mucosae
- Autonomic ganglia in submucosa
- Muscularis externa
- Myenteric plexus
- Serosa

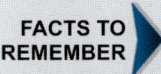

FACTS TO REMEMBER
1. Tongue-shaped villi of different height
2. Diffuse infiltration of lymphocytes in lamina propria
3. No Brunner's glands and no Peyer's patches

Fig. 13.4: *Jejunum. Stain: Haematoxylin-eosin, 100X*

Each follicle consists of lymphocytes, capillary network and dense reticular tissue with spaces. These reticular spaces communicate with larger lymph spaces which in turn are connected to the lacteals.

Surface epithelium overlying the follicles has **'M' cells** for transport of antigens. Aggregated lymphoid follicles or Peyer's patches are maximum around puberty and are antimesenteric in site. Each aggregated follicle is a group of solitary follicles covered with columnar epithelium and M cells; villi are usually absent. These provide B and T lymphocytes for defence of GIT and form part of gut associated lymphoid tissue (GALT).

Functional Aspect

The M cells overlying the surface epithelium sample or taste the antigens, ingest them, reveal them to the lymphocytes which produce specific antibodies against the antigens.

Applied Aspect

- *Cholera*: Occurs due to intake of contaminated water by *Vibrio cholerae*. Toxins produced by the "vibrio" cause severe watery diarrhoea, dehydration and may result in death.
- *Typhoid*: *Salmonella typhi* ingestion with food/fluid invade the lymphoid follicles of small intestine, i.e. Peyer's patches causing ulcers and even perforation of the gut. In enteric fever, typhoid ulceration of the follicles and healing with fibrosis does not cause constriction of the gut.

Tuberculosis: TB of small intestine causes narrowing and obstruction.

LARGE INTESTINE

The large intestine extends from ileocaecal orifice to the anal orifice. On gross examination, it differs from small intestine in having taenia, sacculations and appendices epiploicae.

The differences between small and large intestines are put in Table 13.3.

TABLE 13.3: Differences between small and large intestines

Small intestine	Large intestine
1. Villi are a typical feature, crypts of Lieberkühn seen in lamina propria are fewer and less deep. Goblet cells less in number.	Absence of villi. Crypts of Lieberkühn are deeper and more in number. Goblet cells are preponderant.
2. Longitudinal coat of muscularis externa is uniformly thick.	Longitudinal coat of muscularis externa is thickened to form three taenia coli.
3. No sacculations	Taenia are shorter than the length of large intestine, so sacculations appear.
4. No appendices epiploicae	Peritoneal pouches filled with fat are present. These are called appendices epiploicae

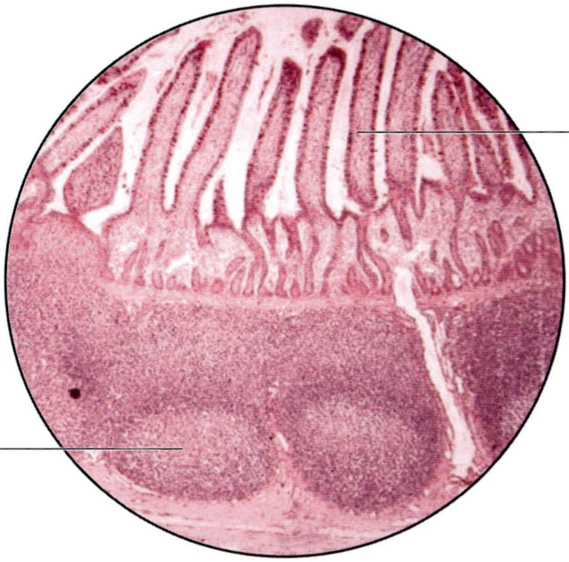

Small and Large Intestines

PHOTOMICROGRAPH

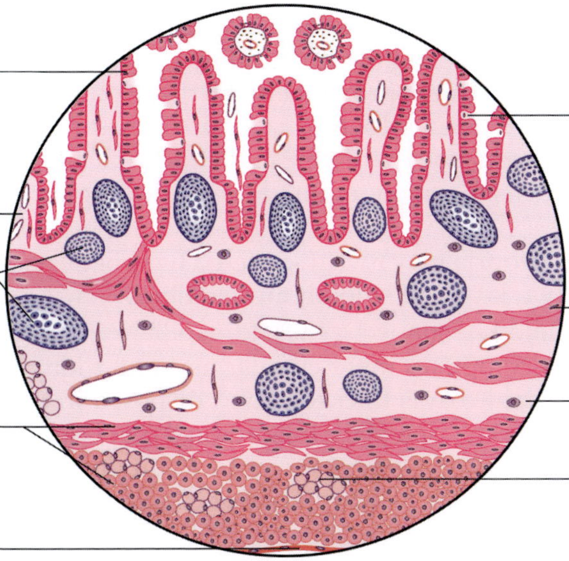

- Villus
- Peyer's patches in submucosa

FIGURE

- Epithelium
- Lamina propria
- Lymphoid follicle in lamina propria and submucosa (Peyer's patches)
- Muscularis externa
- Serosa
- Finger shaped villus with goblet cell
- Interrupted muscularis mucosae
- Submucosa
- Myenteric plexus

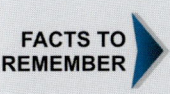

FACTS TO REMEMBER

1. A few thin finger-shaped villi with cut sections of the crypts
2. Aggregation of lymphocytes break through muscularis mucosae to lie in submucosa
3. These aggregations, called Peyer's patches, form typical features

Fig. 13.5: *Ileum. Stain: Haematoxylin-eosin, 100X*

Histologically the large intestine consists of (i) colon, (ii) vermiform appendix, (iii) rectum and anal canal.

PARTS OF LARGE INTESTINE

Colon

Colon helps in the absorption of water, salts and secretions secreted into the gut in its more proximal parts. It also provides an environment for growth of bacterial flora which is essential for digestion and metabolism of organic compounds and supplements vitamin intake.

The structure of caecum, ascending, transverse, descending and pelvic colons is similar. The **mucous membrane** is characterised by the presence of numerous deep *crypts of Lieberkühn* and by *absence of villi* (Figs 13.6 and 13.7).

The surface epithelium consists of (i) columnar absorptive cells with striated border and (ii) abundant goblet cells in between them. (iii) **'M' cells** are present overlying lymphoid follicles in the lamina propria. Many columnar cells have secretory granules. Their secretions are mucoid in nature and are rich in antibodies of IGA types, providing some protection against pathogenic bacteria. Some columnar cells possess an apical tuft of long microvilli and may be sensory in nature.

The lamina propria shows crypts of Lieberkühn. They lie at right angles to the surface, are deep and lined by both absorptive columnar and empty looking goblet cells. The crypts are more closely disposed in large intestine than in small intestine. The goblet cells increase in number from the proximal to the distal parts of large intestine. In the crypts, stem cells and enteroendocrine cells are also present. The secretions of enteroendocrine cells exerts both paracrine and endocrine effects. The crypts increase the surface area for mucus secretion required for lubricating the passage of contents of large intestine.

In addition, lamina propria may reveal scattered lymphatic nodules. The muscularis mucosae consists of two layers of smooth muscle fibres.

Submucosa is made up of connective tissue, capillaries and nerve plexus.

Muscularis externa comprises inner circular and outer longitudinal coat which is different. The longitudinal coat is thickened and disposed in the form of three bands called taenia coli. Between the taenia, the longitudinal coat is much thinner. The circular coat is aggregated in the intervals between the sacculi. In rectum these form a thick layer and in the anal canal these form internal anal sphincter.

The **serous coat** of the colon contains *appendices epiploicae*. These are pendulous projections consisting of adipose tissue. Parts of the colon which have no serosa are covered with adventitia.

Vermiform Appendix

Vermiform appendix in human is the narrowest part of large intestine (Fig. 13.8). In herbivores, the caecum and the appendix constitute a highly important site for digestion of cellulose by symbiotic bacteria.

Its lumen is narrowed irregularly. The epithelium of the mucous membrane is lined by columnar epithelial cells and **'M' cells**, antigen transporting cells. The crypts or glands are few which penetrate deeply into the lymphoid tissue. Lymphoid tissue is

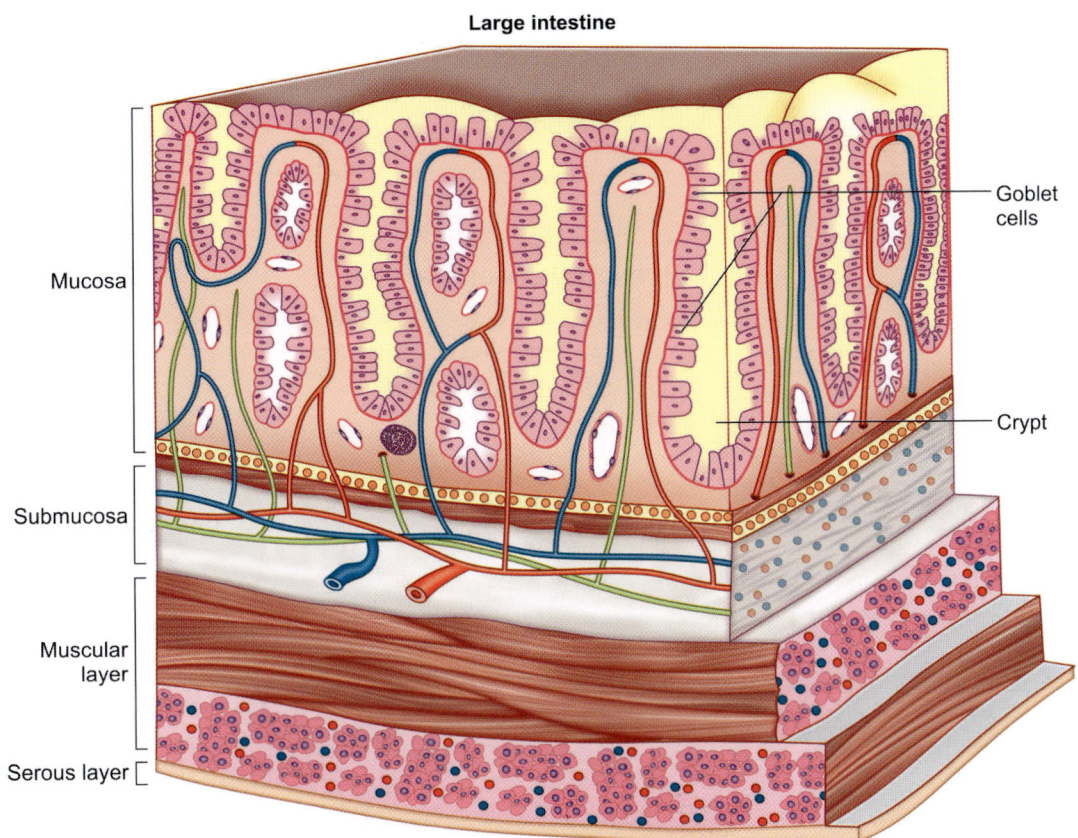

Fig. 13.6: *Various layers of wall of colon (diagrammatic)*

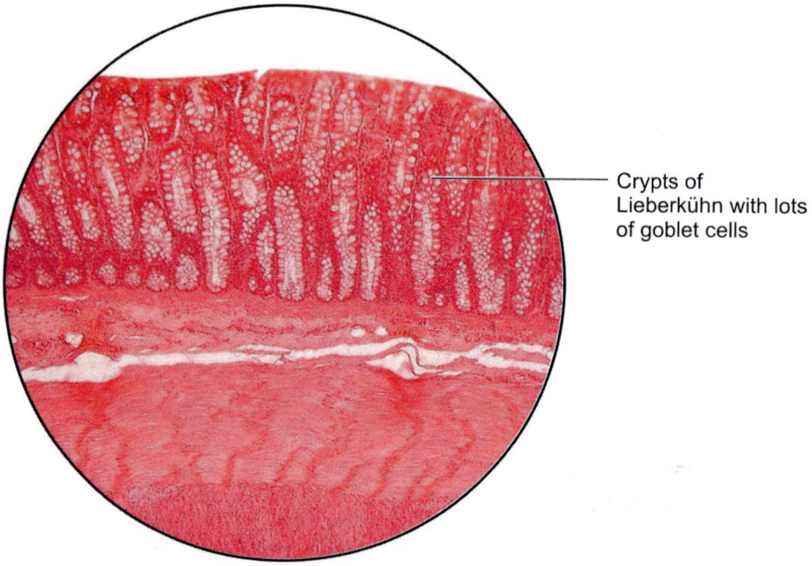

162 Textbook of Histology

| PHOTOMICROGRAPH |

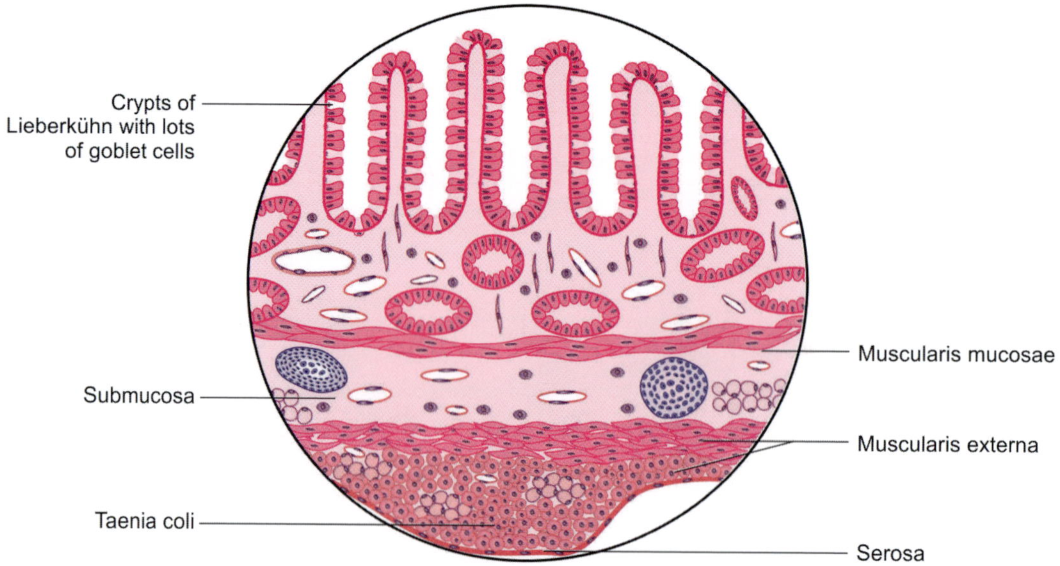

Crypts of Lieberkühn with lots of goblet cells

| FIGURE |

Crypts of Lieberkühn with lots of goblet cells

Submucosa

Taenia coli

Muscularis mucosae

Muscularis externa

Serosa

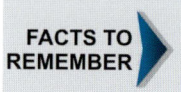 **FACTS TO REMEMBER**
1. Numerous crypts of Lieberkühn. No villi
2. Goblet cells preponderant
3. Longitudinal coat of muscularis externa is thickened at three places to form taenia coli

Fig. 13.7: *Colon. Stain: Haematoxylin-eosin, 100X*

Small and Large Intestines

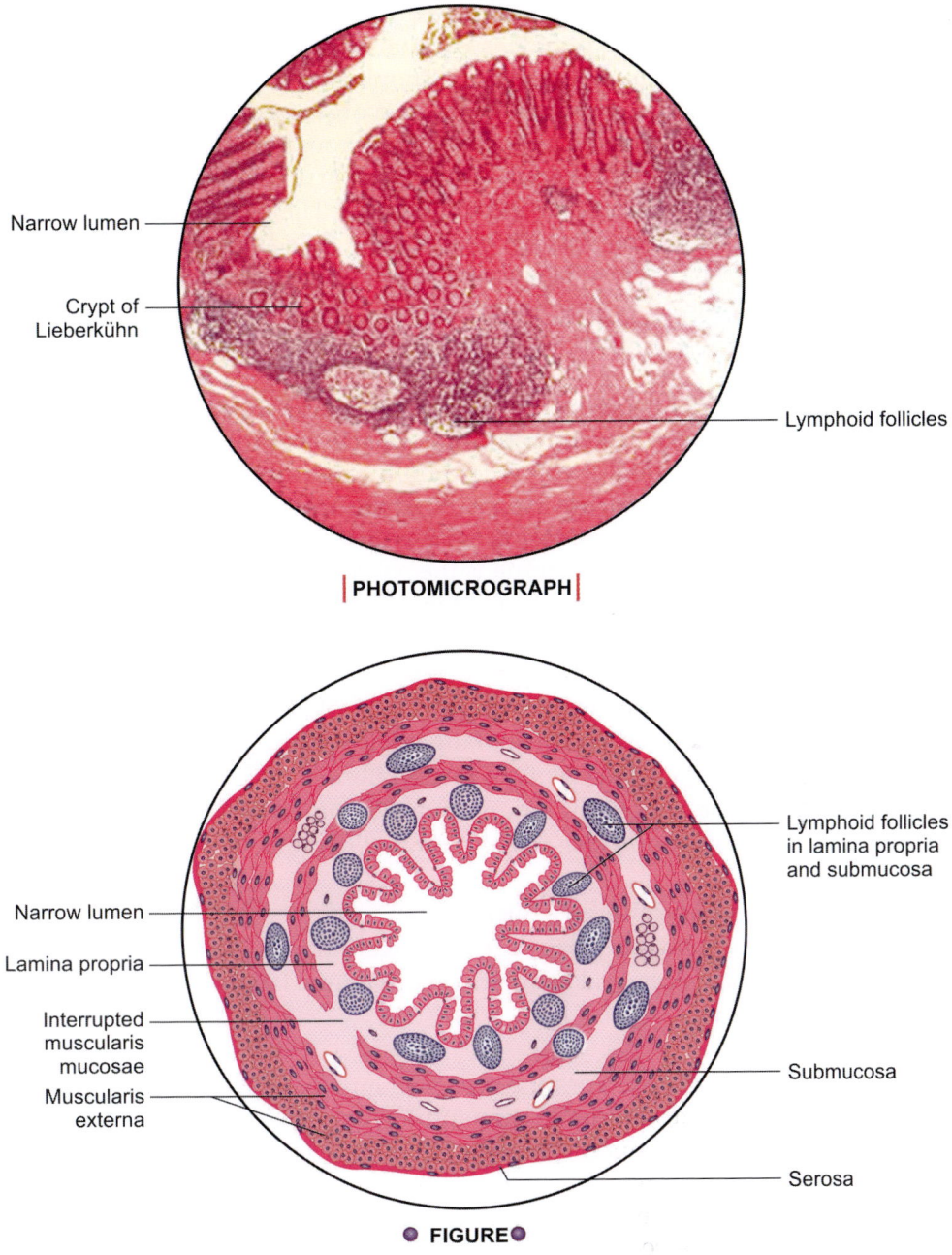

Fig. 13.8: *A vermiform appendix of a child. Stain: Haematoxylin-eosin, 100X*

FACTS TO REMEMBER
1. Whole lumen is seen. The epithelium only shows crypts of Lieberkühn
2. Lymphoid tissue is aggregated as well as scattered
3. Interrupted muscularis mucosae with thin muscularis externa

situated primarily in the lamina propria and extends into the submucosa. The follicular zone containing B and T lymphocytes can be distinguished. Lymphoid tissue is comprised of plasma cells, lymphocytes, eosinophils, mast cells and macrophages in fibrocellular reticulum. The germinal centres are organised like that of *gut associated lymphoid tissue* (GALT) which is an important part of common mucosal immune system. The para follicular zone contains venules for migration of lymphocytes and antibodies.

Muscularis mucosae is ill defined and interrupted. The lymphoid tissue is absent at birth, but accumulates during first ten years of life. In adults, the lymphoid follicles atrophy and are replaced by collagenous tissue. In old age, the lumen of appendix may have fibrous tissue.

Submucosa is well developed with many lymphoid masses which bulge into the lumen.

The **circular muscle** fibres form a thicker layer separated by connective tissue from the outer longitudinal coat. The **longitudinal muscle** coat forms complete uniformly thick layer except over small areas where both muscular coats are deficient, thus bringing the serosa and submucosa in contact. At the base of appendix, the longitudinal coat is thickened to form rudimentary taeniae which are continuous with those of the caecum. Beyond the muscularis externa is the subserous layer of connective tissue.

The **serosa** forms a complete investment in vermiform appendix.

Rectum

The **mucous membrane** is thrown into many large folds. The surface epithelium and crypts both contain abundant empty looking goblet cells.

The lamina propria contains crypts of Lieberkühn.

Muscularis mucosae appears as a thin but well defined layer.

Submucosa contains connective tissue, scattered lymphocytes, nerve fibres and fine blood vessels.

Muscularis externa is uniformly thick.

Serosa is only partly visible in upper part of rectum, rest is covered by adventitia.

Figure 13.9 shows histological comparison of various layers of GIT.

Anal Canal

It is the terminal part of large intestine and is 38 mm long. The mucous membrane is different in upper 15 mm, middle 15 mm and lower 8 mm.

In the upper 15 mm the mucous membrane forms 6–12 vertical columns named as *anal columns*. The lower ends of these anal columns are joined by transverse folds termed the *anal valves*. The epithelium is simple columnar with crypts of Lieberkühn. The muscularis mucosae continues as far as anal columns, where it subdivides and then disappears. Submucosa contains mucus secreting *anal glands*.

The middle 15 mm or transition zone epithelial lining is comprised of *stratified squamous non-keratinised epithelium* and not transitional epithelium. It neither contains sweat gland nor sebaceous gland.

The epithelium of lower 8 mm is true skin and contains all its associated components. The inner circular layer of smooth muscle fibres spans the upper three-fourths of the length of anal canal and is thickened to form the *internal sphincter*. The outer longitudinal

Small and Large Intestines

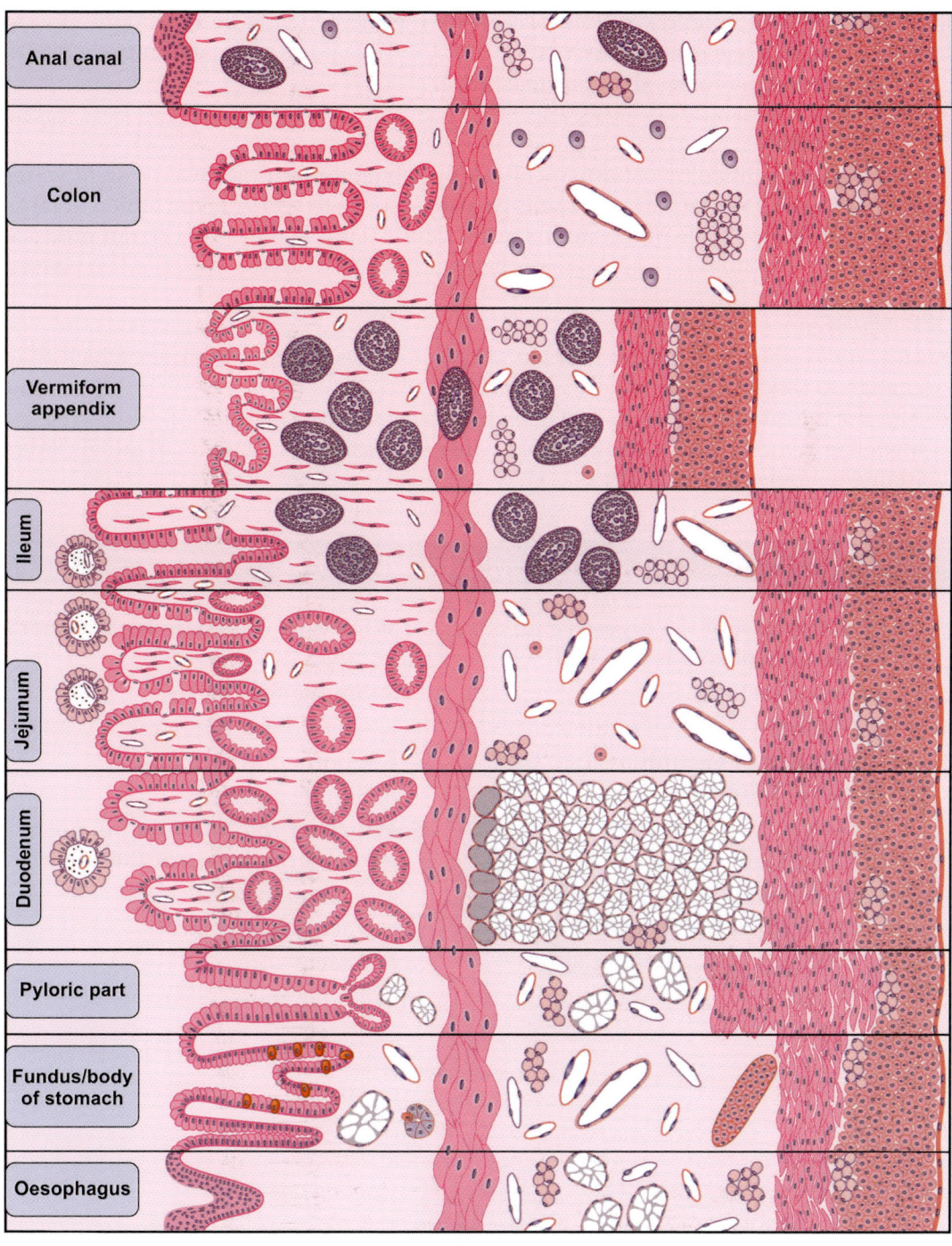

Fig. 13.9: Components of various layers of gastrointestinal tract

layer extends up to the lower limit of transition zone. Outside these smooth muscle layers lies the *external anal sphincter* comprised of three parts of striated muscle fibres.

Tunica adventitia forms the outermost layer.

Functional Aspect

The epithelium is lined by columnar cells with striated border for absorption of water and salts. The preponderant goblet cells produce mucus to lubricate the lumen of large intestine for easy passage of the faecal matter. The cell lining the crypts do not produce any digestive enzymes.

Applied Aspect

- *Ulcerative colitis:* Mucous membrane of colon shows numerous ulcers which may change to cancer.
- *Amoebic dysentery:* Ingestion of *Entamoeba histolytica cysts* with food/fluid, release amoebae in the stomach. The amoebae cause ulcers in colon, leading to mucus laden frequent stools.

MULTIPLE CHOICE QUESTIONS

1. **In which part of the digestive tube Meissner's plexus is situated?**
   a. Oesophagus b. Stomach
   c. Intestine d. All of the above

2. **Which part of gastrointestinal tract contains Brunner's glands?**
   a. Ileum b. Jejunum
   c. Duodenum d. Stomach

3. **Peyer's patches are covered by one of the following types of cells:**
   a. Paneth b. Mesengial
   c. M cells d. Clara cells

4. **What type of glands are Brunner's glands?**
   a. Simple tubular
   b. Compound tubular
   c. Compound racemose
   d. Simple alveolar

5. **Which of the following is not the name of the taenia of the colon?**
   a. Taenia libera
   b. Taenia omentalis
   c. Taenia appendix
   d. Taenia mesocolica

ANSWERS

1. d 2. c 3. c 4. c
5. c

Liver, Gall Bladder and Pancreas

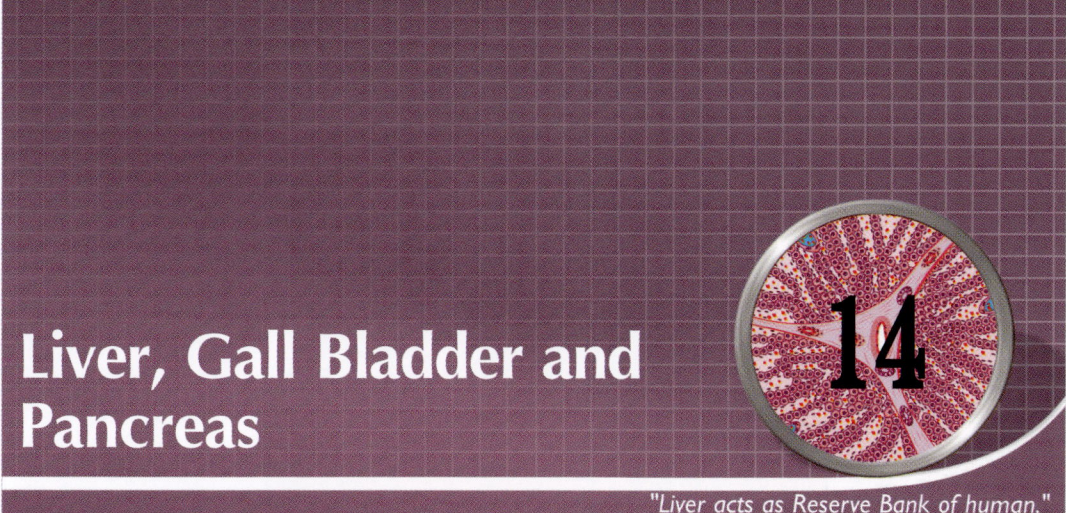

14

"Liver acts as Reserve Bank of human."
"Gall stones have facets and if threaded will form a beautiful necklace."

LIVER

The liver is the largest gland in the body. It functions both as an *exocrine* gland secreting bile through a system of bile ducts into duodenum and an *endocrine* gland synthesising a variety of substances that are released directly into blood stream.

STRUCTURE

The greater part of the liver is covered by peritoneum. Deep to it is a thin capsule of connective tissue called *Glisson's capsule*. At the porta hepatis, it surrounds the entering blood vessels and follows them into the gland forming a framework and dividing the liver substance into innumerable small lobules. Entering the porta hepatis are the proper hepatic artery, the portal vein and fine nerves, whereas leaving it are the two hepatic ducts and lymphatics.

In the pig, each hepatic lobule is completely invested by connective tissue and described microanatomically as consisting of hepatic lobules usually hexagonal in shape (Fig.14.1) with portal radicles or tracts at three to five of its corners. Each tract contains a bile ductule, a branch each of the portal vein, hepatic artery, and a lymphatic duct, enclosed in a common investment of connective tissue. The centre of the lobule contains the central vein. Between the portal tract and central vein lies the liver parenchyma consisting of radiating laminae of hepatic cells.

Each liver cell is hexagonal in shape and has a prominent rounded central nucleus. The liver cells run in many *laminae* which are many cells wide but one cell thick. The bile canaliculus lies in between the adjacent cells of laminae. On one side of the cell is a bile canaliculus and on the other side is a sinusoid and as the laminae branch and anastomose with each other, the sinusoids are also interconnected. Laminae form wall work or *muralium*.

In man, the connective tissue is sparse and the lobular investment is incomplete. It is apparent mainly at points where three hepatic lobules meet (Fig. 14.2) and is known as the *portal lobule*. The portal lobule is triangular to polygonal in shape with portal tract in the centre and three neighbouring central veins on each side of it.

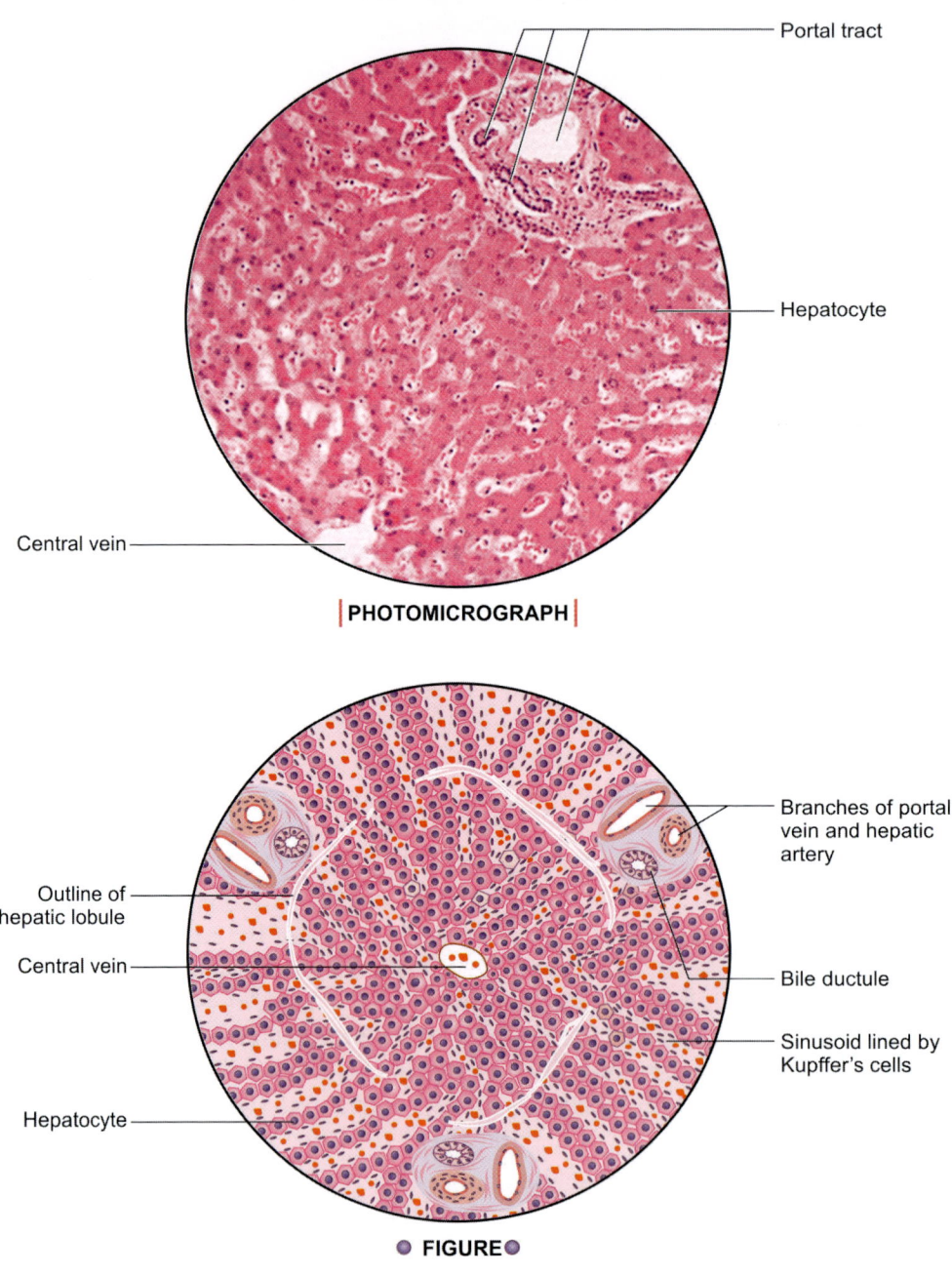

Fig. 14.1: *Liver—hepatic lobule. Stain: Haematoxylin-eosin, 400X*

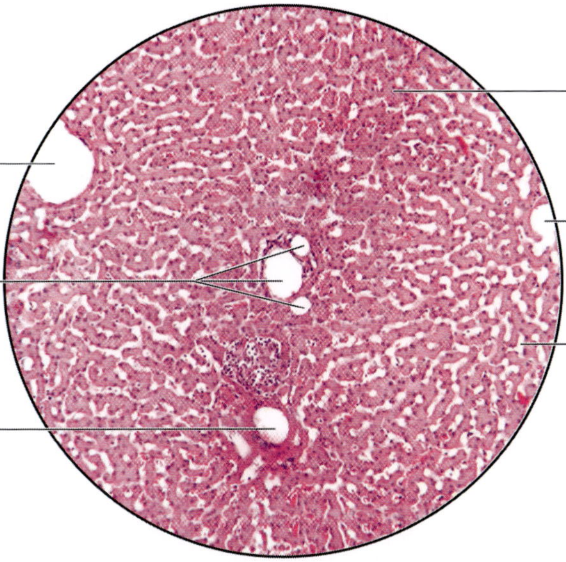

Liver, Gall Bladder and Pancreas

PHOTOMICROGRAPH

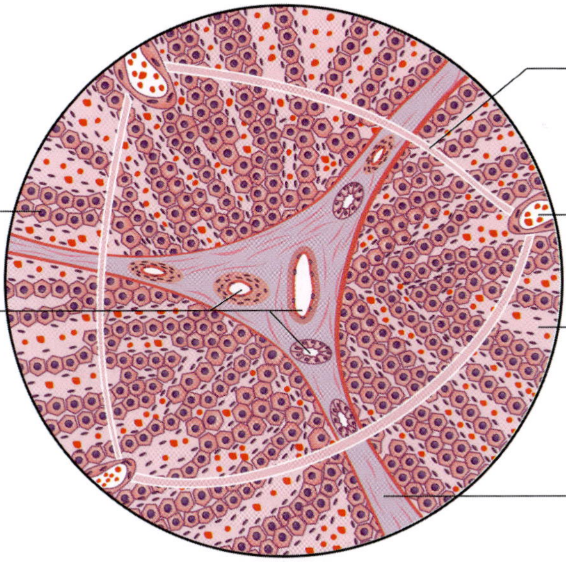

- Central vein
- Portal tract
- Central vein
- Cords of hepatocytes
- Central vein
- Sinusoid

FIGURE

- Plates of hepatic cells
- Interlobular branch of:
  - Portal vein
  - Hepatic artery
  - Bile ductule
- Outline of portal lobule
- Central vein
- Sinusoid
- Interlobular septum

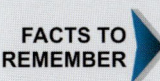

FACTS TO REMEMBER
1. Numerous hepatocytes with prominent central nuclei
2. Portal tract
3. Liver sinusoids lined by Kupffer's cells

Fig. 14.2: *Liver—portal lobule. Stain: Haematoxylin-eosin, 100X*

The liver acinus is defined as the liver parenchyma around a preterminal branch of hepatic arteriole between two adjacent central veins. The peripheral part of liver acinus area 3 (Fig. 14.3) gets affected by anoxia, and the central part (area 1) by toxins. The concept of liver acinus helps to explain gradient zonation in lobule, understand regeneration patterns and genesis of liver cirrhosis.

The liver sinusoids are lined by reticuloendothelial cells called Kupffer's cells. Between the hepatic laminae and sinusoid is a potential space called the *space of Disse*. A similar space is present at the portal tract where lymphatics start and is called the *space of Mall*.

CIRCULATION OF BLOOD THROUGH LIVER

Portal vein brings to the liver blood from large and small intestines, laden with the absorbed products of digestion. Hepatic arterial blood is comparatively less than that of portal vein and is rich in oxygen. Portal vein and hepatic artery together divide into innumerable branches till these reach the level of the liver lobule. At this level the branches of both open into the sinusoids which traverse through the hepatic laminae. The blood courses slowly through these sinusoids, providing nourishment and oxygen to the hepatocytes. Blood finally reaches the central vein of the lobule.

The blood in central vein is devoid of oxygen and nutrients, with the metabolic products of liver added to it. The *central vein* or intralobular veins join to form *sublobular* or *intercalary vein*. Many of these drain into the collecting veins which join to form 2–3 *hepatic veins*. These hepatic veins drain into the inferior vena cava.

Functional Aspect

The liver, like spleen is a haemopoietic organ during foetal life. In adult life, its cells—hepatocytes act both as an endocrine gland and an exocrine gland.

- *Endocrine function*: Liver cells store glucose as glycogen and release it as glucose whenever required. Liver synthesises various plasma proteins. The hepatocytes detoxify various drugs and Kupffer's cells phagocytose the cell debris.
- *Exocrine function*: Liver cells secrete bile which is carried by bile canaliculi, hepatic ducts and cystic duct into gall bladder for temporary storage and concentration.

Applied Aspect

- *Cirrhosis/fibrosis*: Occurs due to malnutrition or chronic alcoholism. Hepatocytes get replaced by fibrous tissue which interferes with circulation of blood through liver, leading to portal hypertension.
- *Jaundice*: Raised serum bilirubin levels due to infection of liver or obstruction to passage of bile.

GALL BLADDER

The gall bladder lies on the undersurface of the liver. Its capacity is 30 to 60 millilitres and it concentrates bile to one-tenth of its amount. Its mucous membrane is thrown

Liver, Gall Bladder and Pancreas

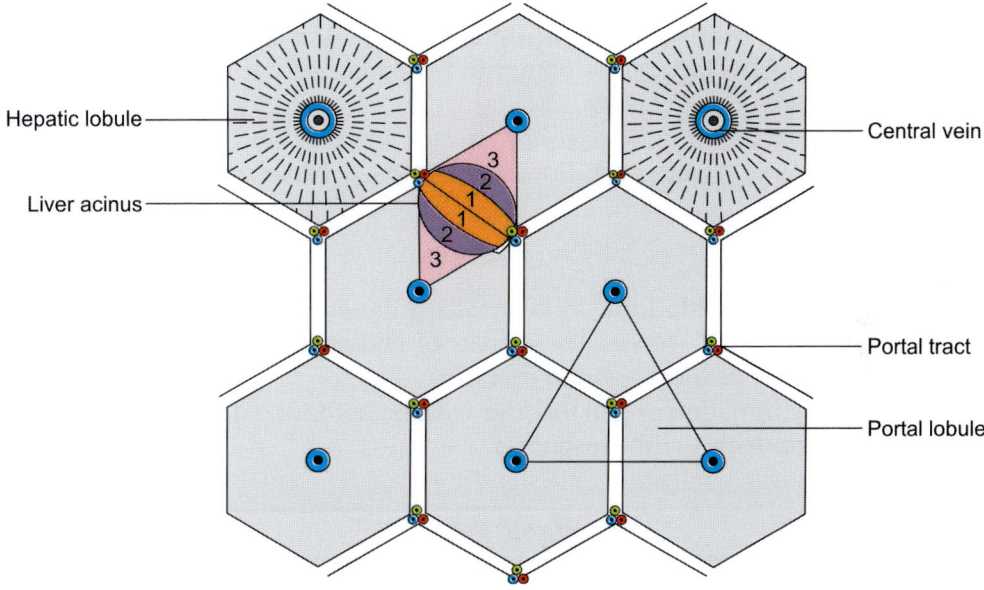

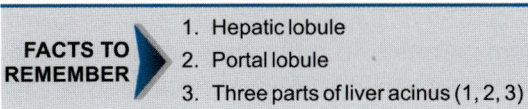

FACTS TO REMEMBER
1. Hepatic lobule
2. Portal lobule
3. Three parts of liver acinus (1, 2, 3)

Fig. 14.3: Liver—Liver acinus, hepatic lobule and portal lobule

into temporary folds. The epithelium consists of a single layer of tall columnar cells. Each cell has basal oval shaped nucleus, and an apical part having a brush border due to the presence of microvilli (Fig. 14.4).

The lamina propria has loose connective tissue with diffuse lymphocytes as well as cut sections of folded epithelium. The muscularis mucosae and glands are absent.

Outside the lamina propria is fibromuscular coat with a few smooth muscle fibres and collagen fibres. This layer rests on a thin fibroareolar coat containing numerous small blood vessels.

The serous coat covers it on its inferior surface whereas thin adventitia envelopes the rest of the surface. At the neck one of the folds is prominent which is spiral in shape.

Applied Aspect

- *Gall stones*: Since gall bladder concentrates bile, some of its constituents may precipitate to form gall stones. These may of cholesterol, or of bile pigments or mixed stones. None of them contain calcium.
- *Cholecystitis*: Inflammation of gall bladder with or without gall stones. There is pain in right hypochondrium with dyspepsia.

PANCREAS

The pancreas is a highly cellular gland composed of an exocrine part secreting pancreatic juice, and an endocrine part called islets of Langerhans, secreting insulin and glucagon (Fig. 14.5).

The exocrine part is divided partially into lobules by very **thin** connective tissue septa containing ducts and blood vessels of various sizes between which lie the serous acini. The ducts to begin with are intercalary which join to form *intralobular, interlobular* and finally the *main pancreatic duct*.

The intercalary duct begins at the *centroacinar cells* which are sometimes seen in the centre of an acinus. The intralobular duct is lined by cuboidal cells, interlobular by columnar cells and the main pancreatic duct by stratified columnar cells. The duct epithelium is better defined than the cells of the acini (Fig. 14.6).

The acini constitute the secretory part of the gland. Each acinus is lined by pyramidal cells which show a very small lumen. The cell have basal basophilia and rounded nuclei which lie close to the bases. The zymogen granules lie in the rest of the cytoplasm. The cytoplasmic granules are the precursors of various enzymes, especially near the luminal end and cause apical eosinophilia in these cells. Between the basement membrane and the cells, a few *myoepithelial* or *basket cells* may be seen. These cause the contraction of the acini. Many capillaries are seen close to the acini.

The islets of Langerhans constitute the endocrine part of the gland. These are lighter areas scattered throughout the acinar tissue. The islets are more or less completely demarcated from the surrounding acinar tissue by a thin layer of reticular fibres.

The islets are ellipsoidal clusters of cells arranged in irregular cords and are paler staining than the acinar cells. There are fenestrated capillaries in between the cells. There are two main types of cells in the islets, α (*alpha*) and β (*beta*) cells. Alpha cells

Liver, Gall Bladder and Pancreas

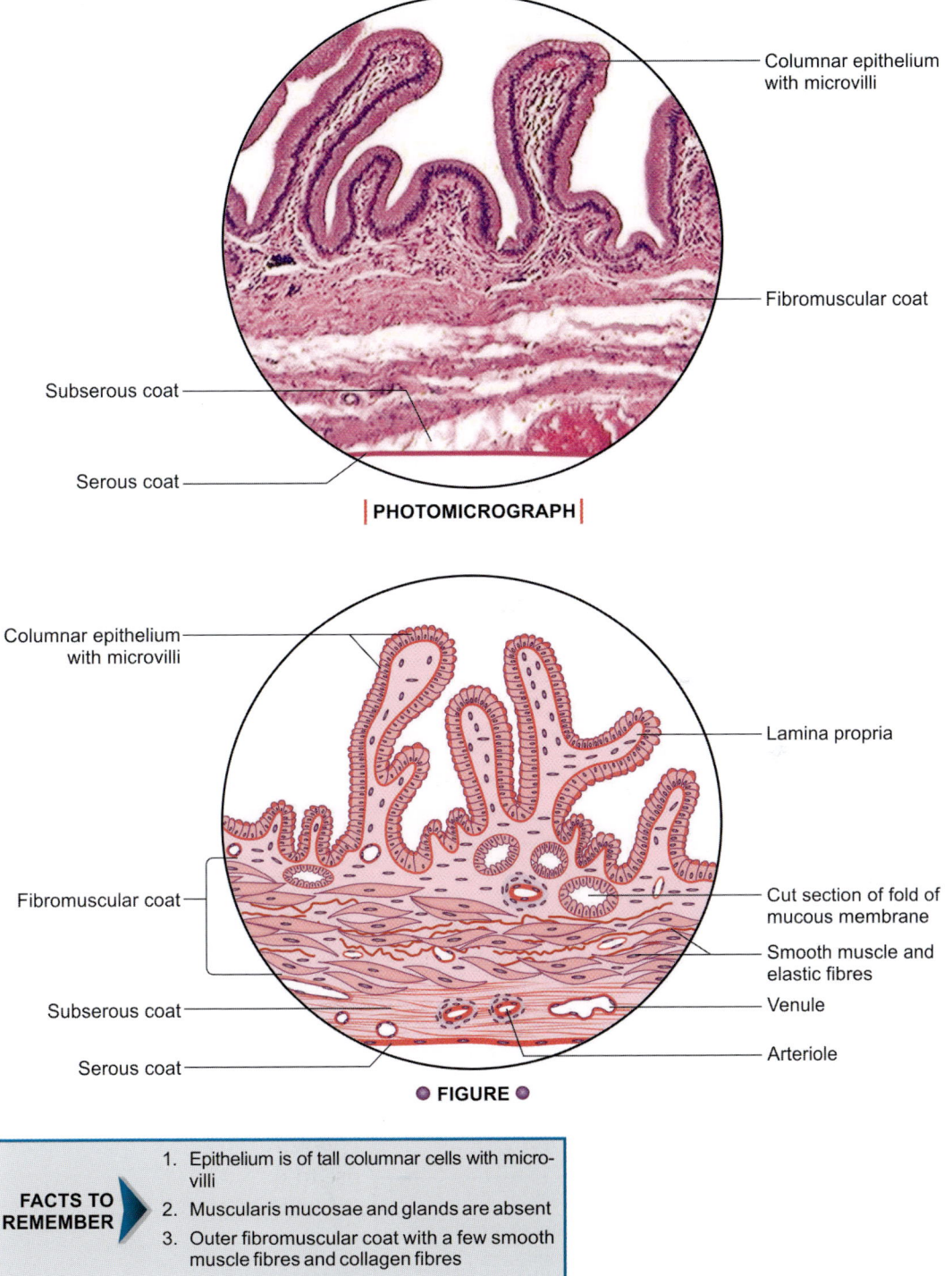

Fig. 14.4: *Gall bladder. Stain: Haematoxylin-eosin, 100X*

FACTS TO REMEMBER
1. Epithelium is of tall columnar cells with microvilli
2. Muscularis mucosae and glands are absent
3. Outer fibromuscular coat with a few smooth muscle fibres and collagen fibres

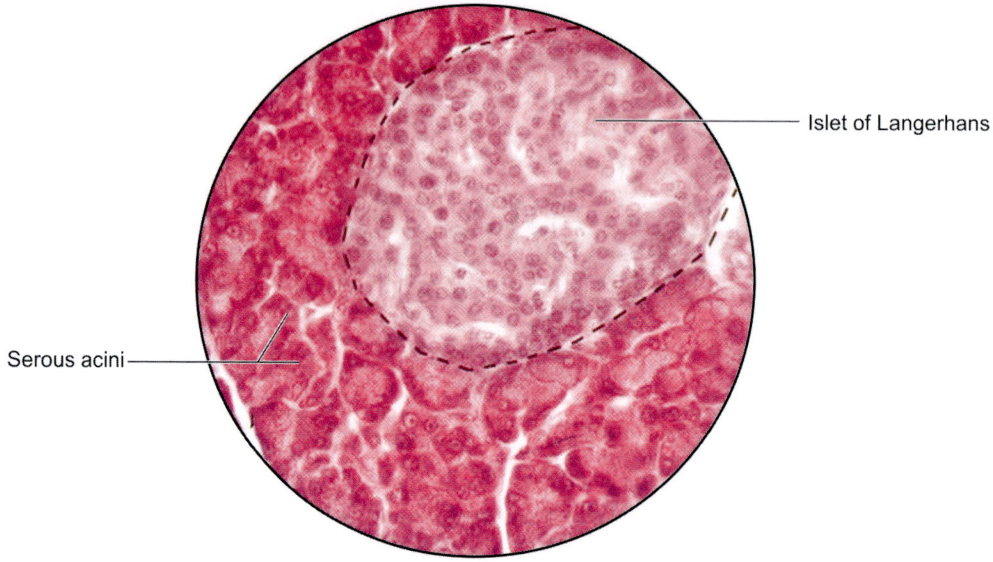

PHOTOMICROGRAPH

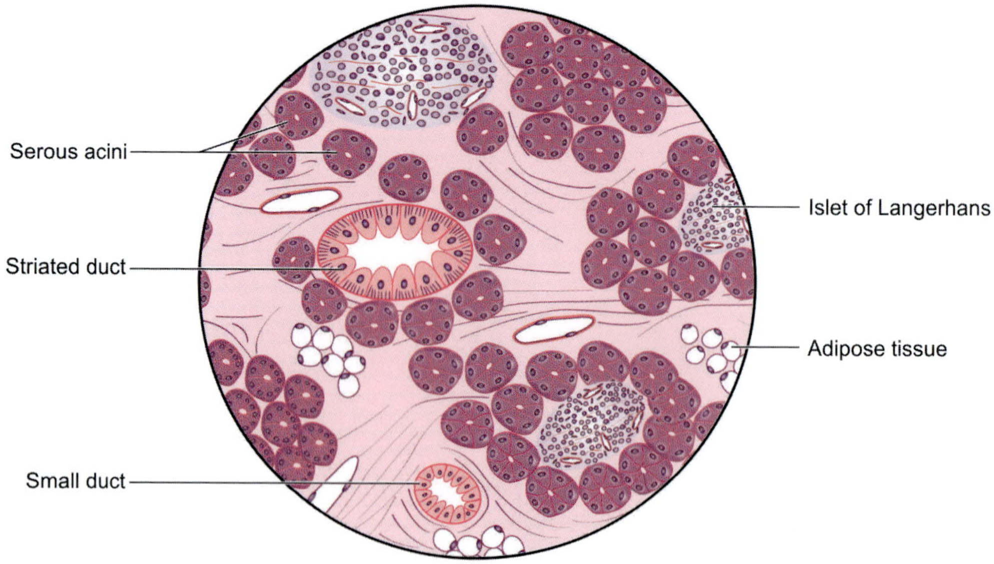

- Islet of Langerhans
- Serous acini

FIGURE

- Serous acini
- Striated duct
- Small duct
- Islet of Langerhans
- Adipose tissue

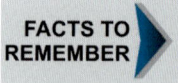

FACTS TO REMEMBER
1. Acini lined by pyramidal cells
2. Lighter islets of Langerhans between the acini
3. Islet contains number of capillaries

Fig. 14.5: *Pancreas. Stain: Haematoxylin-eosin, 400X*

Liver, Gall Bladder and Pancreas

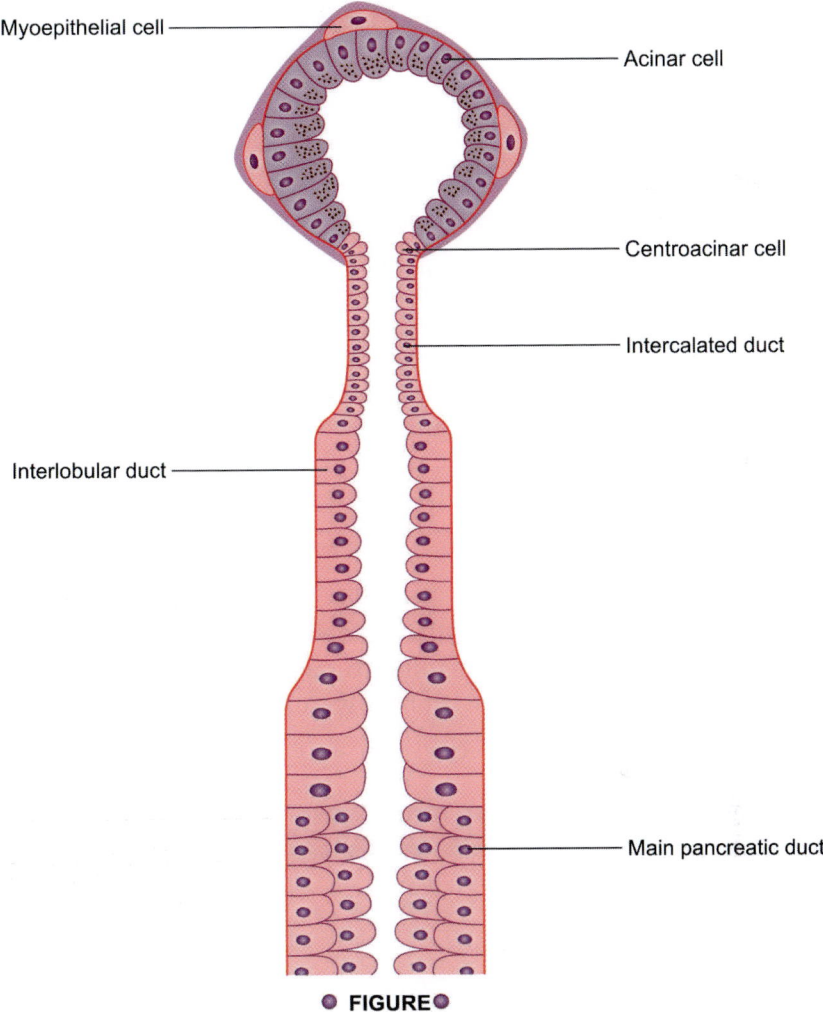

FACTS TO REMEMBER
1. There are no striated ducts in pancreas
2. Centroacinar cells form the intra-acinar portion of the intercalated duct
3. Main pancreatic duct is lined by stratified columnar cells

Fig. 14.6: *Constituents of pancreas. Stain: Haematoxylin-eosin, 400X*

TABLE 14.1: Differences between pancreas and parotid salivary gland

	Pancreas	Parotid salivary gland
1. Connective tissue	Relatively less as septa are few and thin	Relatively more due to numerous thick septa
2. Islets of Langerhans	Present, and are a characteristic feature	Absent
3. Lobes and lobules	Only lobules are present	Both are present

constitute 20 per cent of the total cells and secrete *glucagon*, while beta cells constitute 80 per cent and secrete insulin.

With special stains alpha cells show red granules while beta cells show blue granules. Alpha cell granules are alcohol resistant and water soluble, whereas beta cell granules are soluble in alcohol and are insoluble in water. Alpha cells are present in the peripheral and beta cells in the central part of the islet.

Table 14.1 shows the differences between the pancreas and parotid salivary glands.

Applied Aspect

- *Pancreatitis*: There is blockage of ductules by protein rich plugs. Acini dilate, epithelium degenerates and glandular tissue is replaced by fibrous tissue.
- *Diabetes*: Relative lack of insulin leading to raised blood sugar levels. Diabetes is a metabolic and life style disease with hardly any cure. Frequent small meals are of help.

MULTIPLE CHOICE QUESTIONS

1. Which of the following organs houses the Kupffer's cells?
   a. Spleen   b. Liver
   c. Pancreas   d. Stomach
2. In which organ space of Disse and space of Mall are present?
   a. Pancreas   b. Stomach
   c. Liver   d. Duodenum
3. Which organ is characterised by the presence of centroacinar cells?
   a. Liver   b. Pancreas
   c. Stomach   d. Salivary glands
4. Which organ has "open and closed theories of circulation"?
   a. Pancreas
   b. Spleen
   c. Liver
   d. Lymph node
5. Microvilli are present in which of the following organs?
   a. Liver
   b. Gall bladder
   c. Pancreas
   d. Salivary gland

ANSWERS

1. b   2. c   3. b   4. b
5. b

Urinary System

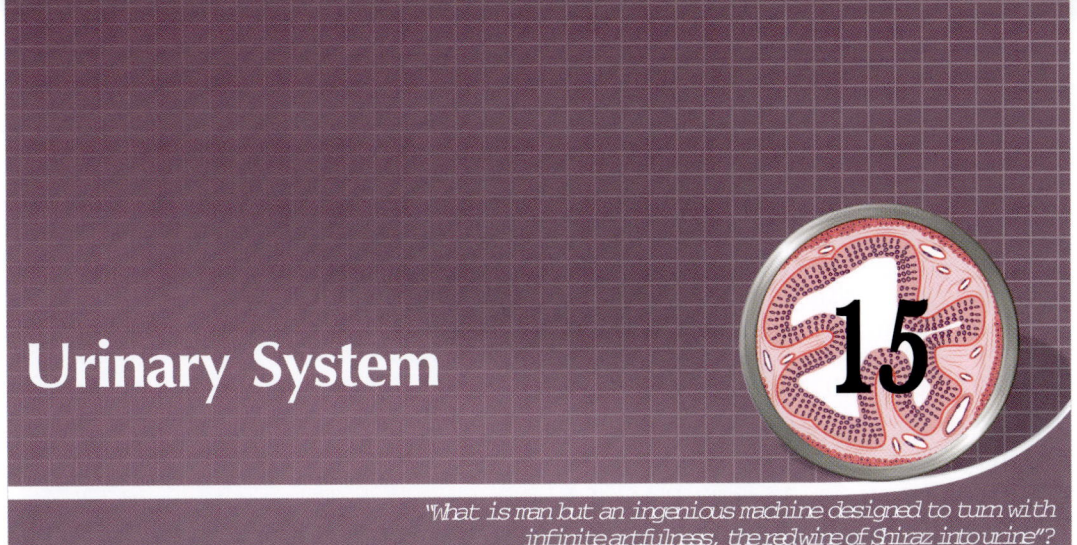

"What is man but an ingenious machine designed to turn with infinite artfulness, the red wine of Shiraz into urine"?

The urinary system consists of a pair of kidneys with corresponding ureters and a single urinary bladder and urethra. The waste products of metabolism are excreted through the urinary system. The kidneys regulate fluid and salt balance of the body. The blood flow through the kidneys is one-fifth of the cardiac output per minute. Thus 1700 litres of blood passes through the kidneys in one day, out of which 170 litres of glomerular filtrate is formed and only about 1.5 litres of urine is excreted. Approximately 168.5 litres of filtrate is reabsorbed into the blood.

KIDNEY

The kidney is covered by a connective tissue capsule and adipose tissue. It is divided into an outer cortex which appears granular in a cut section, and an inner medulla, made up of 8–18 conical masses called *renal pyramids*. The bases of the pyramids are directed peripherally and the apices directed inwards towards the renal sinus, where they form papillae. Each pyramid and the cortical tissue capping it is called *lobe* of the kidney. The extensions of medulla into the cortex are called *medullary rays*. The extensions of cortical tissue into the medulla in between the pyramids are called *columns of Bertini*.

CIRCULATION OF BLOOD THROUGH KIDNEY

The renal arteries are short and broad to maintain hydrostatic pressure for proper filtration of blood. Each renal artery on entering the kidney divides into dorsal and ventral branches. These on subsequent divisions run in between the adjacent pyramids and are termed *interlobar* arteries. At the base of the pyramid, interlobar artery divides dichotomously into branches which run at right angles to the parent stem. These are named as *arcuate* arteries. Both the interlobar and arcuate arteries to each lobe do not anastomose with the adjacent arteries. Arcuate artery gives rise to numerous *straight interlobular* arteries.

Each interlobular artery gives off the *afferent arterioles* for the cortical glomeruli and for the juxtamedullary glomeruli. These break up into capillary plexus of the glomerulus and rejoin to form *efferent arterioles*. Efferent arteriole at cortical glomeruli form cortical *intertubular capillary network*, which drains into *interlobular vein*. This in turn ends into *arcuate, interlobar* and finally *renal vein*. Efferent arteriole of the juxtamedullary glomeruli break up in the medulla into bundles of thin walled veins, the *vasa recta* which make hairpin bends at varying levels and reach back into the cortex. Vasa recta serve as *counter-current exchanges* for the various diffusible substances. These vasa recta drain into interlobular, arcuate, interlobar and finally into the renal vein.

STRUCTURE OF KIDNEY

The kidney is composed of a very large number of tortuous, compactly arranged uriniferous tubules, bound by minimal amount of connective tissue containing blood vessels, lymphatics and nerves. Parts of the uriniferous tubule are *nephron* and *collecting tubule*. Nephron is the secretory component, developing from *metanephros*, while collecting duct is the collecting component arising from the *ureteric bud*.

Nephron comprises the renal corpuscle, i.e. *glomerulus*, meant for **filtration** of blood and the renal tubule which functions for selective reabsorption. The various components of renal tubule are proximal convoluted tubule, descending limb of loop of Henle, loop of Henle which is U-shaped, ascending-limb of loop of Henle, distal convoluted tubule and junctional tubule which finally ends by joining the collecting tubule.

The collecting tubule receives many junctional tubules from numerous glomeruli. Many collecting tubules join to form the *duct of Bellini* which opens into the *minor calyx*.

The glomerulus (Fig. 15.1) is the most characteristic feature of the cortex. It is made up of capillaries which are lined by endothelial cells. The lining of these capillaries is fenestrated. The tuft of glomerular capillaries is enveloped by *Bowman's capsule*, which is double-layered cup lined by squamous epithelium. The layer closely applied to the glomerulus is the *visceral layer* lined by specialised cells called *podocytes* and the outer is the *parietal layer*. Between the two layers is a slit-like space called *capsular space*. The glomerulus with Bowman's capsule is called *renal corpuscle*. The glomerular capillaries connect the afferent and efferent arterioles. The site where afferent and efferent arterioles enter and leave the glomerulus is called *vascular pole*. The afferent arteriole has a thin tunica intima and tunica adventitia, but the cells of the tunica media close to the vascular pole are well developed. The nuclei of these cells are rounded, the cytoplasm is basophilic, granular and they are named *juxtaglomerulus* (JG) cells.

In the region of the JG cells the internal elastic lamina is absent. These cells are close to the *macula densa* of the distal convoluted tubule.

Proximal convoluted tubule is quite tortuous. This segment of the nephron makes up the bulk of the kidney cortex. The cut sections of tubules show a very narrow lumen. The epithelium lining these tubules consists of a single layer of broad-based *cuboidal* cells, resting on a basement membrane. These cells bear a conspicuous brush border of closely packed microvilli. Each cell contains a single spherical nucleus with a nucleolus lying near the base. The cytoplasm of the cells is stained deeply with eosin stain and is granular (Fig. 15.1). The proximal tubule reabsorbs 87.5 per cent of water and sodium from the glomerular filtrate. It also reabsorbs amino acids and glucose.

Loop of Henle

Loop of Henle consists of the *descending limb* of loop of Henle, upper part of which is structurally a continuation of the proximal convoluted tubule. The lower part of

Urinary System

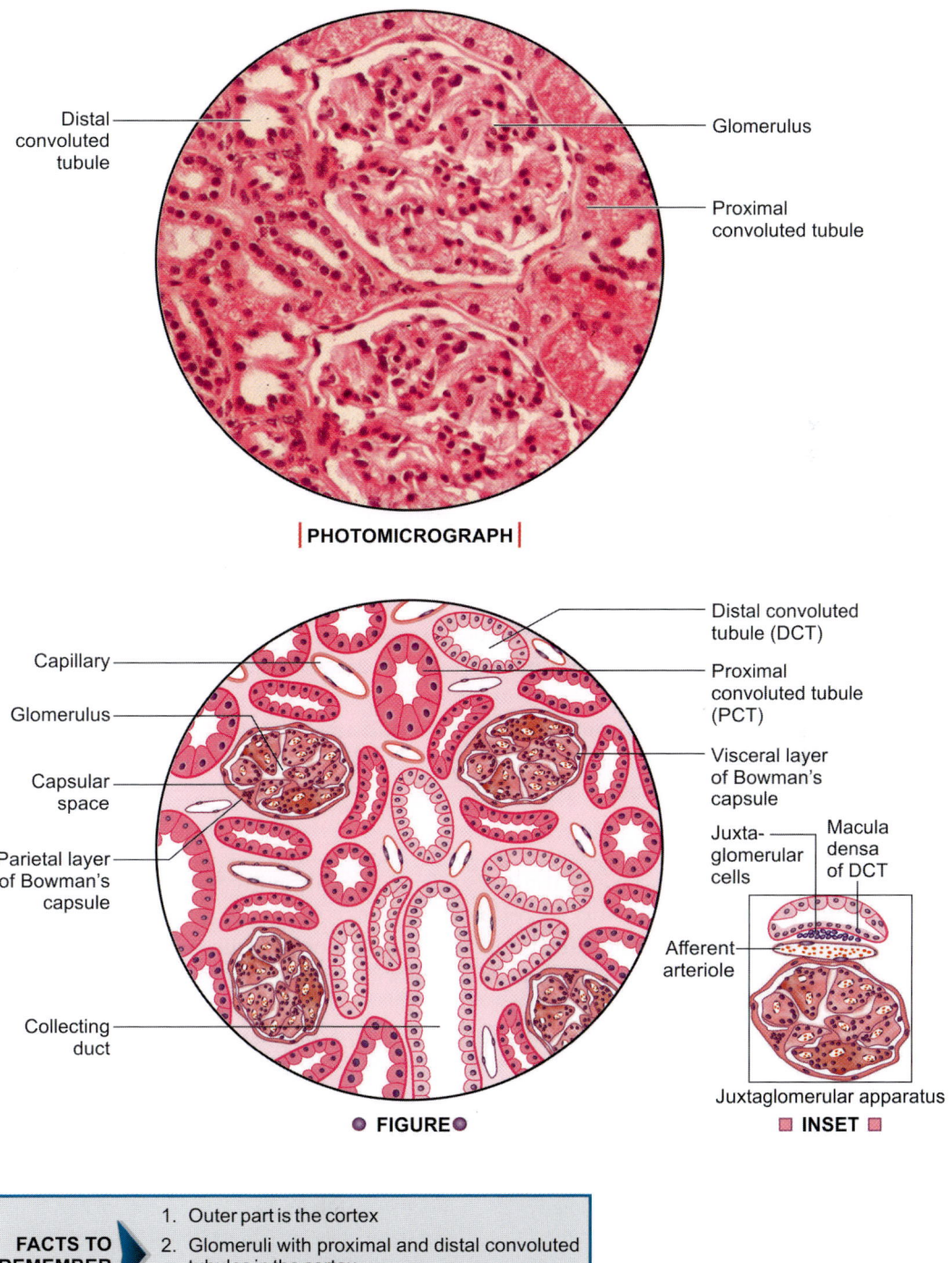

Fig. 15.1: *Kidney–cortex. Stain: Haematoxylin-eosin, 100X*

descending limb is a *thin segment* lined by squamous cells, the nuclei of which bulge into the lumen. The lowest part of descending limb descends into medulla, forms a loop and continues as the *ascending limb* of loop of Henle. The upper part of ascending limb is thicker and is lined by cuboidal cells. It ascends back into the cortex and continues as the distal convoluted tubule.

Distal convoluted tubule is the continuation of the upper part of ascending limb of the loop of Henle. The first loop of this tubule lies close to the vascular pole, particularly to the afferent arteriole in the region of the juxtaglomerular cells. The part of the tubule in contact with the afferent arteriole has a heavily nucleated area. This area is called *macula densa*.

The distal convoluted tubule has many shorter loops. The epithelium of these tubules is *cuboidal* and the lumen is larger than that of the proximal convoluted tubules. The cells rest on a basement membrane. The cells do not have a brush border and the cytoplasm takes up a light eosin stain. It reabsorbs about 14 per cent of water and this function is controlled by the *antidiuretic hormone* (ADH) of the *posterior pituitary gland*. The distal convoluted tubule opens by a small straight tubule into the collecting tubule. Differences between proximal and distal convoluted tubules are depicted in Table 15.1.

Each collecting tubule collects the urine from many distal convoluted tubules. These tubules unite with one another at short intervals and drain into the *ducts of Bellini*, which open on to the summit of a papilla, which in turn drains into a minor calyx.

The cortex of the kidney (Fig. 15.1) shows cut sections of glomeruli, many sections of proximal convoluted tubules, some sections of distal convoluted tubules, a few collecting ducts and capillaries.

A section through the pyramid of medulla of kidney (Fig. 15.2) shows numerous light staining collecting ducts, sections of loop of Henle, i.e. thick and thin segments of descending and ascending limbs, capillaries and connective tissue.

Functional Aspect

- Kidneys maintain homeostasis of the body. Urine formation involves three processes, e.g. filtration, reabsorption and secretion.
- Proximal convoluted tubules are lined by large cuboidal cells with brush border microvilli. These absorb 75–80% of sodium chloride and water from the glomerular filtrate.
- The loop of Henle is important for the production of hypertonic urine.

TABLE 15.1: Differences between the proximal and distal convoluted tubules

Proximal convoluted tubule	Distal convoluted tubule
1. More sections, as it is highly convoluted	Less sections, as it is less convoluted
2. Lining cells are broad based cuboidal with brush border	Lining cells are cuboidal with no brush border
3. Nucleus is large, spherical and basal	Nucleus is smaller and central
4. Lumen hardly visible	Lumen visible
5. Cytoplasm is bright pink	Cytoplasm is light staining
6. Cell outlines are not distinct	Cell outlines are distinct

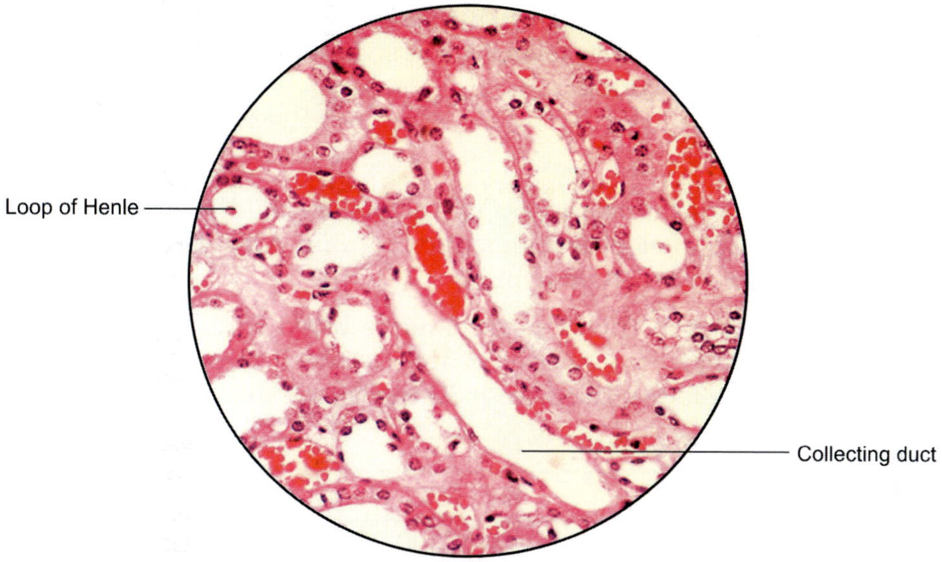

Urinary System

PHOTOMICROGRAPH

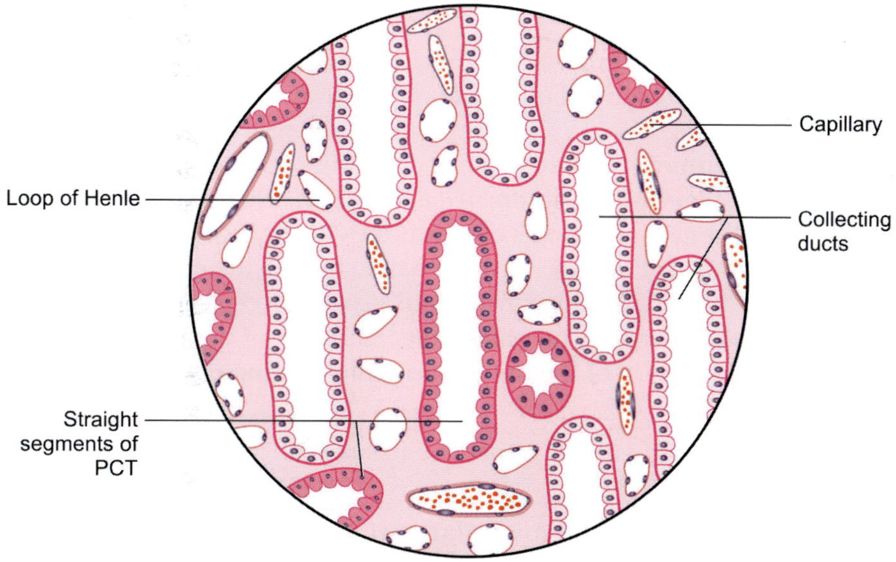

- Loop of Henle
- Collecting duct

FIGURE

- Capillary
- Loop of Henle
- Collecting ducts
- Straight segments of PCT

FACTS TO REMEMBER
1. Sections of collecting ducts
2. Lots of sections of loop of Henle
3. Numerous capillaries

Fig. 15.2: Kidney–medulla. Stain: Haematoxylin-eosin, 100X

- The distal convoluted tubule lined by smaller cuboidal cells reabsorbs sodium ions and excretes potassium or hydrogen ions. The sodium reabsorption is controlled by *aldosterone* of suprarenal cortex.

Applied Aspect

- *Acute glomerulonephritis:* This disease is common in children and young adults, occurring 2–3 weeks after pharyngitis due to group A haemolytic streptococcal infection. Beware of repeated pharyngitis.
- *Tuberculosis of the kidney:* This is usually due to blood spread infection from the lung. Bacilli settle in cortex, caseous foci appear, which spread to medulla, pelvis, ureter and urinary bladder. The disease destroys renal structure.

URETER

The ureter is a muscular tube conveying urine formed by the kidneys to the urinary bladder where it is stored temporarily. The ureter consists of an inner mucous membrane, a middle well developed smooth muscle coat and outer tunica adventitia (Fig. 15.3).

The **mucous membrane** is thrown into 3–5 longitudinal folds giving the lumen a star-shaped appearance. The epithelial lining is of the transitional type. The *transitional epithelium* present in ureter, urinary bladder and proximal urethra is made up of 3–6 layers of cells. The innermost cells are rounded or large cuboidal, stain more deeply than the cells of other layers. These *umbrella-shaped cells* have depression on their undersurface to fit on the *pear-shaped cells* of the underlying layer. The surface membrane known as *cuticle*, seen as a thin eosinophilic band, makes the cells impermeable to urine present in the lumen. The intermediate layers of cells are pear-shaped or irregularly polyhedral in shape. The basal layer is made of cuboidal cells. The cell layers decrease with distention of the organ and relatively increase when the organ is contracted or empty.

The lamina propria is made up of connective tissue with collagen, elastic fibres and lymphocytes.

Unlike that of the intestines, the **muscular coat** in its upper two-thirds has inner longitudinal smooth muscle fibres and outer circular fibres. In the lower one-third there is an additional outer longitudinal coat.

Adventitia forms the outermost coat. The urine passes down the ureter due to the contraction of the muscular coat by its milking action.

Applied Aspect

Calculi in ureter: Small stones or ureteric calculi are seen in ureter. Many of them are formed in kidney, slip down the ureter and get lodged in the constricted parts of ureter. There is acute pain due to blockage in the path of urine.

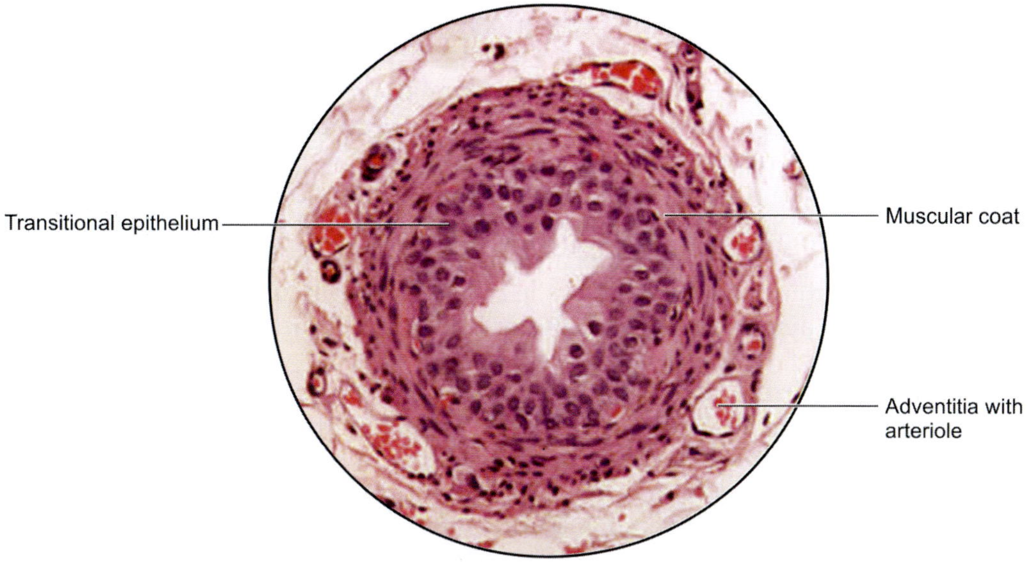

Urinary System

| PHOTOMICROGRAPH |

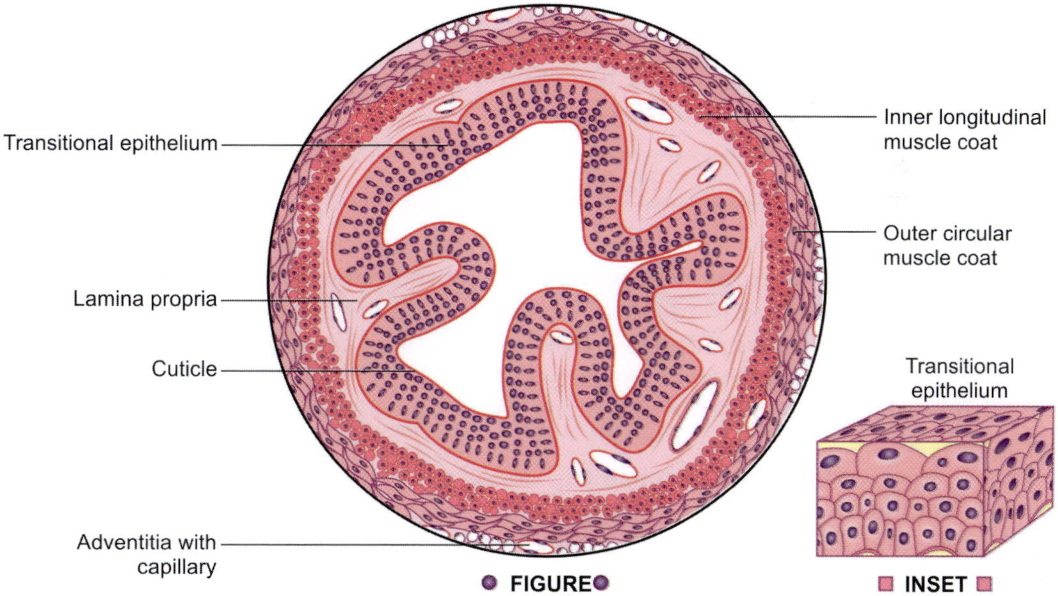

Transitional epithelium — Muscular coat — Adventitia with arteriole

| FIGURE |

Transitional epithelium — Lamina propria — Cuticle — Adventitia with capillary — Inner longitudinal muscle coat — Outer circular muscle coat

| INSET | Transitional epithelium

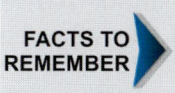
FACTS TO REMEMBER
1. Star-shaped lumen
2. Lining epithelium of transitional variety
3. Inner longitudinal and outer circular layer of smooth muscle fibres

Fig. 15.3: *Ureter. Stain: Haematoxylin-eosin, 100X*

URINARY BLADDER

The urinary bladder is a temporary waterproof storehouse of urine. Its wall is thicker and lumen is much bigger than that of ureter. It also comprises inner mucous coat, middle muscular coat and outer fibrous coat (Fig. 15.4).

The *mucosa* is thin and adherent to the underlying musculature in the region of trigone of urinary bladder. The epithelium is of the *transitional* variety and is made up of three to six layers in the empty bladder and of lesser number of layers in the distended bladder. It has the same characteristics as the transitional epithelium of the ureter. The lamina propria contains collagen and elastic fibres, capillaries and many nuclei of fibroblasts.

The *muscular coat* of urinary bladder known as *detrusor* muscle is made up of smooth muscle fibres running in all directions, i.e. transverse, longitudinal and oblique, with abundant interstitial connective tissue in between the bundles of muscle fibres. The circular layer is thickened at the internal urethral orifice to form the *internal sphincter*.

Only part of the bladder is covered with a mesothelial lining of peritoneum, the rest of it has an **adventitial coat**.

Applied Aspect

- **Stones in urinary bladder**

Urinary bladder may lodge calculi passed down the ureter. These can increase in size in the bladder. Stones may get formed in the urinary bladder if there is chronic inflammation or urethral obstruction.

FEMALE URETHRA

The female urethra is a muscular passage which conducts urine to be voided from the urinary bladder. The **mucous membrane** has longitudinal folds. The epithelium close to the urinary bladder is of transitional variety, near the external opening it is *stratified squamous* and in the remainder it is *pseudostratified columnar*. The lamina propria has plenty of elastic fibres and venous plexuses.

The **muscular coat** consists of inner longitudinal and outer circular smooth muscle fibres.

In the region of the external sphincter, smooth muscle fibres are supplemented by the striated muscle fibres.

The male urethra is described with the male reproductive system.

Functional Aspect

- The luminal cells of the transitional epithelium are larger, being attached to each other by *zonula occludens* and desmosomes. These cells provide osmotic barrier between the *hypertonic* urine in the lumen of urinary bladder and the subjacent connective tissue.
- The remaining layers of cells are unique, as their cell membranes have thick regions called *plaques* connected by thin regions called *interplaque* regions. When the bladder is empty the interplaque regions permits folding of the cell membrane. When the bladder gets full, these folds are effaced.

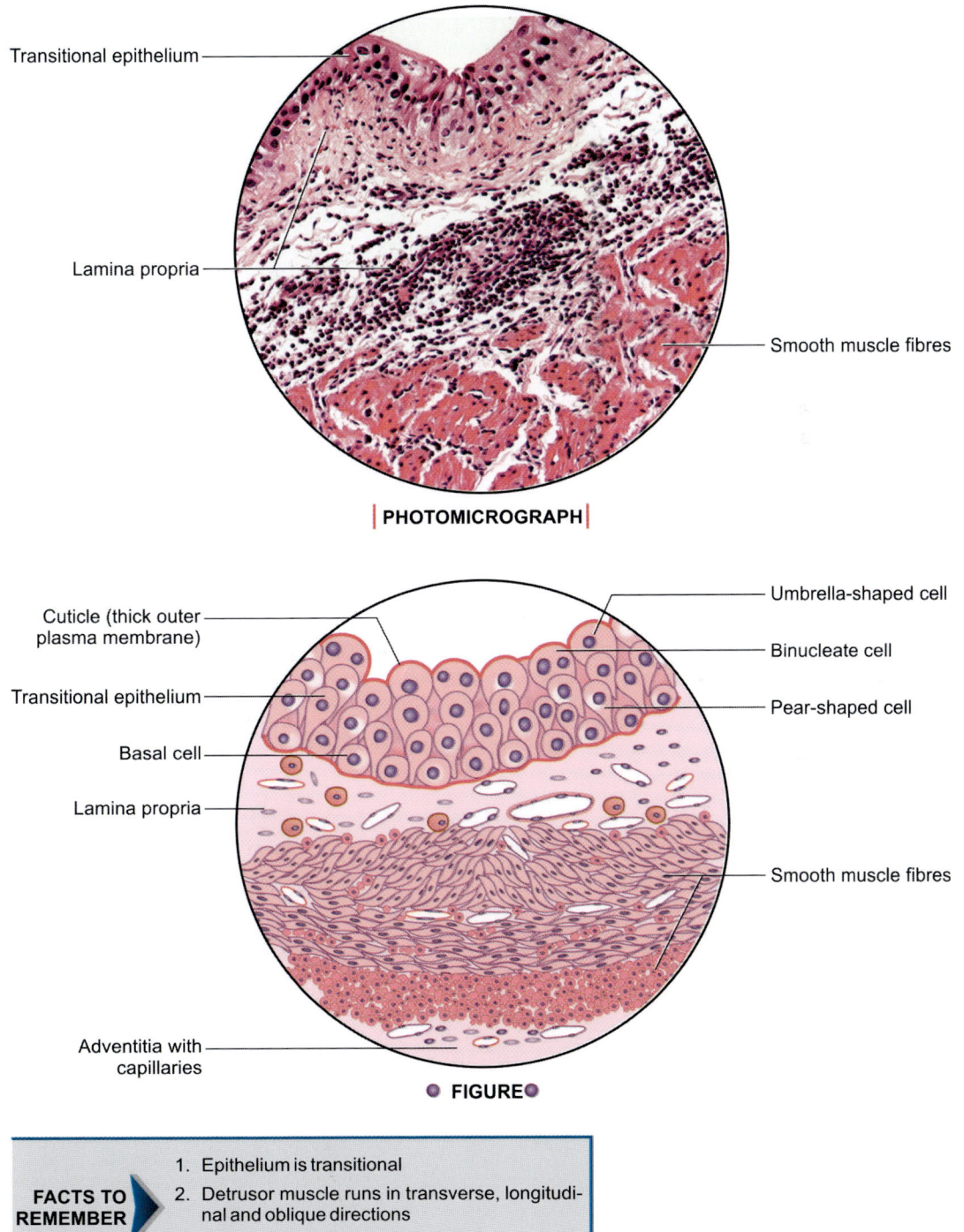

Fig. 15.4: *Urinary bladder. Stain: Haematoxylin-eosin, 400X*

MULTIPLE CHOICE QUESTIONS

1. **Podocytes are present in which part of the nephron?**
   a. Glomerulus
   b. Duct of Bellini
   c. Proximal convoluted tubule
   d. Loop of Henle
2. **Where is macula densa present?**
   a. Afferent arteriole
   b. Efferent arteriole
   c. Distal convoluted tubule
   d. Proximal convoluted tubule
3. **Ducts of Bellini are present in:**
   a. Liver
   b. Pancreas
   c. Kidney
   d. Ureter
4. **Lining of ureter is one of the following:**
   a. Stratified columnar
   b. Columnar
   c. Transitional
   d. Squamous
5. **Juxtaglomerular cells are present in which of the following part?**
   a. Efferent arteriole
   b. Afferent arteriole
   c. Loop of Henle
   d. Proximal convoluted tubule

ANSWERS

1. a   2. c   3. c   4. c
5. b

Male Reproductive System

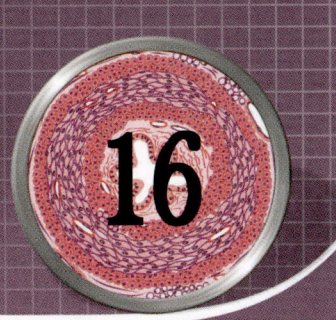

"It is not because things are difficult that we do not dare; it is because we do not dare that they are difficult."

Male reproductive system: It consists of the following:
1. A pair of sex glands, the testes.
2. Conducting tubes like epididymis, ductus deferens and ejaculatory ducts, including accessory glands like prostate and seminal vesicles.
3. Copulatory organ, the penis, containing urethra.

The male sex cells or spermatozoa are produced by the testis, conducted by the various tubes and ejected through the urethra. The fluid vehicle is produced by the secretions of the glands, which nourish the spermatozoa during the passage. The secretions of the glands together with the spermatozoa is a whitish viscous fluid known as *seminal fluid* or *semen*. The process of expulsion of semen from urethra is called *ejaculation*.

TESTIS

The testis is covered by a thick fibrous capsule, the *tunica albuginea*, which is made up of dense collagen fibres. From the tunica, thin fibrous septa extend inwards dividing the testis into various lobules. Each lobule contains one to four highly convoluted *seminiferous tubules*. The convoluted tubule becomes continuous with a straight tubule. The straight tubules open into a network of channels lying in the *mediastinum testis* called the *rete testis*, which are continued into efferent ductules of the testis.

The seminiferous tubules (Fig. 16.1) seen are cut in various planes—transverse, oblique and longitudinal. Each is lined by *stratified epithelium* 4–8 layers thick in a fully functioning testis. It is composed of two major categories of cells, which are the *supporting cells* and the *spermatogenic cells*.

Supporting cells known as *cells of Sertoli*, are slender and elongated cells extending from the basement membrane to the lumen of the tubules. The cytoplasm is well stained, nucleus is pale staining, ovoid or triangular and may vary in position in different cells. The cells of Sertoli provide mechanical support and protection for the developing germ cells and participate in their nutrition and maturation. These also synthesise *androgen binding proteins* and provide *blood testis barrier* (Fig. 16.2).

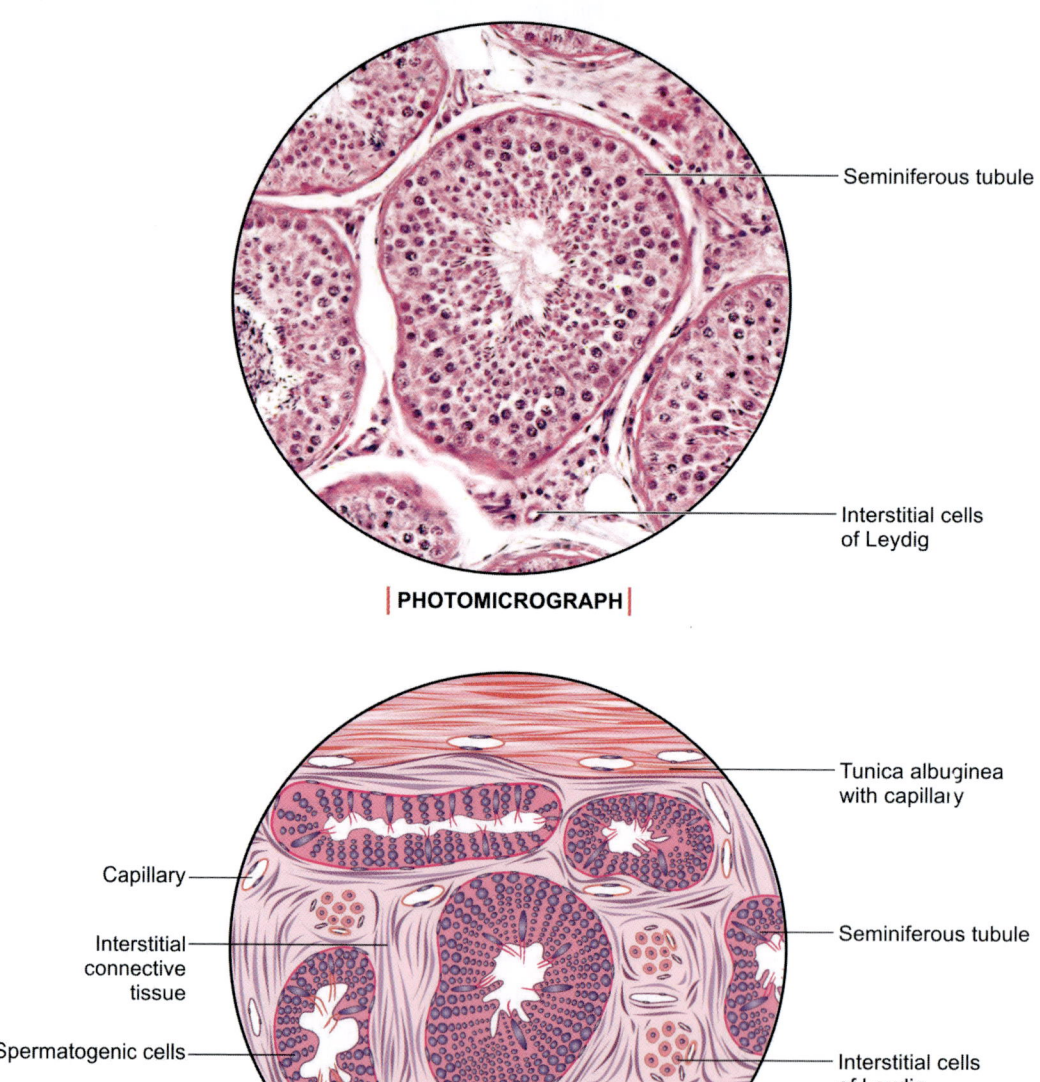

Fig. 16.1: *Testis. Stain: Haematoxylin-eosin, 100X*

Male Reproductive System

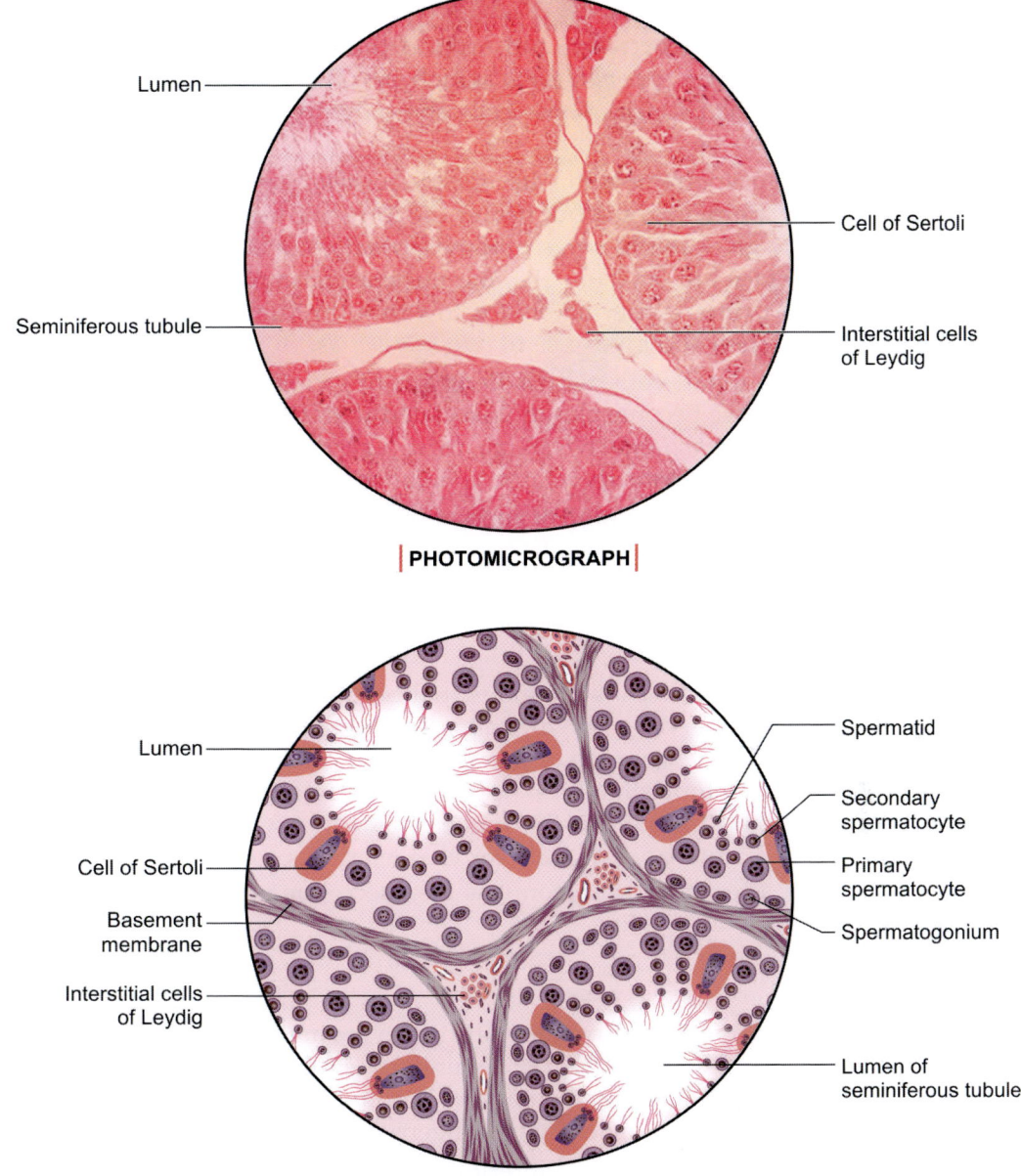

Facts to Remember
1. Spermatogonia rest on the basement membrane
2. Reduction division occurs between primary and secondary spermatocyte stage
3. Cells of Leydig secrete testosterone

Fig. 16.2: *Seminiferous tubule. Stain: Haematoxylin-eosin, 400X*

SPERMATOGENIC CELLS

These are arranged in rows between and around the cells of Sertoli. The parent spermatogenic cells are the *spermatogonia* which lie on the basement membrane supported by thin lamina propria. These cells show lightly stained cytoplasm and round or ovoid nuclei.

By **mitotic division** of spermatogonia the *primary spermatocytes* (44 + XY) are formed which lie adjacent to spermatogonia but nearer the lumen. By **meiotic division** each primary spermatocyte gives rise to two *secondary spermatocytes* (22 + X or 22 + Y). The secondary spermatocytes are smaller cells, the nuclear chromatin is less dense and these lie next to the primary spermatocytes towards the lumen. Each secondary spermatocyte divides soon and gives rise to two *spermatids*.

The spermatids are small cells which lie in groups close to the lumen of the seminiferous tubule. These become closely associated with the cytoplasm of the cells of Sertoli and undergo *metamorphosis* to form *spermatozoa*. This process of metamorphosis of spermatid into spermatozoa is called *spermiogenesis*.

The whole process of transformation of spermatogonia to spermatozoa is known as *spermatogenesis* and takes about 64 days. The spermatozoa lie in the lumen of the tubule and each consists of a deep staining *head*, constricted *neck*, *body* and *tail*.

LEYDIG'S CELLS

Between the seminiferous tubules is the interstitial connective tissue which contains fibroblasts, blood vessels, nerves and lymphatics. In addition are present special cells called *interstitial cells of Leydig* in small groups. These cells are large, rounded or polygonal in shape. The cytoplasm is eosinophilic, granular, and the nucleus is ovoid. The interstitial cells secrete the male sex hormone or *androgen*, which is responsible for the development and maintenance of male sex characteristics.

These cells are **not** affected by vasectomy as their secretion is poured directly into the blood.

Functional Aspect

- *Sertoli cells* support, protect and provide nutrition to the maturing spermatid. These release the spermatozoa in the lumen of seminiferous tubule. These cells produce *androgen binding protein* (ABP) as well as the hormone *inhibin*. Sertoli cells form *blood testis barrier*, preventing the entry of antigens.
- *Follicle stimulating hormone (FSH)* of anterior pituitary monitors the secretions of ABP by Sertoli cells.
- *Inhibin* inhibits the secretion of FSH by negative feedback. The *luteinising hormone* (LH) of anterior pituitary causes production of *testosterone* from interstitial cells of Leydig. Spermatogenesis requires a cooler temperature (by 2–3°C). This is attained by pampiniform plexus around the testicular artery, making arterial blood cooler by 2–3°C.

Applied Aspect

- *Orchitis:* Inflammation of testis is called **orchitis**.

- *Carcinoma of testis:* For example, seminoma and teratoma are common.
- *Syphilitic lesion:* In its tertiary stage, lesions are common in testis.

EPIDIDYMIS

The epididymis is a highly convoluted tube resting upon and on the side of the testis. A transverse section through this tube shows the tubules of various sizes and shapes which are surrounded by connective tissue. It consists of an *epithelial lining*, resting on a basement membrane and a thin layer of smooth muscle fibres disposed circularly, which helps to move the sperms along the ducts. Movement of the sperms is also by vacuum created by the absorption of fluid and cell debris (Fig. 16.3).

The epithelium is of the *pseudostratified columnar* variety. There are columnar cells and a few basal cells, the nuclei of which lie at different levels but all the cells rest on the basement membrane. On their free surface, the columnar cells carry a tuft of long *nonmotile stereocilia* (branching microvilli like processes).

These columnar cells are secretory. The secretion passes along the stereocilia to the centre of the lumen of the tube and nourishes the spermatozoa present in the lumen of the tubules. The lumen frequently contains spermatozoa.

Functional Aspect

- The columnar cells lined by stereocilia absorb testicular fluid. These cells also remove any degenerating sperm cells.
- The columnar cells secrete a glycoprotein which inhibits capacitation of sperms in the male reproductive system.
- The epididymis stores the sperms and helps in their maturation.

Applied Aspect

- *Tuberculosis of epididymis* is common. The process may spread along vas deferens to seminal vesicles, prostate and bladder.

DUCTUS DEFERENS

The ductus deferens is a thick muscular tube which conducts the spermatozoa from the epididymis to the base of the urinary bladder. There, the duct joins the duct of the seminal vesicle to form the *ejaculatory duct* which opens into the prostatic part of the urethra. The entire outer wall can be seen in single low power field of microscope. Ductus deferens comprises the following:

i. Inner mucous membrane (Fig. 16.4)
ii. Middle muscular coat
iii. Outer fibrous coat/adventitia

The lumen of the ductus deferens is narrow. Depending upon the region of the duct, the **epithelium** varies from *ciliated columnar epithelium* to *pseudostratified* epithelium.

The lamina propria contains an extensive elastic network, which throws the epithelium into folds.

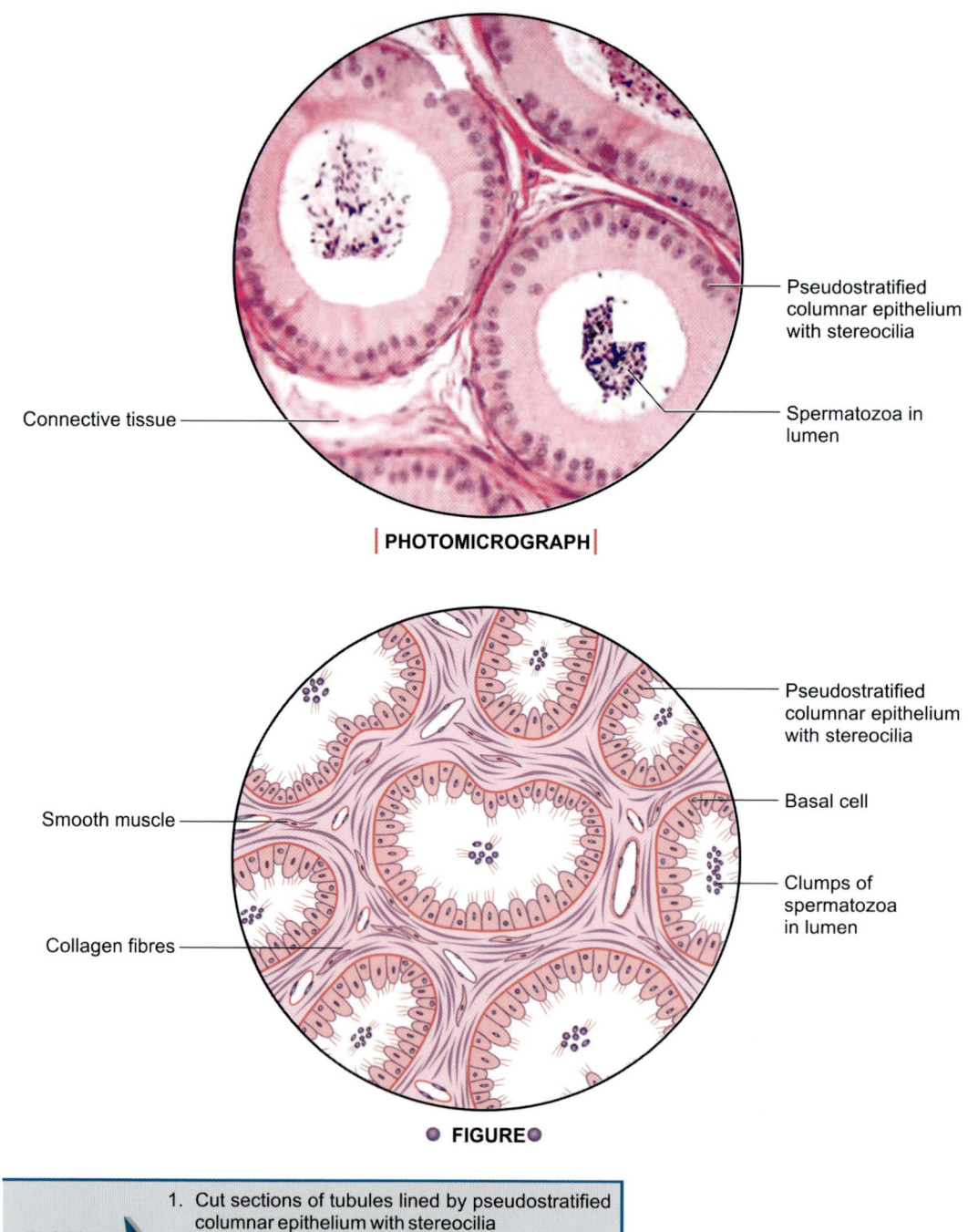

Fig. 16.3: *Epididymis. Stain: Haematoxylin-eosin, 100X*

Male Reproductive System

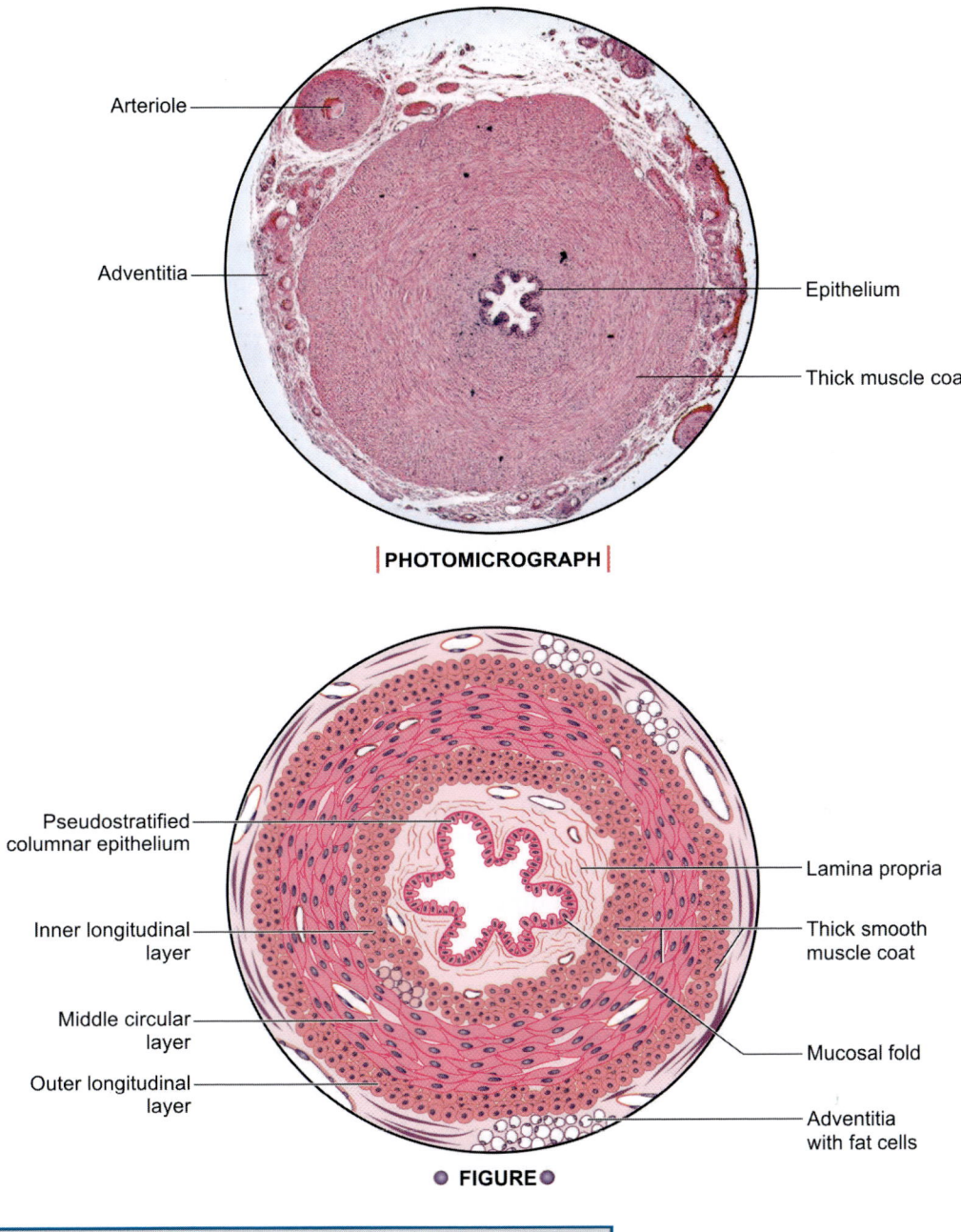

Fig. 16.4: *Ductus deferens. Stain: Haematoxylin-eosin, 100X*

FACTS TO REMEMBER
1. Lumen is small
2. Lining varies from ciliated columnar to pseudo-stratified columnar epithelium
3. Thick muscle in three layers, outer and inner longitudinal and middle circular

The **smooth muscle coat** is thick and three layered. The inner and outer layers consist of longitudinal muscle fibres and a powerful intermediate layer is made of circular muscle fibres. The contraction of smooth muscle fibres is under the control of *autonomic nerves*.

The **adventitia** is a thin layer of connective tissue and contains abundant blood vessels and nerves.

Applied Aspect

Vasectomy is done for family welfare. Recanalisation of vas is possible if required.

PROSTATE GLAND

The prostate gland is about the size of a chestnut and guards the urethra at its beginning at the neck of the urinary bladder. It is a compound tubuloacinar gland The glandular tissue is embedded in a fibromuscular stroma. Thus, it is a **fibromuscular glandular organ** (Fig. 16.5).

The gland is covered by a thin capsule containing collagen and smooth muscle fibres. The stroma consists of abundant collagen fibres and smooth muscle fibres which run in various directions:

The acini of the gland are irregular in shape, the epithelial lining is highly folded and at many places extends into the lumen of the glandular acini. The epithelial lining is of tall columnar cells and is secretory. The basement membrane is indistinct and the glandular epithelium rests upon a layer of connective tissue with dense elastic network. The lumen of the acini may contain small colloid masses known as *amyloid bodies* or *corpora amylacea* in old age. Between the prostatic acini are a few ducts which are lined by *bilaminar epithelium*, having an inner columnar layer and an outer cuboidal layer.

The prostate is traversed by the urethra which in its prostatic part is lined by *transitional epithelium*. Sometimes opening of one or both ejaculatory ducts may be seen in a section, the epithelium of the ducts being either columnar or pseudostratified.

The secretion of the prostate is thin, opalescent fluid with a slightly acidic reaction and is rich in an enzyme called *acid phosphatase* in addition to *fibrinolysin* and *prostaglandins*. The secretion nourishes the spermatozoa.

Testosterone increases the activity of prostate, while oestrogen suppresses its activity. So oestrogen is given in cancer of prostate gland.

AGE CHANGES IN PROSTATE

At birth	:	Stroma forms the bulk of the gland. The duct system is embedded in this stroma. Follicles are represented as end buds on the ducts. The ducts show hyperplasia due to action of maternal oestrogens. Changes last for 6–8 weeks.
9th year	:	Hyperplasia of duct epithelium and division of duct system. There is slow and continuous increase in size of the prostate.
At puberty	:	There is rapid increase in size of gland due to development of follicles. There is relative increase in glandular tissue as compared to stroma. This is due to secretion of testosterone in blood.

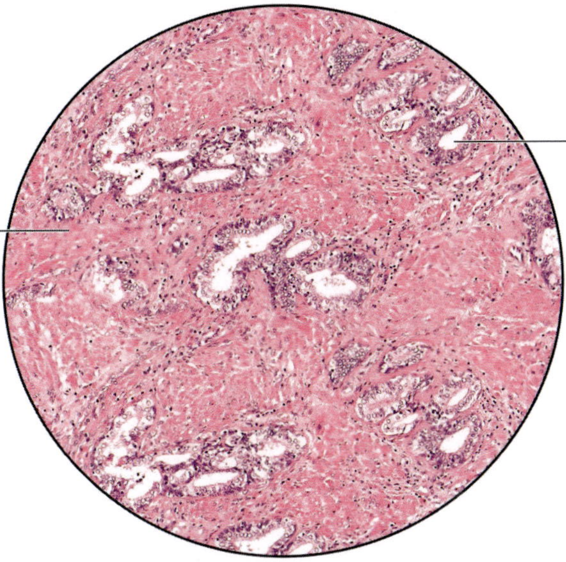

Male Reproductive System

PHOTOMICROGRAPH

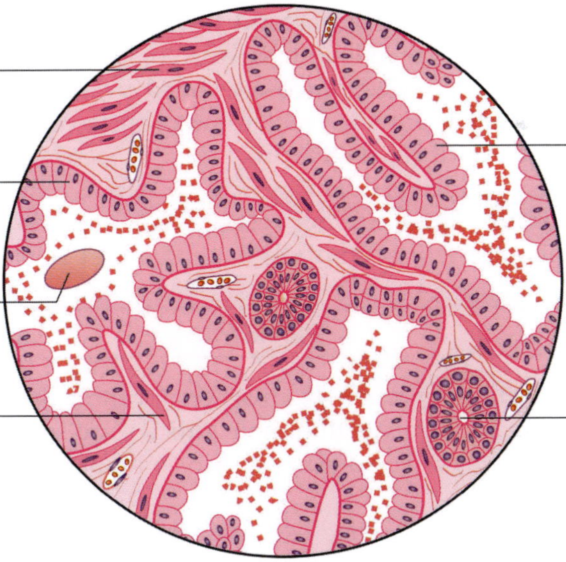

- Fibromuscular stroma
- Acinus of the gland

FIGURE

- Smooth muscle fibres
- Acinus lined by columnar epithelium
- Corpora amylacea
- Fibromuscular stroma
- Glandular epithelium
- Duct

FACTS TO REMEMBER
1. Acini lined by columnar epithelium
2. Fibromuscular stroma
3. Corpora amylacea may be present

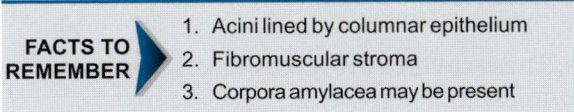

Fig. 16.5: *Prostate gland. Stain: Haematoxylin-eosin, 100X*

20–30 years : Glandular epithelium shows infoldings into the lumen of follicles.
30–50 years : Infoldings of epithelium disappear so that outlines of follicles are more regular and amyloid bodies increase in number.
After 50 years : Either it undergoes benign hypertrophy or gradual atrophy.

Functional Aspect

Prostate gland secretes a thin watery, slightly acidic secretion. This secretion is rich in acid phosphatase, amylase and citric acid. The semen is the secretion of prostate, seminal vesicles and bulbourethral glands mixed with millions of spermatozoa. These secretions provide necessary nourishment to sperms. These also neutralise the acidity of the vaginal canal.

Applied Aspect

- **Benign prostatic hyperplasia** may cause compression of urethra, with retention of urine.
- **Cancer of prostate** is very common cause of death in men.

SEMINAL VESICLE

The two seminal vesicles are situated behind the urinary bladder. Each consists of highly tortuous tube about 15 cm in length. In histological sections, the tube is seen in different planes. The highly folded mucosa is lined by pseudostratified columnar epithelium rich in secretory granules. The lamina propria contains elastic fibres and thin layer of smooth muscle fibres (Fig. 16.6).

The seminal vesicles produce yellowish viscid secretion, rich in fructose providing energy for sperm motility. These are not reservoirs for spermatozoa. The height of epithelial cells and their secretory activity is dependent on level of testosterone.

PENIS

The penis is the male copulatory organ. It subserves for the passage of both semen and urine. The skin covering the penis is thin, hair follicles are seen only at the root, the distal part being devoid of hair. The dermis of skin contains smooth muscle fibres and dilated venous spaces.

Penis consists of three cylindrical bodies of erectile or cavernous tissue. Two *corpora cavernosa* lying dorsally and a single *corpus spongiosum* situated on the ventral aspect.

Each corpus cavernosum consists of the following:
 i. Outer fibrous covering named *tunica albuginea.*
 ii. Trabeculae comprised of connective tissue and smooth muscle fibres enclosing spaces or **caverns**.
 iii. Caverns are lined by endothelial cells. These caverns are fed by arterioles, branches of helicine arteries and drained by venules.

In the corpus spongiosum, the trabeculae are finer and branches of helicine arteries are narrow. Corpus spongiosum is traversed throughout its length by the spongy part of urethra (Fig. 16.7).

Male Reproductive System

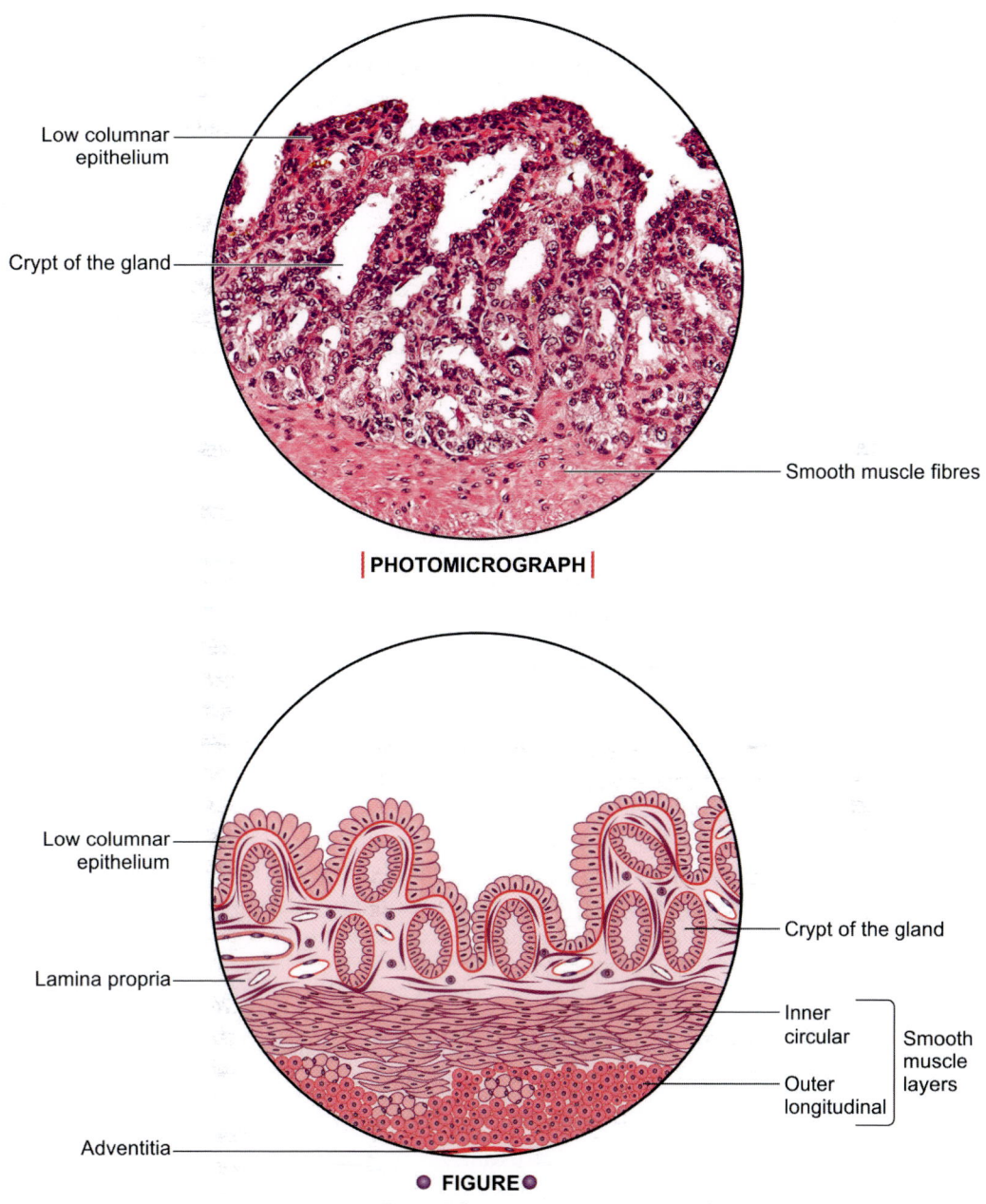

Fig. 16.6: *Seminal vesicle. Stain: Haematoxylin-eosin, 100X*

FACTS TO REMEMBER
1. Folds lined by low columnar epithelium
2. Many crypts seen as sections of the folds
3. Smooth muscle layers and adventitia form the outer layers

Functional Aspect

The penis, male copulatory organ, is normally in the flaccid state. During erotic stimulation, the corpus spongiosum and two corpora cavernosae get distended with blood. The filling up of vascular spaces greatly enlarges the size of penis, make it hard and erect. After ejaculation, the blood from the cavernous vascular spaces returns, bringing the penis back to its flaccid state.

Applied Aspect

- *Phimosis* is non-retraction of foreskin of glans penis for which circumcision is done.
- *Syphilis:* Lesions of early syphilis are seen on the penis.

MALE URETHRA

Male urethra is about 18–20 cm long and consists of two main parts: Short posterior urethra and long anterior urethra. Posterior urethra comprises (i) preprostatic, prostatic and membranous segments, (ii) long anterior part comprises bulbar or perineal and penile or spongy segment.

i. *Preprostatic and prostatic parts:* These are lined by *transitional epithelium*. The lamina propria has a rich plexus of capillaries. The muscle layer consists of inner longitudinal and outer thick circular layer.

   Membranous part: It is the *shortest* part of urethra, which is lined by *pseudostratified columnar* cells with some smooth muscle fibres in the lamina propria. The sphincter urethrae is within the wall of urethra.

ii. *Long anterior part:* It is the longest part of the urethra. The lining epithelium of bulbar and penile segments is of *pseudostratified columnar* epithelium. In the navicular fossa the lining is *stratified squamous* non-keratinised which is continuous with the *stratified squamous keratinised* epithelium of the glans penis.

Applied Aspect

- There may be obstruction in male urethra due to prostate enlargement.
- Catheter is introduced carefully into the urinary bladder through long urethra for relieving the obstruction till the operation.
- Infection of urethra may lead to urethritis.

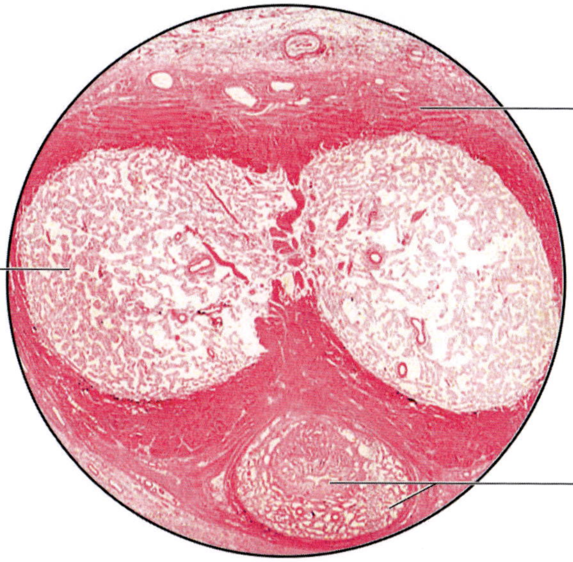

Male Reproductive System

PHOTOMICROGRAPH

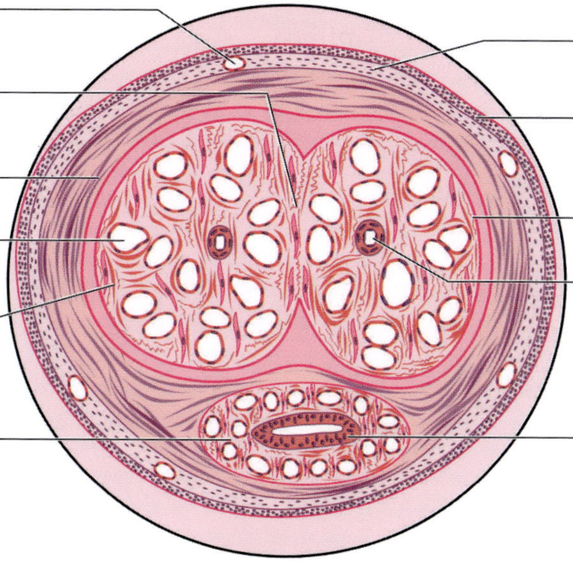

Labels: Dartos muscle; Corpus cavernosum; Corpus spongiosum with urethra

FIGURE

Labels: Venule in superficial fascia; Median septum; Dartos muscle; Caverns lined by endothelial cells; Trabeculae; Corpus spongiosum; Tunica albuginea; Epidermis; Corpus cavernosum; Deep artery; Urethra

FACTS TO REMEMBER
1. Two corpora cavernosa
2. One corpus spongiosum traversed by penile urethra
3. Dartos muscle, dermis and epidermis outside

Fig. 16.7: Penis. Stain: Haematoxylin-eosin, 20X

MULTIPLE CHOICE QUESTIONS

1. **Which one of the following cells form the blood–testis barrier?**
   a. Primary spermatocyte
   b. Spermatid
   c. Interstitial cells
   d. Sertoli cells
2. **Which layer is not present in the testis?**
   a. Tunica albuginea
   b. Tunica vasculosa
   c. Tunica vaginalis
   d. Tunica adventitia
3. **What is the lining of the epididymis:**
   a. Columnar
   b. Stratified columnar
   c. Pseudostratified columnar
   d. Stratified squamous non keratinised
4. **One of the following organs are devoid of tunica albuginea:**
   a. Ovary
   b. Testis
   c. Epididymis
   d. Penis
5. **"Fibromuscular glandular" organ structure is present in one of the following organs:**
   a. Penis
   b. Prostate
   c. Testis
   d. Ovary

ANSWERS

1. d   2. d   3. c   4. a
5. b

Female Reproductive System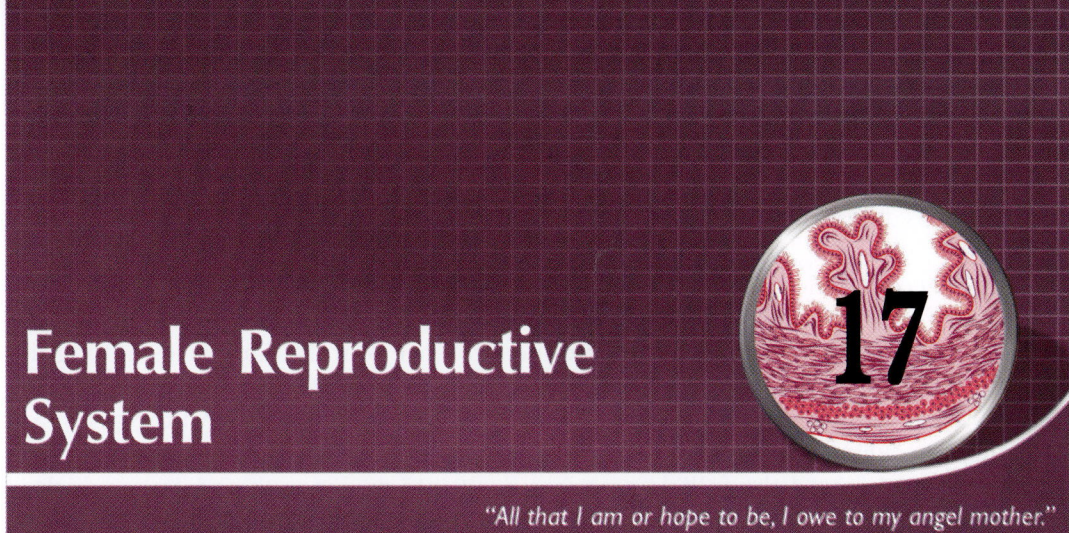

"All that I am or hope to be, I owe to my angel mother."

The female reproductive system consists of a pair of *ovaries*, a pair of *fallopian tubes* or oviducts, a *uterus, cervix,* and *vagina*. Accessory reproductive organs are the *mammary glands*, *placenta* and *umbilical cord*. In the sexually mature female the ovaries and uterus undergo marked changes in their structure and functional activity in relation to the menstrual cycle and pregnancy.

OVARY

The surface of the ovary is covered by *cuboidal epithelium* (modified peritoneal lining) known as the surface epithelium. Beneath this is a thin layer of connective tissue called *tunica albuginea*. The ovary consists of a thick peripheral or outer cortex which surrounds the inner *medulla* (Fig. 17.1).

Cortex consists of ovarian follicles in various stages of development and a connective tissue stroma. The stroma is highly cellular. Its cells and fibres run in a whorl-like manner.

Medulla consists of loose connective tissue, elastic fibres, numerous blood vessels and a few smooth muscle fibres.

The functions of ovary, i.e. production of ova and secretion of hormones are governed by the follicle stimulating hormone (FSH) and the luteinising hormone (LH) of the anterior pituitary. Ovarian follicles in the cortex of ovary after puberty can be classified as:

i. *Primordial follicle:* It consists of a *primary oocyte* surrounded by a single layer of flattened cells.
ii. *Primary follicle:* Each primary follicle has a *primary oocyte* surrounded by single layer of cuboidal cells. The primary oocyte has a large nucleus, with prominent nucleolus and pale chromatin. The cytoplasm is also pale and granular.
iii. *Secondary follicles:* The follicular epithelial cells proliferate and become many layered. The *primary oocyte* also increases in size. As the oocyte grows a thick non-cellular membrane called *zona pellucida* develops around it. After fertilisation of the mature ovum and during its division into the morula and the blastula, the rigid **zona pellucida** prevents increase in the diameter of the dividing zygote, to ensure its

easy passage through the narrow isthmus of the fallopian tube into the cavity of the uterus, and probably helps in nutrition of the developing ovum.

iv. *Graafian follicle* (Fig. 17.2): In the multiplying follicular cells which are known as *granulosa cells*, little irregular spaces filled with clear fluid, known as *liquor folliculi*, appear. The increase in amount of this follicular fluid is associated with further increase in the size of the follicle, and a confluence of irregular spaces among the granulosa cells form a single crescentic cavity, the *antrum*. At this stage the primary oocyte lies on one side of the cavity. Follicular cells which surround the ovum are called the *cumulus oophorus*.

The stroma around the follicle arranges itself into an inner *theca interna* which is vascular as well as cellular, and an outer theca externa which is fibrous. The cells of theca interna secrete estrogens. The follicle bulges onto the surface of the ovary. Such a follicle is called *mature Graafian follicle*.

The primary oocyte undergoes first meiotic division and becomes the *secondary oocyte* and in this state it bursts from the follicle. The follicular cells which still surround the secondary oocyte are called *corona radiata* cells. The rupture of follicle, with liberation of secondary oocyte is called *ovulation* and occurs nearly 14 days before the onset of next cycle.

Thus, the first meiotic division occurs just prior to ovulation and second meiotic division occurs at fertilization.

v. *Atretic follicle:* Many follicles do not develop fully, but degenerate and are called atretic follicles. These follicles secrete estrogens.

CORPUS LUTEUM

After the rupture of the follicle and liberation of **secondary oocyte** the **granulosa** or follicular and **theca interna** cells get thrown into folds. The granulosa cells become enlarged, accumulate lipid and are transformed into pale staining polygonal cells called *lutein cells*. The **theca interna** cells are smaller, fewer and dark staining. These are termed as **prolutein** cells. Capillaries and fibroblasts grow into these cells and the follicle is called *corpus luteum*. It secretes hormones chiefly **progesterone** and **some oestrogens** for 10–12 days if there is no pregnancy and for three months if there is pregnancy. After its function is over, the cells of the corpus luteum shrink in size and leave a white scar which is known as *corpus albicans*. Changes involving formation of ovarian follicles till the degeneration of corpus luteum constitute the *ovarian cycle*.

Functional Aspect

- Ovarian follicles undergo cyclical changes between puberty and menopause. The follicles grow in size and mature as well. This occurs under the effect of follicle stimulating hormone of anterior pituitary, which is controlled by gonadotrophin releasing hormone (GnRH) of hypothalamus. **Theca interna** cells of the maturing follicles secrete oestrogens. The peak of oestrogen occur just before ovulation. The high level of oestrogen causes **surge of LH** release as well as release of small amount of FSH. Both these, especially **LH surge** causes completion of first meiotic division, followed by ovulation and release of secondary oocyte, which is **viable for only 24 hours**. Second meiotic division occurs only at fertilization just prior to the penetration of the spermatozoon.

Female Reproductive System

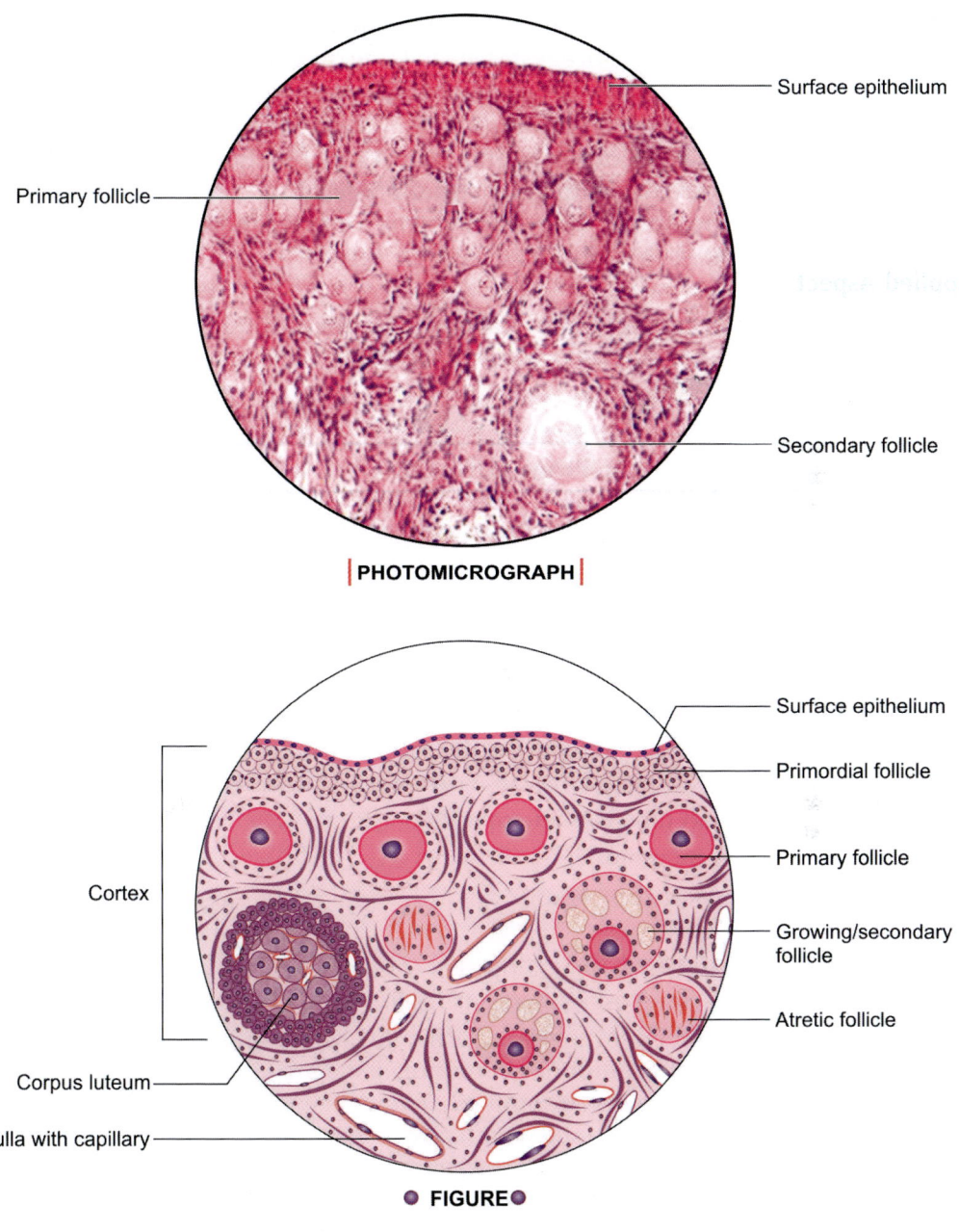

Fig. 17.1: *Ovary. Stain: Haematoxylin-eosin, 100X*

- After ovulation, LH modifies granulosa and theca interna cells into lutein and prolutein cells which secrete progesterone in large quantities and oestrogen in small amounts for preparation of endometrium. High levels of progesterone inhibit both hypothalamus and anterior pituitary.
- If oocyte is not fertilised, corpus luteum shrinks and its hormone secretion stops. The lack of hormones causes the menstrual phase of the uterine cycle. In case of fertilisation of oocyte, corpus luteum functions for three months.

Applied Aspect

There may be single or multiple follicular cysts, i.e. **theca lutein cysts**. Many types of tumours, usually malignant ones occur in the ovary. These quickly spread to distant regions.

FALLOPIAN TUBE OR OVIDUCT

Fallopian tube is the part of female reproductive tract that receives the secondary oocyte, provides the appropriate environment for its fertilisation and transports it to the uterus. Several segments along its length are identified.

The part of the tube traversing the wall of uterus is called *intramural part*.

The narrow medial third near the uterine wall is the *isthmus*.

The expanded intermediate segment is the *ampulla.*

The funnel shaped abdominal opening is the infundibulum, the margins of which are drawn into numerous tapering fringe like processes, the *fimbriae*.

The wall of the fallopian tube is made up of:
 i. Innermost mucous membrane,
 ii. Middle smooth muscle coat, and
 iii. Outermost serous coat.

   i. *The mucous membrane* (Fig. 17.3) is thrown into many longitudinal folds, so much so that the lumen may not be visualised. The folds reveal branching but there is no anastomosis. The epithelium consists of a single layer of cells resting on a basement membrane. The cells are columnar in nature, some are ciliated especially near the fimbria and ampulla, others are non-ciliated. A few *clear cells* lying close to the basement membrane may also be seen. The cilia beat towards the uterus and create a current of fresh fluid in the oviduct towards the uterus. The height of these cells varies according to the menstrual phase.

   The lamina propria consists of loose connective tissue with less differentiated fibroblasts. In *ectopic pregnancy*, these fibroblasts change to *decidual cells.*

   Muscularis mucosae is absent.

  ii. The *muscle coat* is made up of inner circular and outer longitudinal layers. The contraction of these muscle fibres pushes the ovum towards the uterus. The isthmus has the thickest muscle coat (Fig. 17.3).

  iii. The *serous coat* is the outermost layer, which is lined by mesothelial cells of the peritoneum.

Female Reproductive System

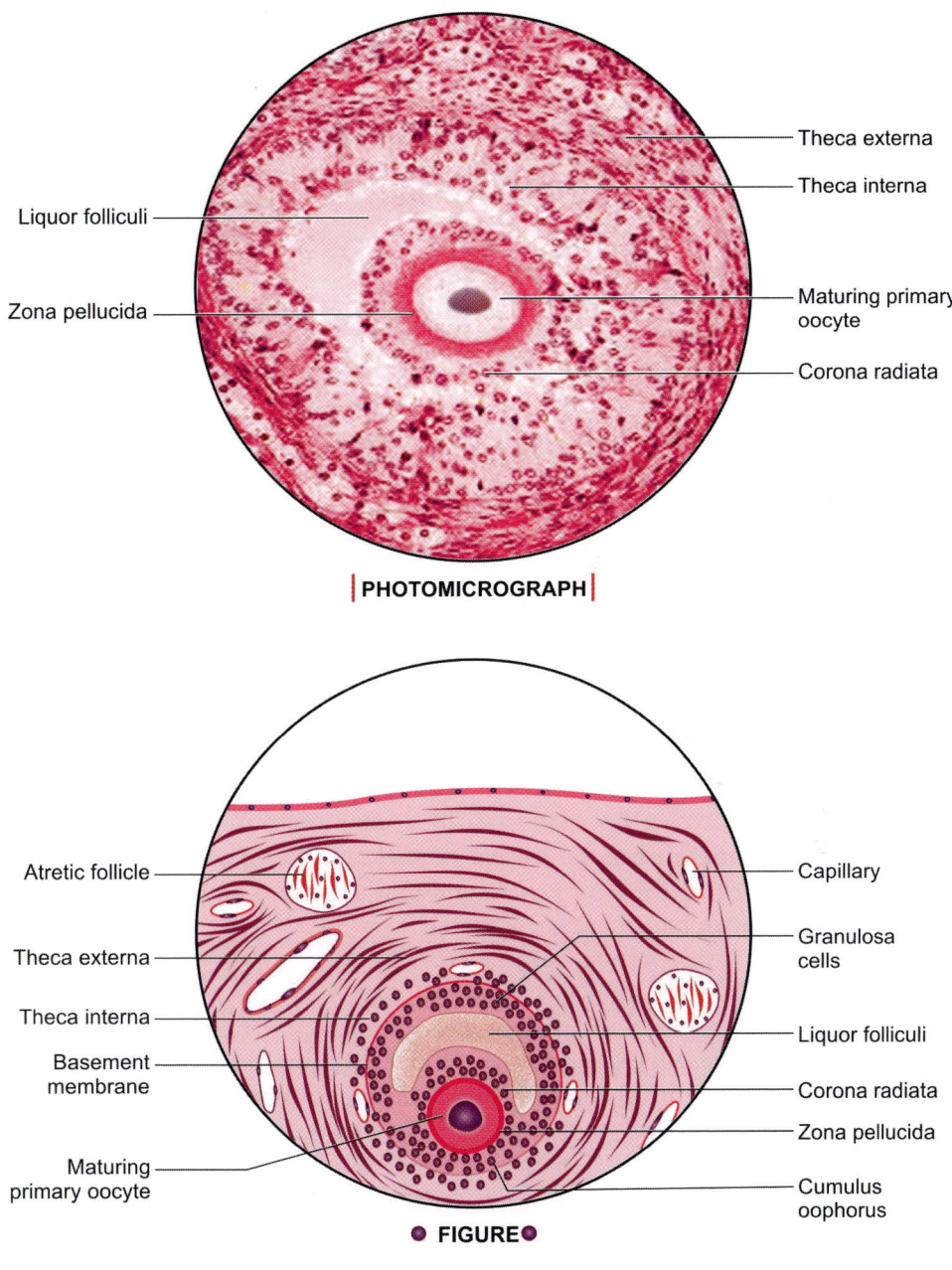

Fig. 17.2: *Graafian follicle. Stain: Haematoxylin-eosin, 400X*

Functional Aspect

- The epithelium of fallopian tube undergoes cyclic changes. When the levels of oestrogens are high in proliferating phase the height of the epithelium is greatest. The fimbria of the fallopian tube "catch" the secondary oocyte with the help of cilia and smooth muscles in its wall. The cilia and contraction of muscles transfer and transport the zygote to the uterus. The non-ciliated cells provide nutrition during the "journey". Fertilisation, if it has to take place, occurs in the ampullary part of the tube.
- During tubectomy, parts of the tubes are ligated, removed and sections seen by microscope.

Applied Aspect

- *Ectopic pregnancy:* At times, implantation of morula occurs in fallopian tube, which ruptures within 2–3 months.
- *Salpingitis:* Chronic infection of the tubes may be tubercular in nature. TB salpingitis leads to infertility.

UTERUS

The uterus is the organ of the reproductive tract that receives the fertilised ovum from the fallopian tube, provides attachment and establishes vascular relations necessary for sustenance of the embryo and foetus throughout its development. Wall of the uterus consists of the following three layers:

i. Innermost is the lining with a glandular mucous membrane called *endometrium*.
ii. Middle layer is made of smooth muscle fibres known as *myometrium*.
iii. Outermost is a serous lining of *peritoneum* made up of a single layer of flattened cells resting on a thin basement membrane.

ENDOMETRIUM

Beginning at puberty till menopause, the uterine endometrium undergoes monthly cyclic changes in structure, in response to rhythmic variations in the secretion of ovarian hormones. The endometrium is divisible into a basal one-third called the *stratum basale* and superficial two-thirds known as *stratum functionalis*, the latter being shed during the menstrual flow.

The cyclic activity of the non-pregnant uterus may be divided into three phases of the endometrium:

a. Follicular or proliferative or reparative or oestrogenic phase,
b. Progestational or progravid or secretory phase, and
c. Menstrual phase.

a. Proliferative Phase

The lining consists of a single layer of columnar cells resting on the basement membrane.

The lamina propria or endometrial stroma contains simple tubular glands, lined by a single layer of columnar cells. The deep part of the endometrium shows cut sections

Female Reproductive System

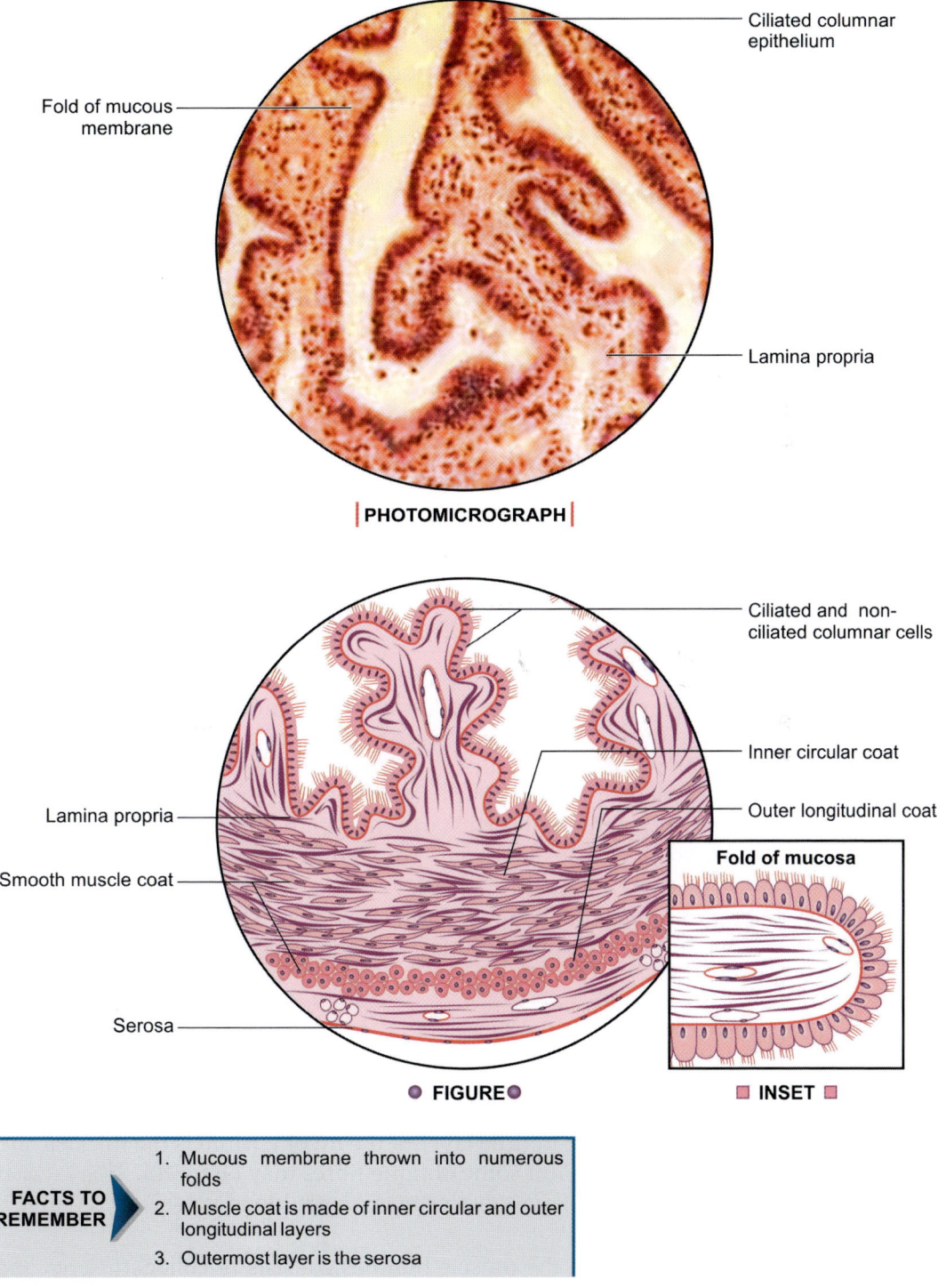

Fig. 17.3: *Fallopian tube. Stain: Haematoxylin-eosin, 100X*

of the glands, the bases of which extend to the myometrium. The deeper layer of endometrium shows sections of coiled arteries.

The connective tissue stroma made up of fibroblasts and reticular fibres is much more than the glands. This phase lasts from the fifth to the fourteenth day of the menstrual cycle (Fig. 17.4).

b. Progestational or Secretory Phase

The endometrium becomes much thicker due to secretion of glands and oedema of the uterine stroma.

In the lamina propria, glands get dilated and there is accumulation of secretion in them. There is large amount of stored glycogen in the basal part of the cytoplasm of the cell and the nucleus gets displaced towards the apical part of the cell. The glands continue to grow in size, become tortuous and ultimately develop marked sacculations, resulting in a wide lumen of irregular outline, filled with a carbohydrate rich secretion (Fig. 17.5).

The convolutions of coiled arteries continue and these extend up to the superficial portion of the endometrium. This lasts from the fifteenth to the twenty-eighth day of the menstrual cycle.

The endometrium is subdivided into a narrow *stratum compactum*, a large *middle stratum spongiosum* and a *basal third named the stratum basale*.

c. Menstrual Phase

Nearly two weeks after ovulation, the stimulation of endometrium by ovarian hormones *declines*. The coiled arteries constrict so that the superficial zone of the endometrium is ischaemic for a few hours at a time. The glands stop secreting. The walls of vessels get necrosed and blood pours into the stroma and soon breaks through into the uterine lumen and menstrual flow starts. The epithelium is lost and the inner wall is covered by blood clots. The blood cells are seen in the stroma as well as in the glands.

The superficial two-thirds of the endometrium is shed off. The basal one-third with straight arteries remains. The endometrium starts regenerating in the next proliferative phase (Fig. 17.6).

MYOMETRIUM

This is the thickest coat of the uterus. It consists of three layers. Outer and inner layers are thinner and muscle fibres are predominantly longitudinal but some oblique and circular bundles are also seen. The middle layer of the myometrium is the thickest and has predominantly circular fibres but some oblique fibres may be found. This layer is also called *stratum vasculare* because it contains many large blood vessels which give it a spongy appearance.

The connective tissue between the muscle bundles consists of collagen fibres and fibroblasts. During pregnancy, there is increase in size of the muscle fibres as well as their new formation from the connective tissue in between the muscles, under the effect of estrogen hormone.

Female Reproductive System

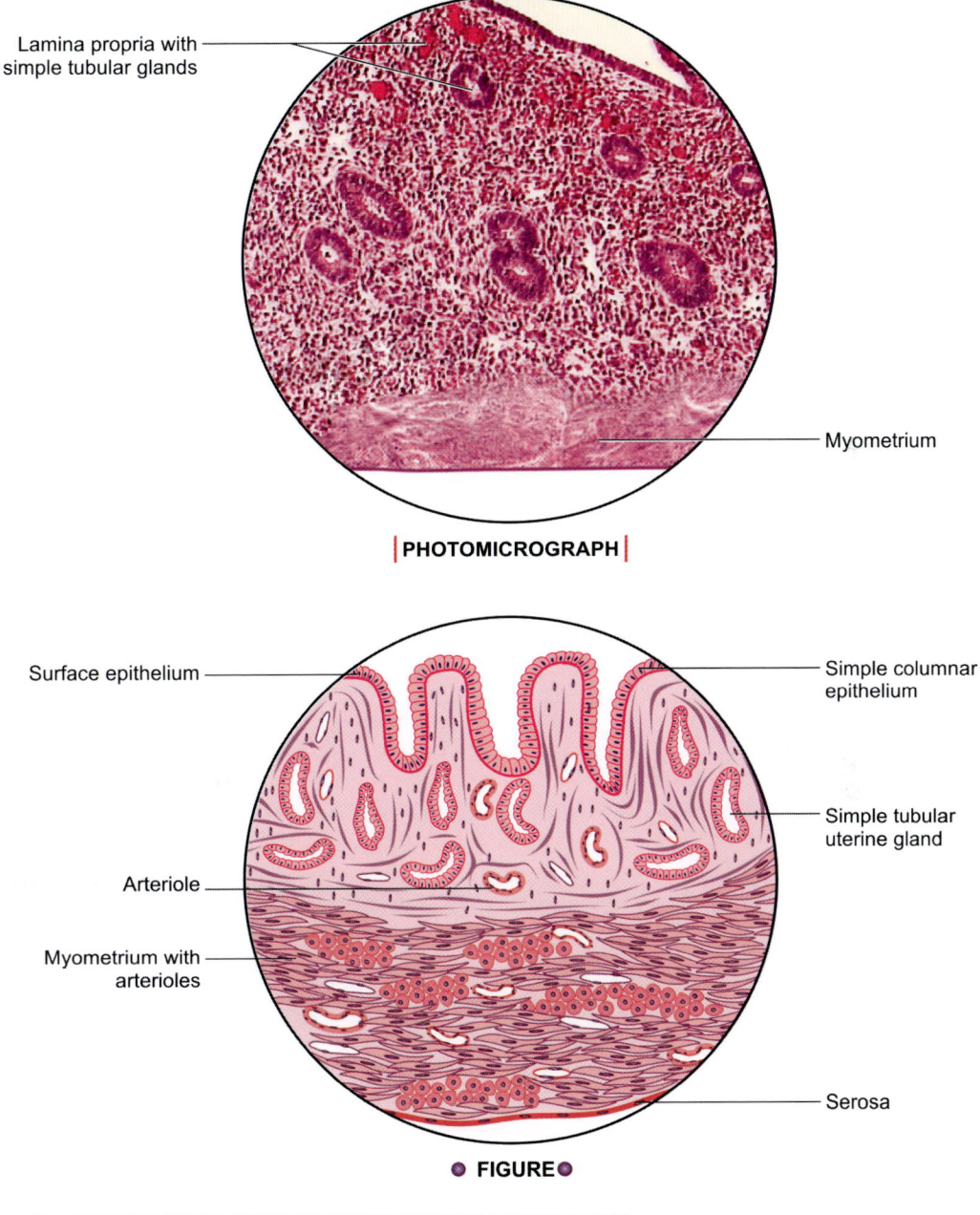

Fig. 17.4: *Uterus—proliferative phase. Stain: Haematoxylin-eosin, 100X*

FACTS TO REMEMBER
1. Endometrium lined by single layer of columnar cells
2. Lamina propria contains simple tubular glands
3. Thick myometrium with arterioles

PHOTOMICROGRAPH

FIGURE

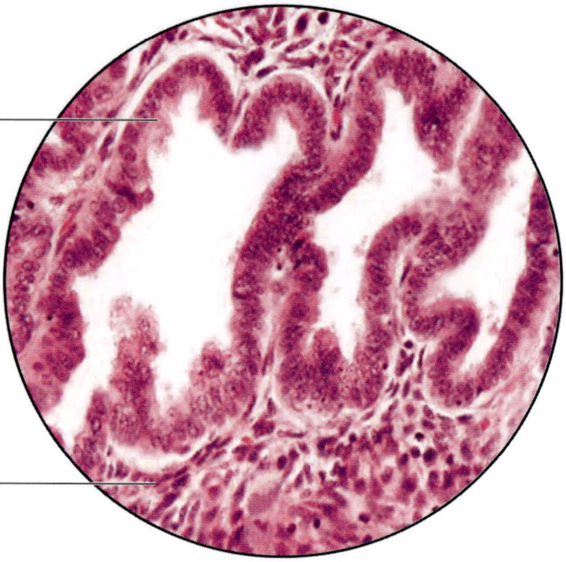

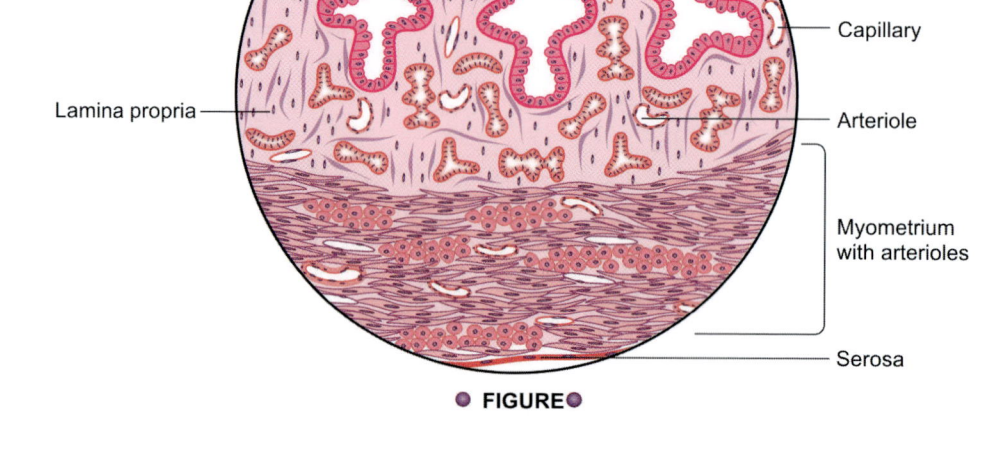

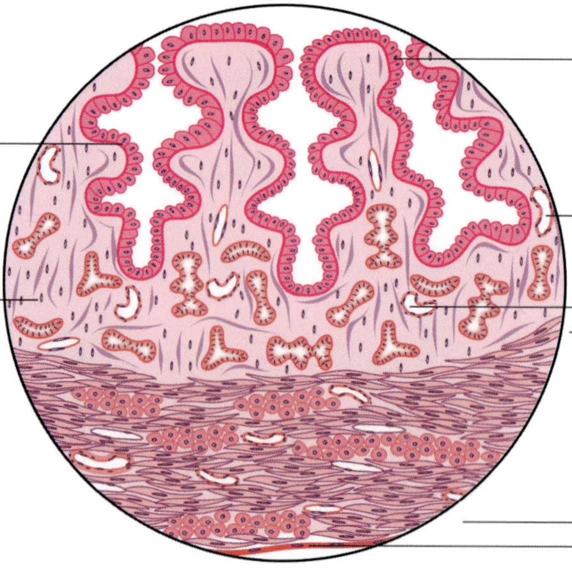

FACTS TO REMEMBER

1. Thick endometrium due to secretion of glands
2. Tortuous uterine glands and coiled arteries
3. Columnar cells line the glands

Fig. 17.5: *Uterus—progestational phase. Stain: Haematoxylin-eosin, 100X*

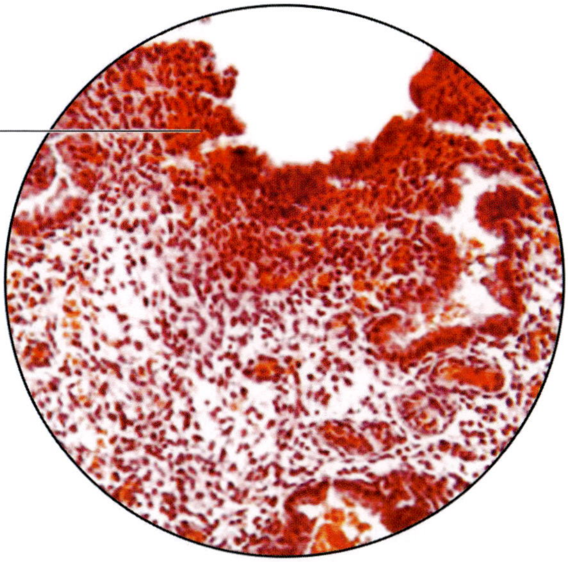

Female Reproductive System

PHOTOMICROGRAPH

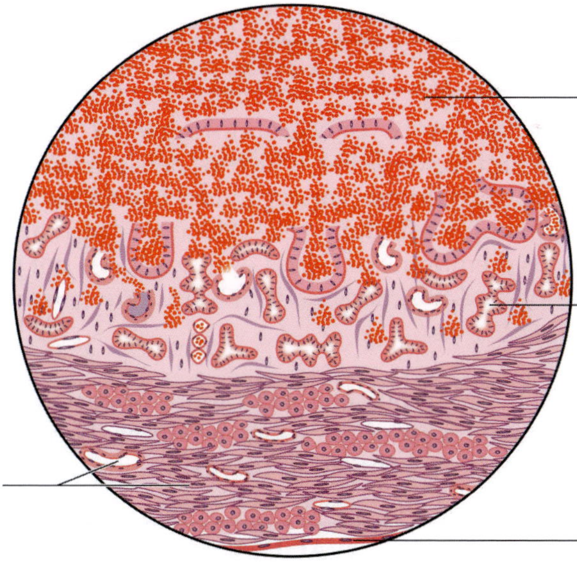

- Blood in lumen

FIGURE

- Blood in lumen
- Basal part of uterine gland
- Myometrium with arteriole
- Serosa

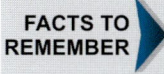

FACTS TO REMEMBER
1. Denuded epithelium with blood in lumen
2. Superficial 2/3rd of endometrium is shed off
3. Outer myometrium

Fig. 17.6: *Uterus—menstrual phase. Stain: Haematoxylin-eosin, 100X*

SEROSA

Peritoneal or serous coat consists of single layer of squamous cells.

Functional Aspect

The uterine endometrium prepares itself for the "welcome", i.e. implantation of blastocyst. First it is done by estrogen of the maturing ovarian follicles. This occurs from 5th–14th day of the cycle. From 15th to 28th day further preparations of the endometrium start. These are under the control of progesterone.

If fertilization occurs, it is followed by *implantation*, uterus is "happy" and continues to grow in size providing optimum environment to the developing embryo and foetus. In case, fertilisation does not occur, most of the endometrium is shed off in the form of menstrual flow, lasting from day 1 to day 4 of the cycle.

Applied Aspect

- *Fibroid of uterus:* Tumour derived from smooth muscle of uterus. The fibroids may be single or multiple. It usually leads to infertility.
- *Tubercular endometritis:* This is due to infection spreading from the fallopian tube. This usually leads to infertility due to small infrequent glands and thin atrophic epithelium as part of the disease.

CERVIX

The external surface of the cervix (ectocervix) is covered with stratified squamous non-keratinised epithelium, underlying which is dense irregular connective tissue. The epithelium changes to columnar variety in cervical erosion. The internal surface (endocervix) is lined by simple columnar cells. Mucous glands are seen in the centre of the section. The mucous membrane of cervix of uterus does not take part in the cyclic changes of menstruation and pregnancy (Fig. 17.7).

Applied Aspect

Carcinoma of cervix: The squamous cell carcinoma of cervix is the very common malignant tumour of female reproductive system. Cervix becomes hard, later a large fungating mass is formed. It may spread to uterus, vagina and other pelvic organs.

VAGINA

Vagina is a fibromuscular passage extending from the cervix of the uterus to the vestibule. It comprises:
- Inner mucous membrane
- Middle muscular coat
- Outer fibrous coat/adventitial coat

The **mucous membrane** consists of epithelium and an underlying lamina propria. The epithelium is of the *stratified squamous non-keratinised* variety resting on dense connective tissue which is thrown into papillae. The thickness of the epithelium depends upon the level of oestrogen in the blood.

Female Reproductive System

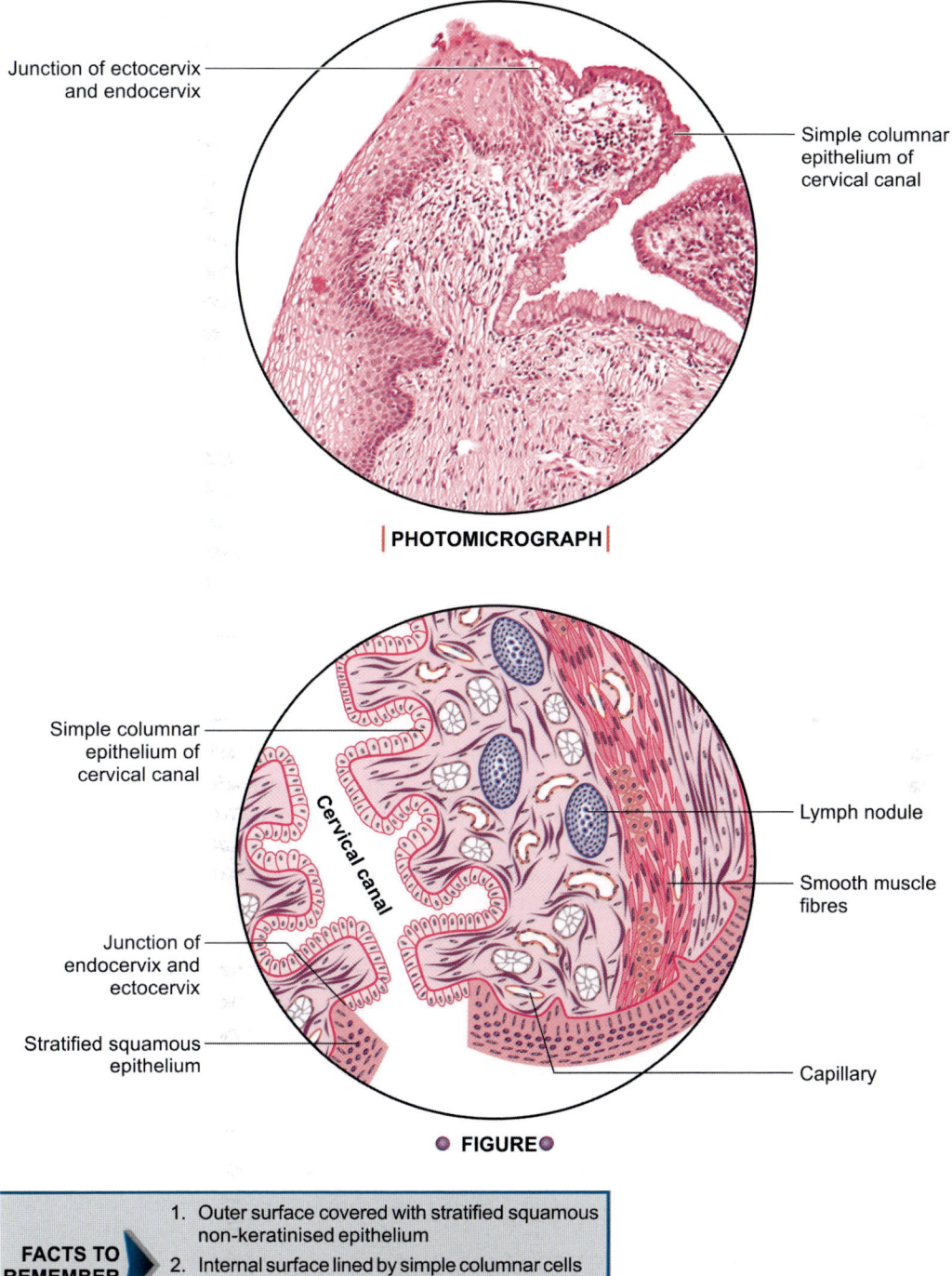

Fig. 17.7: Cervix. Stain: Haematoxylin-eosin, 100X

FACTS TO REMEMBER
1. Outer surface covered with stratified squamous non-keratinised epithelium
2. Internal surface lined by simple columnar cells
3. A few mucous acini and smooth muscle fibres seen

The lamina propria is made up of dense connective tissue with elastic fibres. Accumulation of lymphocytes is abundant and sometimes lymph nodules are present. There are no glands in the lamina propria. The vaginal epithelium is kept moist by secretions of glands in the cervix of the uterus. The deeper layer contains plexus of veins.

The **middle layer** consists of a fibromuscular coat, with circular and longitudinal smooth muscle fibres, intermingled with elastic fibres.

Outermost is the **adventitial coat.** The posterior wall in its uppermost part is covered by a serous coat. Vaginal cytology is done for detection of cancer and for hormonal status of the patient (Fig. 17.8).

Functional Aspect

The epithelium of vagina thickens under the influence of estrogens. The epithelial cells synthesise and accumulate glycogen. Then these cells get desquamated into the lumen of vagina. Bacteria in the vagina metabolise glycogen and release lactic acid, thus helping to increase the acidity of the vagina.

Applied Aspect

- *Leukoplakia* are the white patches in the region of external genitalia. These patches may be precancerous.
- *Rape:* Sexual intercourse without consent.

MAMMARY GLANDS

The mammary glands are specialised accessory glands of the skin, which have evolved in mammals to provide nourishment to the young ones. Mammary gland consists of 15–20 lobes with the same number of ducts. Each lobe is madeup of many lobules containing acini. Histologically only lobules are discernible in the gland.

Resting Phase in Non-pregnant Adult Female

The mammary gland in this phase consists mainly of ducts and their branches (Fig. 17.9). The stroma has connective tissue and fat cells.

The intralobular ducts are usually lined by *low columnar epithelium* resting on a basement membrane. The intralobular connective tissue which is derived from the papillary layer of the dermis is more cellular, containing fibroblasts.

The interlobular connective tissue, which lies between the ducts of adjacent lobules, is derived from the reticular layer of the dermis, and is more fibroreticular in nature. It contains fat lobules. Each fat cell is round or oval with a flattened peripheral nucleus. With haematoxylin and eosin stain, the cytoplasm looks empty. Only a few blood vessels are seen in the stroma.

The differences between resting and lactating phases of the gland are depicted in Table 17.1.

Lactating Phase

The gland is full of acini with minimum amount of connective tissue. Some acini are lined by tall columnar cells, others by normal columnar cells. The nucleus may be

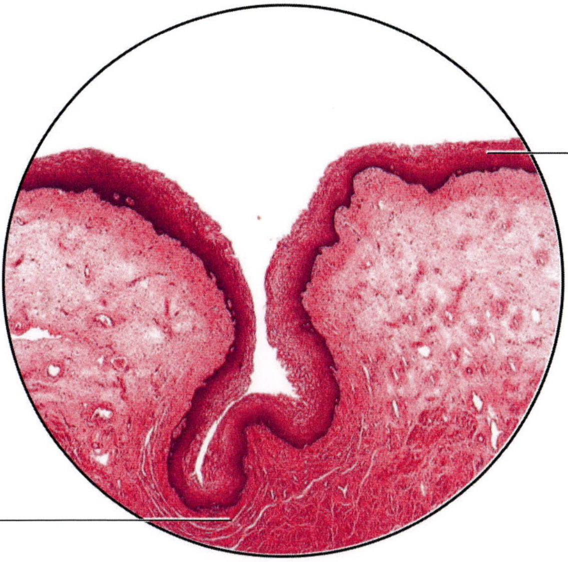

Female Reproductive System

PHOTOMICROGRAPH

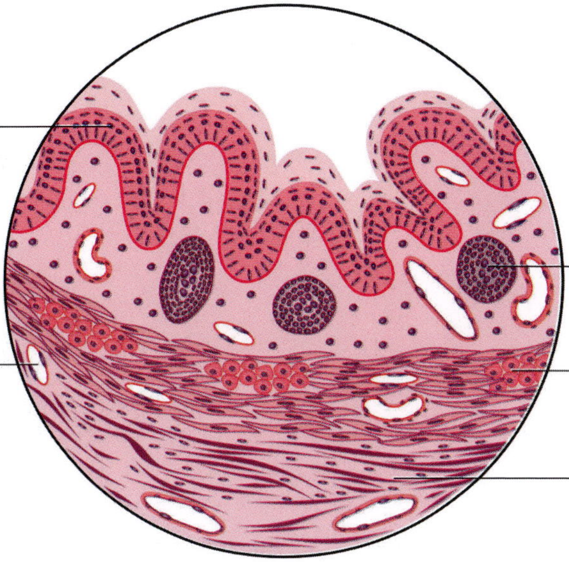

- Stratified squamous epithelium
- Fibromuscular coat

FIGURE

- Stratified squamous non-keratinised epithelium
- Capillary
- Lymph nodules
- Fibromuscular coat
- Adventitia

FACTS TO REMEMBER
1. Mucous membrane lined by stratified squamous non-keratinised epithelium
2. Elastic fibres in lamina propria
3. Fibromuscular coat covered by adventitia

Fig. 17.8: *Vagina. Stain: Haematoxylin-eosin, 100X*

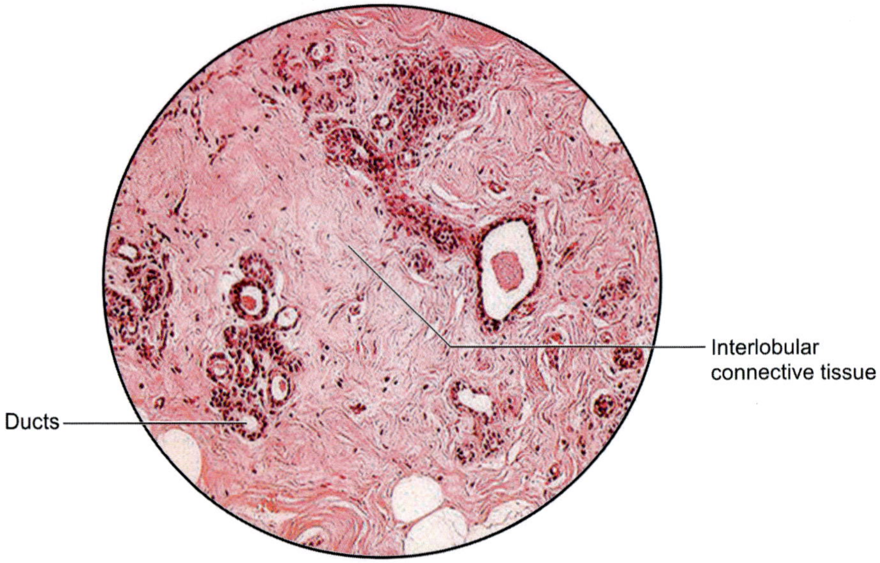

PHOTOMICROGRAPH

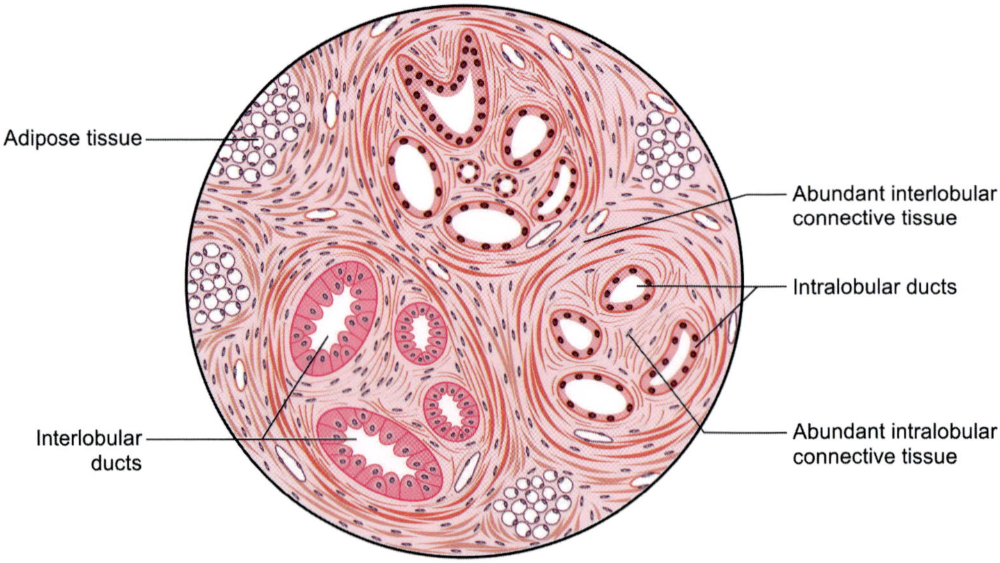

- Ducts
- Interlobular connective tissue

FIGURE

- Adipose tissue
- Abundant interlobular connective tissue
- Intralobular ducts
- Abundant intralobular connective tissue
- Interlobular ducts

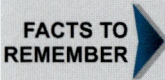

FACTS TO REMEMBER
1. Abundant interlobular connective tissue
2. Ducts of different size
3. Plenty of fat cells, lobules ill defined

Fig. 17.9: *Mammary gland—resting phase. Stain: Haematoxylin-eosin, 100X*

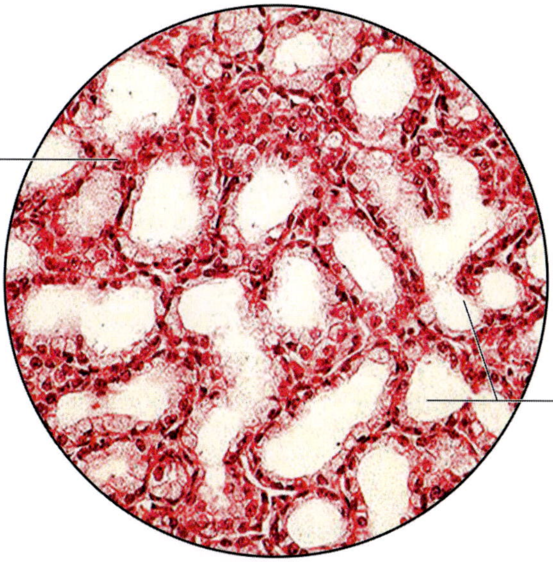

Female Reproductive System

PHOTOMICROGRAPH

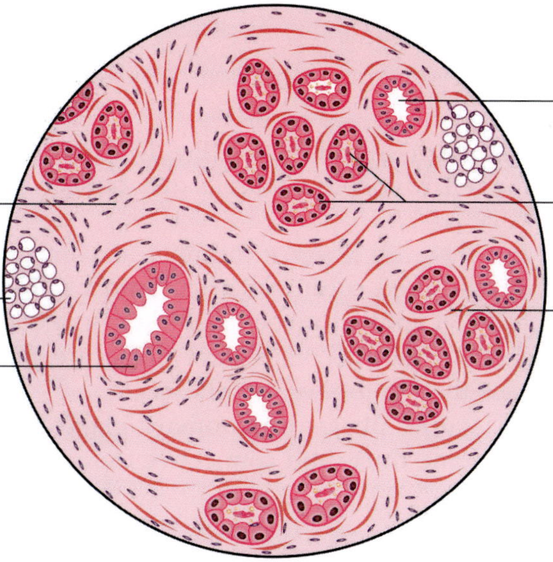

Labels:
- Scanty interlobular connective tissue
- Numerous secretory acini

FIGURE

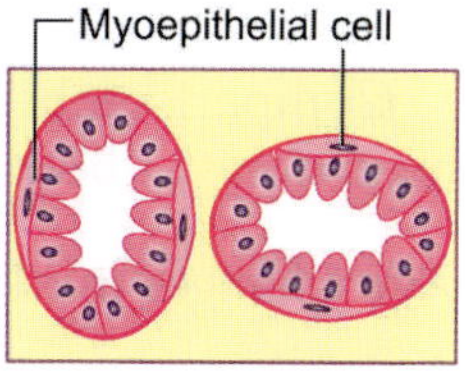

Labels:
- Intralobular duct
- Scanty interlobular connective tissue
- Numerous secretory acini
- Fat cell
- Scanty intralobular connective tissue
- Interlobular duct

INSET

- Myoepithelial cell

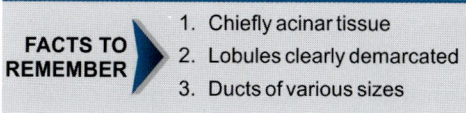

FACTS TO REMEMBER
1. Chiefly acinar tissue
2. Lobules clearly demarcated
3. Ducts of various sizes

Fig. 17.10: *Mammary gland—lactating phase. Stain: Haematoxylin-eosin, 100X*

TABLE 17.1: Differences between resting and lactating phases of the gland

Resting or non-lactating phase	Lactating phase
• Predominantly comprised of ducts and fibrofatty tissue	Comprised chiefly of acini
• Lobules ill defined	Lobules clearly demarcated
• Intralobular connective tissue contains fibroblasts	It contains fibroblasts, lymphocytes, plasma cells and eosinophils

TABLE 17.2: Comparison of lactating mammary gland and prostate gland

Lactating mammary gland	Prostate gland
1. No smooth muscle fibres around the acini	Abundant smooth muscle fibres around the acini
2. Presence of fat cells	Absence of fat cells
3. The epithelium of acini does not show infoldings	The epithelium is infolded in many acini. It may be pseudostratified
4. More ducts visible	Less number of ducts
5. Interlobular connective tissue is thinned out. Acini may show secretions, i.e. milk	Connective tissue is seen around the acini. These may show concretions formed by calcified coagulated secretion
6. Only ducts seen	May show the opening of urethra and two ejaculatory ducts

round or oval and is seen in the middle of the cell (Fig. 17.10). Droplets of fat accumulate near the free surface of the cell. Myoepithelial cells may be seen between the basement membrane and secretory cells.

Ducts are also seen but they are fewer in number as compared to the acini. The bigger ducts are lined by stratified columnar or columnar epithelium and secretion may be seen in the ducts. Duct epithelium stains darker than the acinar epithelium.

The interlobular connective tissue becomes scanty in nature. Blood vessels are many more in the lactating phase than in the resting phase.

Comparison between lactating phase of mammary gland and prostate gland has been done as both contain acini, ducts and connective tissue in (Table 17.2).

Age Changes in Mammary Gland

At birth	: A few ducts are present.
Childhood	: Only ducts are present. No sex difference.
Puberty	: There is deposition of fat and ducts multiply in number. Sometimes fat deposition may be seen in boys also.
Menstrual cycle	: The mammary gland is continuously affected by the hormones of the ovary. There is multiplication of ducts and deposition of fat. Due to continuous attack of hormones, the breast may develop adenoma or other tumours.
Pregnancy	: Mammary glands are very active during pregnancy, as these are preparing themselves for the secretion of milk for the

		newborn under the effect of hormones. There is further proliferation of ducts during first trimester. These terminal ends of ducts acquire acini during second trimester. These acini increase and begin to secrete watery fluid during the third trimester. **Colostrum** is secreted during the end stage and must be given to the infant, as it is rich in proteins and antibodies as well.
Lactation	:	Acini secrete the milk which is of vital importance to the newborn. For first three to six months, the infant can be brought up "exclusively on breastfeeding". Mother must take nutritious diet during this period. Lactation is also hormone-dependent.
Post lactation	:	The acini gradually disappear. During 2nd pregnancy, the acini appear again.
Menopause	:	Approximately at 45–50 years of age, the menstrual cycle gradually comes to an end. Concomitantly the acini and ducts also involute. Mainly fibrofatty tissue remains.

Functional Aspect

- The acini and ducts of mammary gland grow under the effects of oestrogen and progesterone produced initially in pregnancy by corpus luteum and later by placenta.
- Additional growth of the gland occurs due to prolactin of anterior pituitary gland.
- After birth, the milk secretion occurs due to conjoint actions of prolactin and oxytocin. The latter causes contraction of *myoepithelial cells* around the secretory acini. Decreased suckling causes decrease secretion of milk.

Applied Aspect

- *Breast abscess:* Acute inflammation of acini of breast with pus formation may occur during lactation.
- *Carcinoma of breast* is most common malignant tumour in the female. It is felt as localised hard, painless unilateral mass, usually fixed. The carcinoma spreads via lymphatics to axillary and parasternal lymph nodes of same side and later to the opposite side. Secondaries may appear in liver, lung and vertebral column. **Self examination of breasts** for early detection of any mass must be impressed on all females.

PLACENTA

Placenta starts forming immediately after implantation and is fully formed and functional by three months of pregnancy. The placenta from a foetus at five months of pregnancy shows cut sections of several chorionic villi. The trophoblastic epithelium of the villi is composed of an external layer of *syncytiotrophoblast* and an inner layer of *cytotrophoblast*.

The cells of the cytotrophoblast are bigger and pale staining with only slightly basophilic cytoplasm whereas the cytoplasm of syncytial cells is strongly basophilic. In the interior of the villus, there is embryonic connective tissue and foetal blood vessels which are branches of umbilical blood vessels. These are lined by endothelial cells resting on a basement membrane, and contain both nucleated and non-nucleated erythrocytes. The villi lie in the maternal blood which contains non-nucleated erythrocytes (Fig. 17.11).

The chorionic villi of the placenta at full term show the chorionic epithelium only as syncytial trophoblast whose syncytial character gets more pronounced (Fig. 17.12). Cytotrophoblast starts disappearing after five months of pregnancy and the foetal capillaries increase in number.

Placental barrier is constituted by:

i. Thin syncytiotrophoblastic cells
ii. Basement membrane of cytotrophoblastic cells
iii. Basement membrane of foetal capillaries
iv. Thin endothelial cells

Functional Aspect

Placenta is the "God" of foetus. Syncytiotrophoblast secrete chorionic gonadotrophins, which stimulates corpus luteum to secrete estrogen and progesterone for 3 months. Placenta secretes many other hormones to maintain pregnancy. It acts like respiratory, gastrointestinal, excretory and endocrine system for the foetus.

Applied Aspect

- *Hydatidiform mole:* The uterus is partially or fully filled by benign cysts of varying size. The cysts are enlarged chorionic villi.
- *Choriocarcinoma:* This is malignant tumour of trophoblast and spreads early to the lung.

UMBILICAL CORD

The umbilical cord approximately 50 cm long at full term connects the placenta to the foetus. It is the **lifeline of foetus**.

It consists of an outer covering of flattened amniotic epithelial cells, containing in its interior a mass of mesoderm, which is transformed into a viscid mucoid connective tissue known as *Wharton's jelly*. It has widely spaced fibroblasts separated by fine collagen fibres and ground substance.

Traversing the cord are two umbilical arteries and only one (left) umbilical vein (Fig. 17.13). The arteries are provided with a thick muscular coat. The internal elastic lamina is folded, thus there is considerable narrowing of the lumen. The vein shows a wide lumen, which is often collapsed.

Female Reproductive System

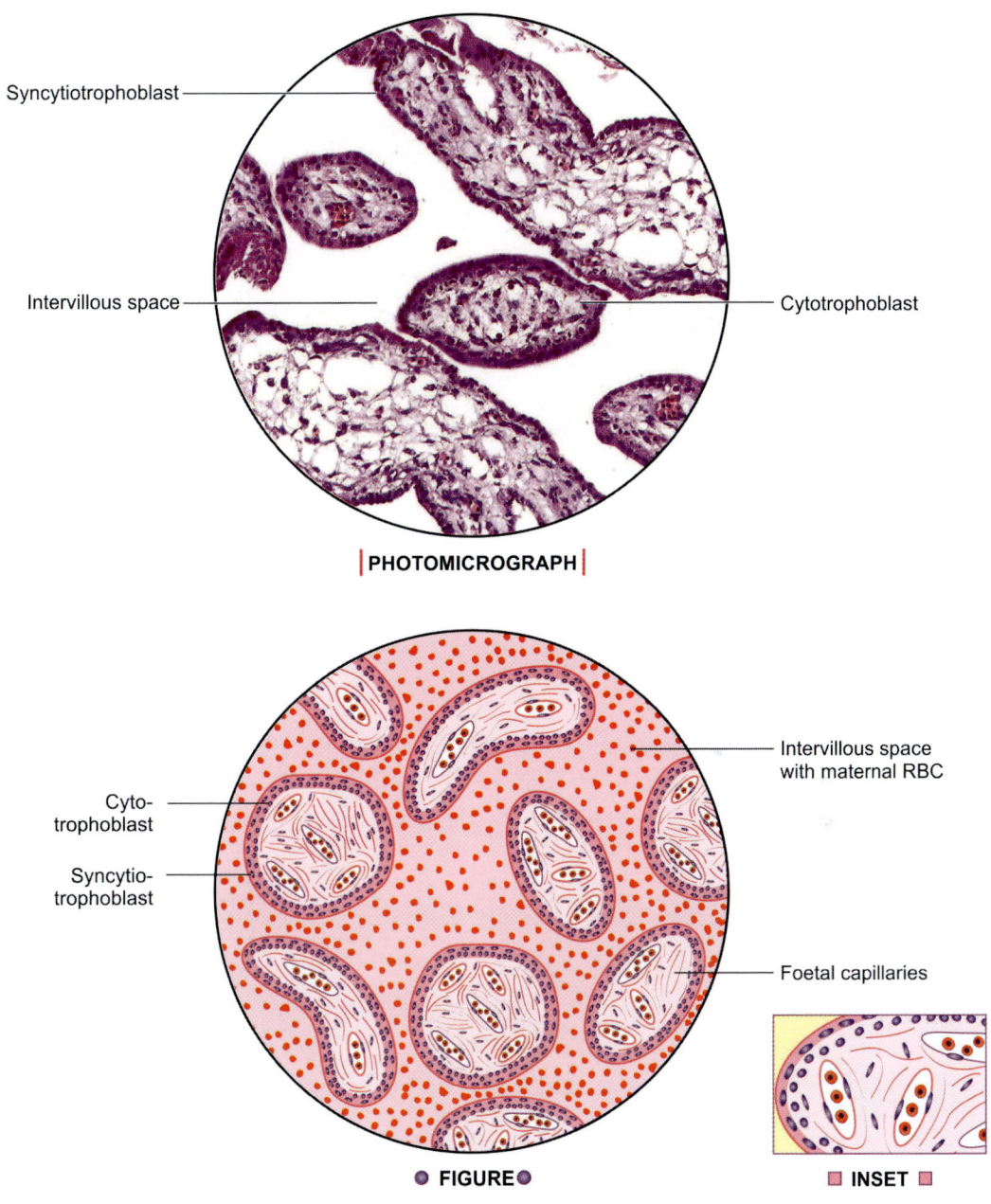

Fig. 17.11: *Placenta at 5 months. Stain: Haematoxylin-eosin, 100X*

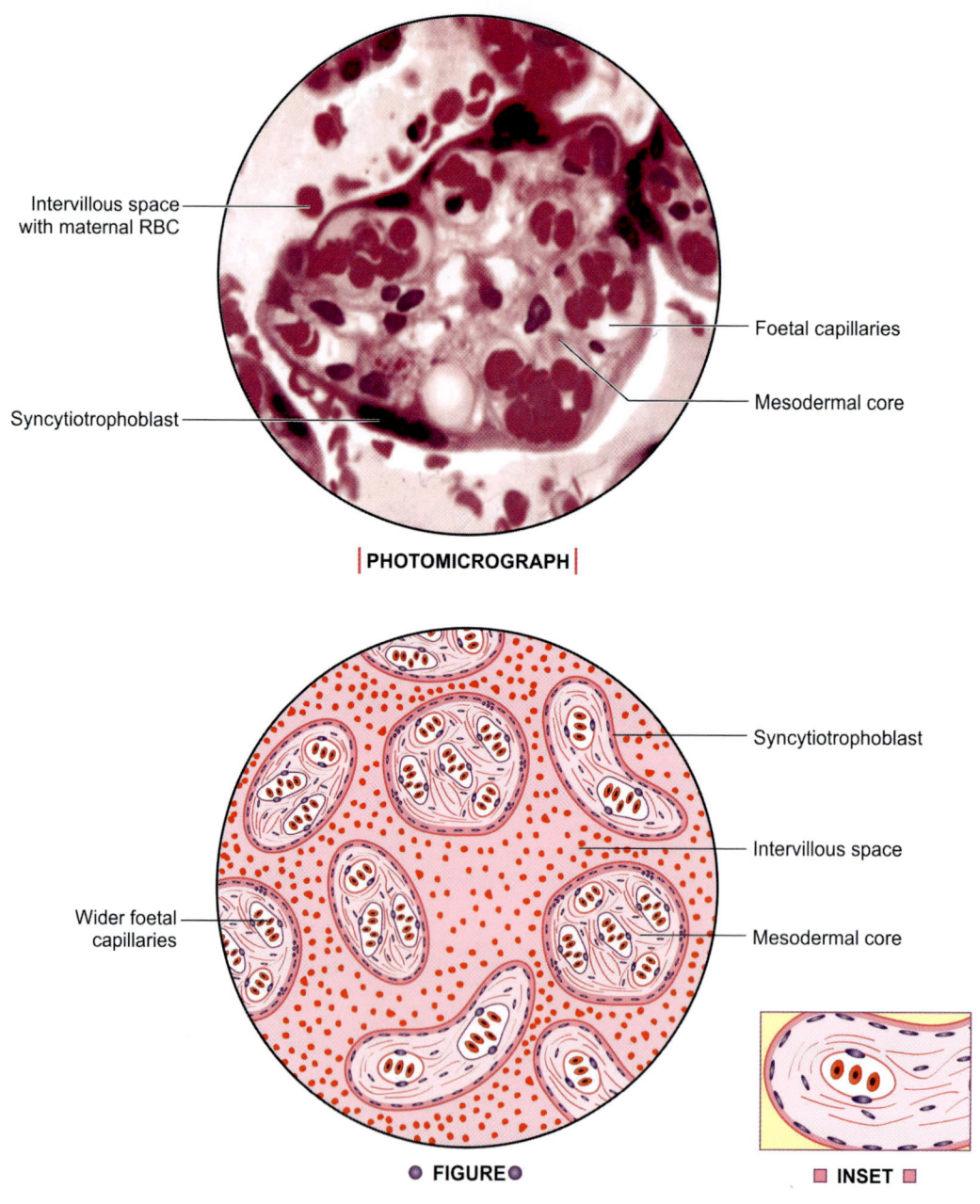

Fig. 17.12: Placenta—full term. Stain: Haematoxylin-eosin, 100X

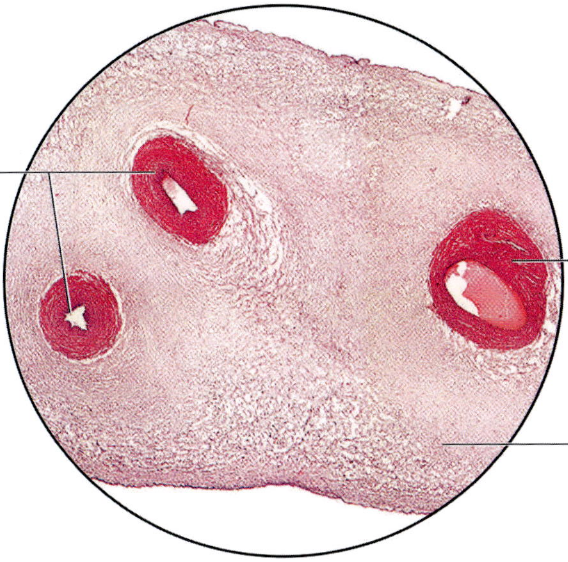

Female Reproductive System

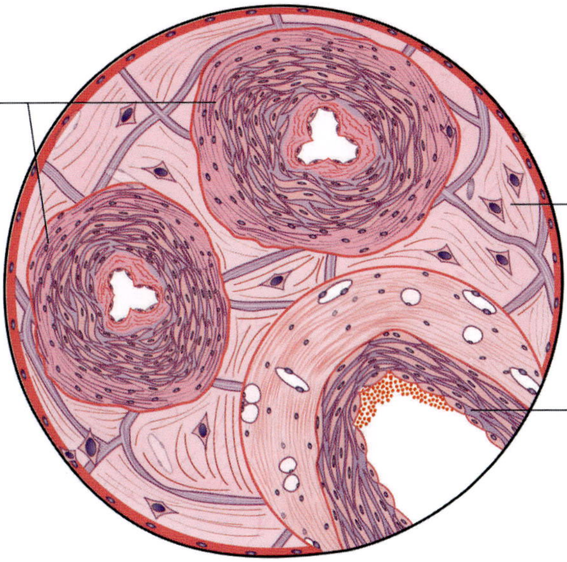

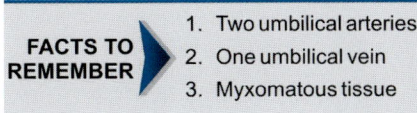

Fig. 17.13: *Umbilical cord. Stain: Haematoxylin-eosin, 100X*

MULTIPLE CHOICE QUESTIONS

1. Which of the following cells is liberated at the time of ovulation?
   a. Mature oocyte
   b. Primary oocyte
   c. Secondary oocyte
   d. Oogonium
2. How much period does the corpus luteum of pregnancy remains active?
   a. 2–3 weeks   b. 3–4 months
   c. 9 months   d. 6 months
3. Lining of endometrium is:
   a. Simple columnar
   b. Cuboidal
   c. Stratified columnar
   d. Pseudostratified columnar
4. Lining of vagina is:
   a. Pseudostratified columnar
   b. Stratified squamous non-keratinised
   c. Stratified squamous keratinised
   d. Stratified columnar
5. Which hormone is exclusively present in female?
   a. Oestrogen
   b. Testosterone
   c. Progesterone
   d. Luteinising hormone

ANSWERS

1. c   2. b   3. a   4. b
5. c

Endocrine Glands

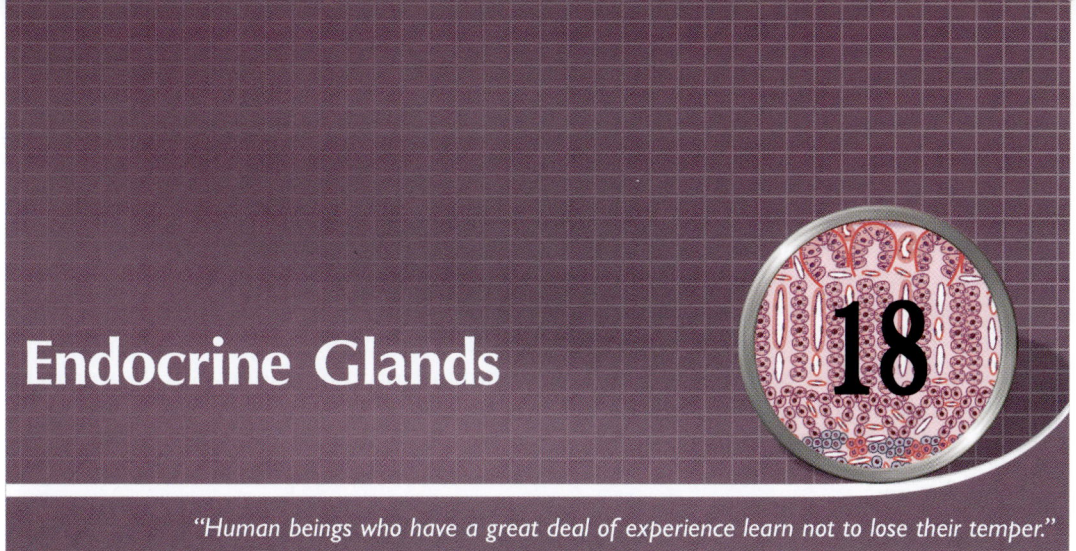

"Human beings who have a great deal of experience learn not to lose their temper."

The endocrine or ductless glands are situated in various regions of the body. They are devoid of ducts and the secretions are poured directly into the blood through the capillaries and numerous sinusoids draining and irrigating the gland. These have rich blood supply. Each of the gland secretes specific hormones with distinct functions. The principal endocrine glands are the hypophysis, thyroid, parathyroid, suprarenal, pineal glands and parts of pancreas, testis and ovary.

HYPOPHYSIS CEREBRI

The hypophysis cerebri lies in the cranial cavity and is attached to the base of the brain by the stalk or infundibulum. The hypophysis has two major divisions; the *neurohypophysis* which develops as a process growing downward from the floor of the diencephalon, and the *adenohypophysis* which originates in the embryo as a dorsal outpouching from the roof of the mouth. The neurohypophysis is also known as the posterior lobe.

There are three subdivisions of the adenohypophysis, the *pars distalis* or anterior lobe, *pars intermedia* and *pars tuberalis* (Fig. 18.1).

PARS DISTALIS

Pars distalis forms the largest subdivision of the hypophysis cerebri. It is composed of glandular cells arranged in irregular cords or clumps. These are intimately related to the extensive system of thin walled capillaries and sinusoids. The glandular cells are:
  i. Chromophobes which form 50 per cent of the total cell population.
  ii. Chromophils, forming the rest of the 50 per cent of the cell population.
     Chromophils are of two types: Acidophils or alpha cells and basophils or beta cells.

Chromophobes

Chromophobes are small cells, with homogeneous light staining cytoplasm. Nuclei are pale and lie in the centre of the cells. The cells are frequently arranged in groups or clumps. These cells are believed to give rise to chromophils or are fatigued secretory cells (Fig. 18.2).

Chromophils

Chromophils are larger than the chromophobes and contain granules in their cytoplasm. These cells are usually present at the periphery of the clump. Chromophils consist of *alpha* or acidophilic cells and *beta* or basophilic cells. Acidophilic cells can be further distinguished by differential histochemical stains into type A acidophil and Type B acidophil. Type A acidophil secretes somatotropin hormone (STH) or growth hormone and type B acidophil secretes lactogenic/luteotropic hormone (LTH). Similarly basophils can be differentiated into beta basophils, responsible for the secretion of thyrotropic hormone (TSH) and adrenocorticotrophic hormone (ACTH) and Delta basophils which elaborate gonadotropins (FSH, LH and ICSH).

PARS INTERMEDIA

The pars distalis is separated from the neurohypophysis by a cleft lined on the juxtaneural side by a multilayered epithelium of basophilic cells comprising the pars intermedia. The cells here are low columnar in shape and are basophilic in their staining properties. The cells are arranged in the form of vesicles which are lined by low columnar cells and contain colloid in their cytoplasm. The only hormone secreted by the pars intermedia is the *melanocyte stimulating hormone*.

PARS NERVOSA

Pars nervosa consists of terminal portions of axons of extrinsic secretory neurons (supraoptic and paraventricular nuclei) whose cell bodies are located in the hypothalamus and an intrinsic population of modified neuroglial cells called the *pituicytes*. These cells are highly variable in size, shape and have cytoplasmic processes. Throughout the neurohypophysis are spherical masses that stain deeply with chrome-alum haematoxylin stain and are called *Herring bodies*. These are believed to be local accumulations of neurosecretory material in the axoplasm of the *hypothalamo-hypophyseal tract*, to be discharged into the sinusoids present therein. Hormones secreted by pars nervosa include *oxytocin, and antidiuretic hormone vasopressin*.

BLOOD SUPPLY OF HYPOPHYSIS

The blood supply of hypophysis is related to the secretory activity of the gland. Two *inferior hypophyseal arteries* from cavernous part of internal carotid supply the posterior lobe and to a lesser extent anterior lobe of the gland. Many *superior hypophyseal arteries* arise from internal carotid and posterior communicating branch of circle of Willis and supply capillaries to median eminence of hypothalamus and base of pituitary. The blood from these regions is collected by long and short portal veins which open into a second set of sinusoidal capillaries in the anterior lobe of hypophysis. The veins from here drain into cavernous sinus. This type of circulation is called *hypothalamo-hypophyseal portal circulation*.

The functional aspects of hypophysis cerebri are given in Table 18.1.

Applied Aspect

- *Gigantism:* Excess of growth hormone of pituitary before puberty causes person to be very tall, i.e. gigantism.

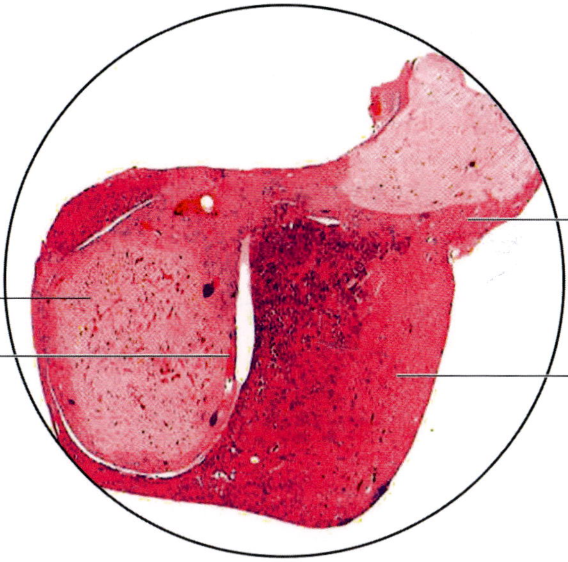

Endocrine Glands

PHOTOMICROGRAPH

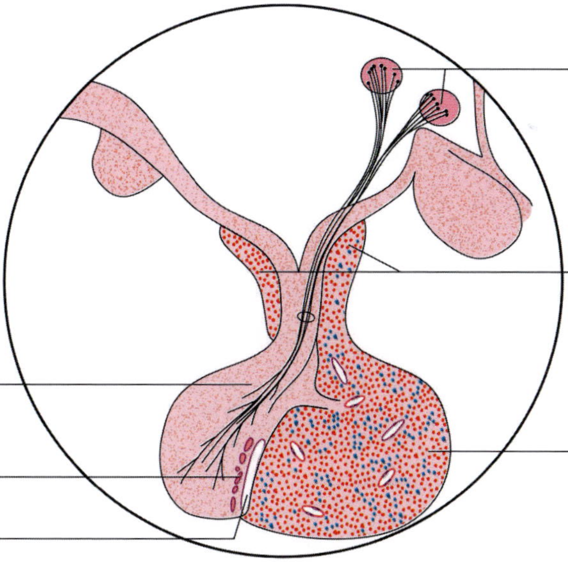

Labels: Pars nervosa, Pars intermedia, Pars tuberalis, Pars anterior

FIGURE

Labels: Supraoptic and paraventricular nuclei, Pars tuberalis, Pars anterior, Pars nervosa with axons, Pars intermedia, Cleft

FACTS TO REMEMBER
1. Pars anterior with lots of cells
2. Pars intermedia
3. Pars nervosa with nerve fibres

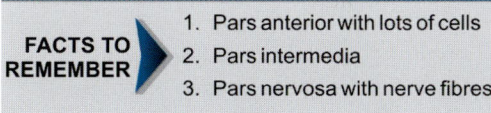

Fig. 18.1: *Hypophysis cerebri. Stain: Haematoxylin-eosin, 20X*

TABLE 18.1: Functional aspects of the hypophysis cerebri

Cell type	Releasing hormone	Hormone secreted	Physiological actions
ADENOHYPOPHYSIS			
ACIDOPHIL:			
Somatotrope	Somatotropin releasing hormone	Somatotropin	Stimulates growth of long bones, uptake of amino acids and protein synthesis
Mammotroph	Prolactin releasing hormone	Prolactin	Stimulates secretion of milk
BASOPHIL:			
Thyrotrope	Thyrotropin releasing hormone	Thyrotropin	Stimulates thyroid hormone synthesis and its release
Corticotrope	Corticotropin releasing hormone	Corticotropin	Stimulates release of hormone of adrenal cortex
Gonadotrope	Gonadotropin releasing hormone	Follicle stimulating hormone (FSH) and Luteinizing hormone (LH)	Stimulates development of ovarian follicles in females and spermatogenesis in males
PARS INTERMEDIA			
Cells	Melanocyte stimulating hormone in amphibians and fishes. Pars intermedia is not developed in human	—	Increase pigmentation of skin
NEUROHYPOPHYSIS			
Cells		Vasopressin or antidiuretic hormone	Increase permeability of collecting ducts and reabsorbs water
Cells		Oxytocin	Increases contraction of smooth muscle fibres of uterus during parturition. During suckling also, this hormone causes contraction of myoepithelial cells around secretory acini of mammary gland

Endocrine Glands

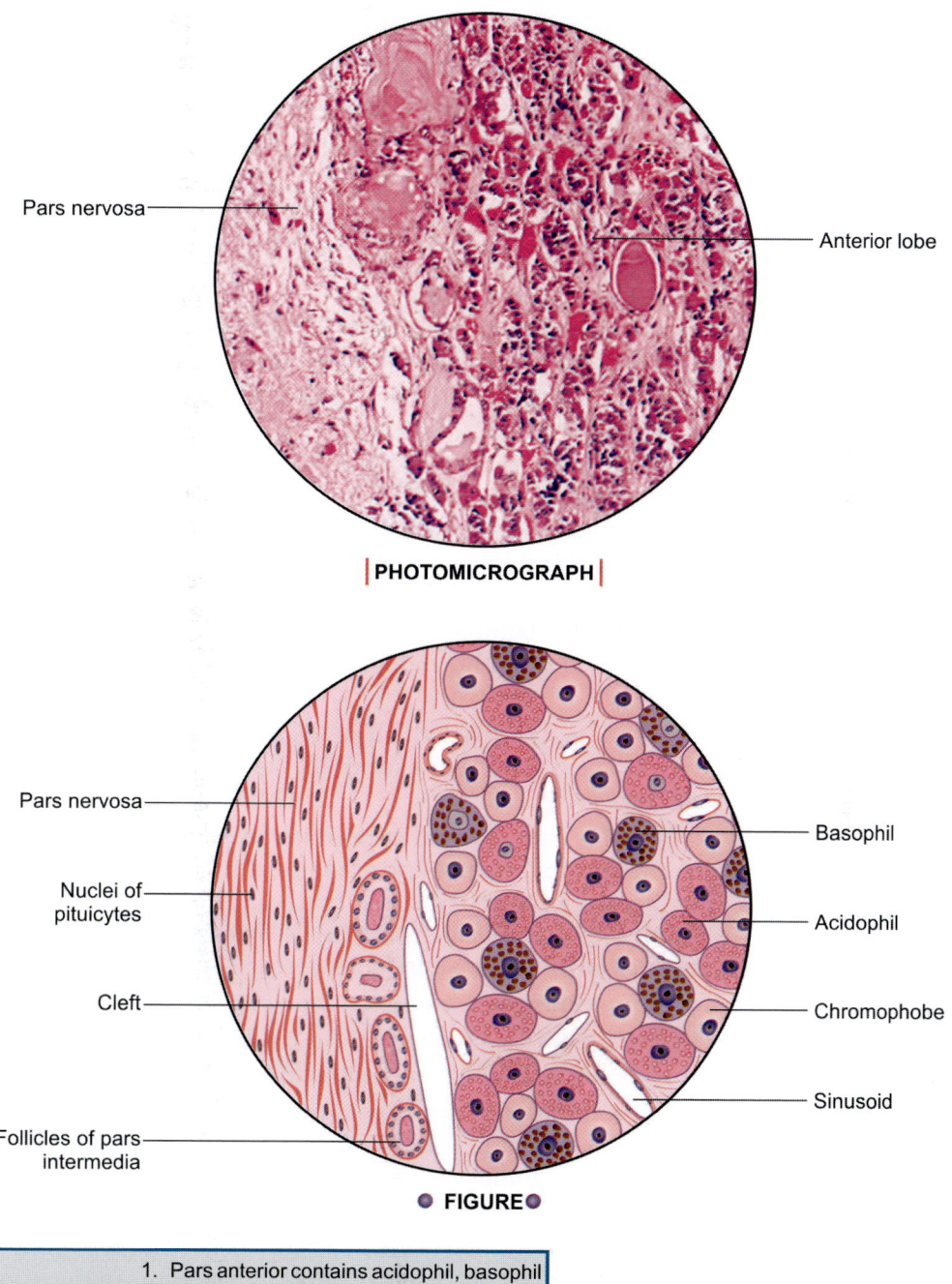

Fig. 18.2: *Hypophysis cerebri. Stain: Haematoxylin-eosin, 400X*

- *Acromegaly:* If the same occurs after puberty, the condition is called acromegaly with large jaw, large hands and large feet.

THYROID GLAND

Thyroid gland is responsible for maintaining the *basal metabolic rate* of the body by means of tetraiodothyronine (thyroxine) and tri-iodothyronine elaborated by the follicular cells. Another smaller number of cells called the *parafollicular cells* lower the calcium in the blood by means of *thyrocalcitonin*.

Thyroid gland is covered by the false capsule derived from pretracheal fascia. Its true capsule is comprised of collagen fibres. This capsule sends connective tissue septa into the gland to form lobes and lobules. These septa provide support to the abundant fenestrated capillaries present in the gland.

The structural and functional unit of thyroid gland is a *follicle*. Each follicle is an oval or round space lined by single layer of epithelial cells. The epithelial cells vary in size according to activity of the gland. The epithelium is cuboidal in normal functioning area, columnar in hyperactive stage and low cuboidal in resting phase. Different areas of gland show variance in height of cells (Fig. 18.3).

The epithelial cells rest on a basal lamina. The sparse connective tissue is rich in capillaries of blood and lymph, as thyroid hormones are absorbed both by blood and lymph capillaries.

The lumen of the follicles contains colloid which represents the stored product of the secretory activity of the gland and takes up acidophilic stain. Its main constituents are *thyroglobulin* and *iodothyroglobulin*.

In addition to the follicular cells, another smaller population of cells are seen. These are lighter in colour, bigger in size and are present amongst the follicular epithelium, situated between the basement membrane and the epithelial cells or between the follicles. These cells are termed as *parafollicular* or *'C' cells*. These secrete a hormone named **thyrocalcitonin** or **calcitonin** responsible for lowering blood calcium level.

Synthesis and release of thyroid hormones:

i. Iodide circulating in blood is selectively taken up by the follicular cells. Iodine is liberated from iodide by peroxidase which enters the lumen of follicle.

ii. Follicular cells synthesise protein molecules from amino acids especially tyrosine. Carbohydrate is added to this protein molecule forming thyroglobulin which is also pushed into the lumen of the follicle.

iii. Iodine already present in the lumen combines with the tyrosine radicle of thyroglobulin to form mono and di-iodotyrosine which further combine to generate tri-iodothyronine and tetra-iodothyronine (thyroxine). All this occurs in the lumen.

iv. According to the requirements of the body, iodothyroglobulin is taken by the follicular cells from the lumen of the follicle. It is acted upon by enzymes present in these cells and tri- and tetra-iodothyronine are released from the basal aspects of follicular cells.

Tri-iodothyronine is quick and short lasting in action, whereas thyroxine is slower and long lasting in its effects on the various tissues of the body.

Endocrine Glands

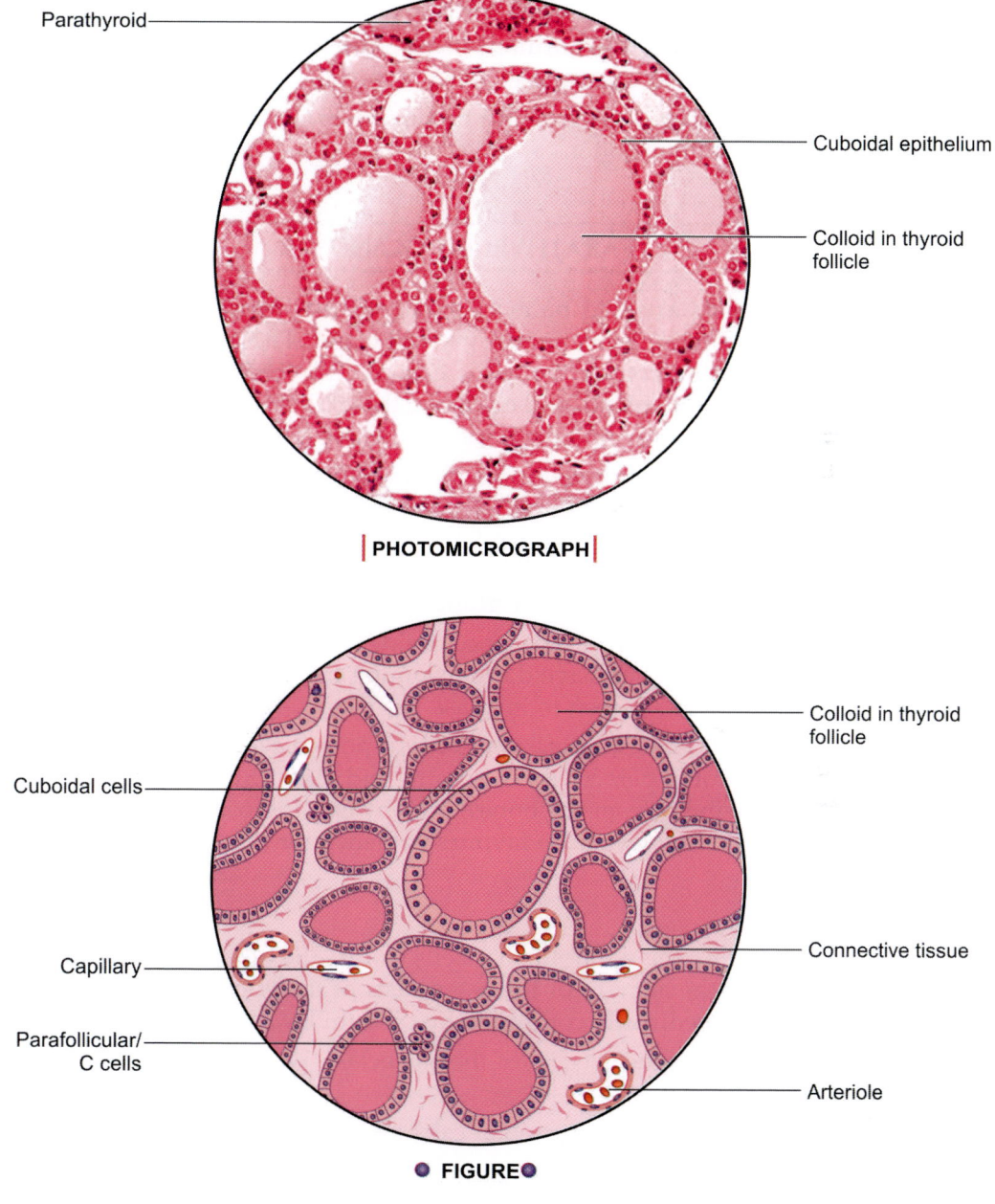

FACTS TO REMEMBER	1. Thyroid follicles lined by cuboidal to columnar cells containing colloid 2. Scanty connective tissue with capillaries 3. C cells in connective tissue or within the follicles

Fig. 18.3: *Thyroid gland. Stain: Haematoxylin-eosin, 100X*

Applied Aspect
- *Myxoedema:* Insufficient thyroid hormone in newborn and children leads to *cretinism*, while in adults, it leads to *myxoedema*.
- *Exophthalmic goiter:* Excessive thyroid hormone causes protrusion of the eyeball and is known as exophthalmic goiter.

PARATHYROID GLAND

The parathyroid glands are two pairs of small, yellow brown bodies intimately connected with the posterior aspect of the thyroid gland. These glands are separated from the thyroid by a thin connective tissue capsule. The capsular connective tissue extends into the parathyroid gland, and it is along these trabeculae that larger branches of blood vessels, nerves and lymphatics enter and leave (Fig. 18.4).

The reticular tissue forms framework of the parathyroid gland. The parenchyma consists of *principal cells* and *oxyphilic cells*. Principal cells or chief cells are arranged in sheets with numerous sinusoids and capillaries traversing them. The principal cells are polygonal or round with a centrally placed vesicular nuclei and a pale staining acidophilic cytoplasm. These cells show granules with special stains.

Oxyphilic cells are a few in number, occur singly or in small groups. These are larger than principal cells. They have darkly staining nuclei and strongly acidophilic cytoplasm. Oxyphilic cells are seen to increase with age.

The principal or chief cells secrete *parathormone* responsible for maintaining the blood calcium level. In cases of hyperactivity of parathyroid gland, blood calcium level gets elevated by withdrawing it from the bones, thereby causing osteoporosis or fracture of bones. Increased calcium level also favours tendency for renal stone formation.

Functional Aspect
- Calcitonin secreted by the parafollicular cells lowers the blood calcium levels. It is done by increasing the activity of the osteoclasts of the bones. The secretion and release of calcitonin is directly controlled by calcium levels of the blood.
- Parathormone increases the activity of the osteoclasts which releases calcium from the bones.
- Parathormone facilitates reabsorption of calcium from distal convoluted tubules. It also promotes the kidneys to form the hormone, calcitriol which enhances absorption of calcium from intestine. The control of parathormone is dependent on blood calcium levels.

Applied Aspect
- *Hypoparathyroidism:* Lack of parathormone causes tetany, i.e. twitchings and spasms of the hand.
- *Hyperparathyroidism:* Excess parathormone causes repeated kidney stones and repeated fracture of the bones.

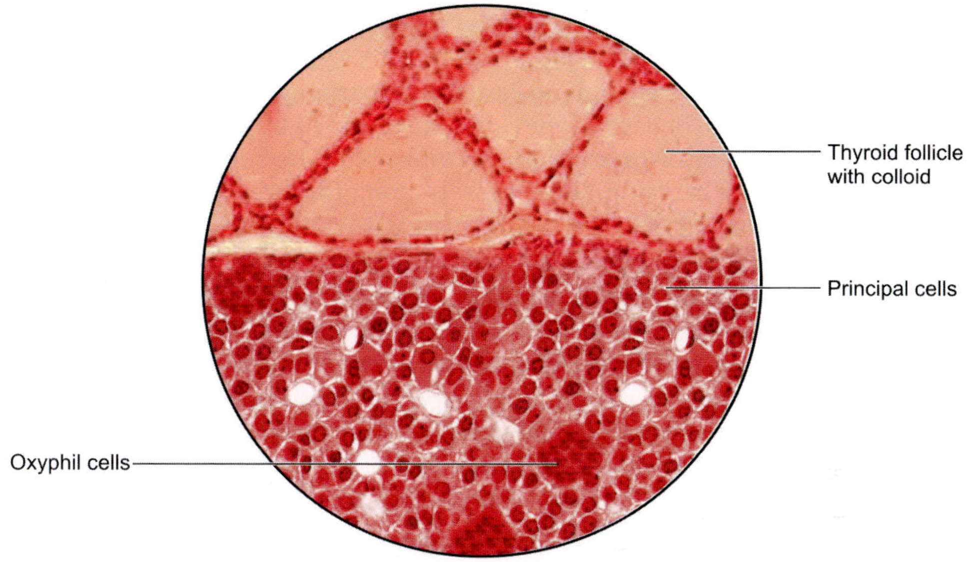

Endocrine Glands

PHOTOMICROGRAPH

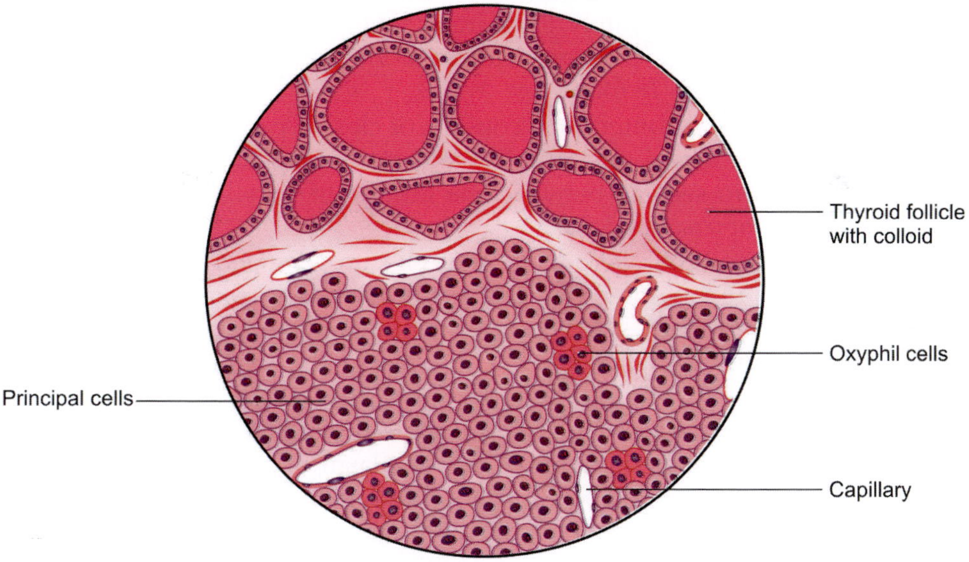

- Thyroid follicle with colloid
- Principal cells
- Oxyphil cells

FIGURE

- Thyroid follicle with colloid
- Oxyphil cells
- Principal cells
- Capillary

FACTS TO REMEMBER
1. Principal cells
2. Oxyphil cells
3. Capsule separating the parathyroid from thyroid tissue

Fig. 18.4: *Parathyroid gland. Stain: Haematoxylin-eosin, 100X*

SUPRARENAL OR ADRENAL GLAND

The paired suprarenal or adrenal glands are roughly triangular or semilunar flattened glands, at the cranial pole of each kidney. It is surrounded by a thick capsule in which are branches of main vessels, nerves and lymphatics. The septa penetrate from the capsule into the interior carrying blood vessels along them.

Each gland is comprised of outer yellow cortex surrounding the inner dark brown medulla. Medulla appears to be the "filling" of a sandwich formed by the cortex.

Cortex develops from the *coelomic epithelium* (mesoderm) whereas medulla originates from *neural crest cells* (ectoderm). Cells of medulla are comparable to sympathetic ganglion cells as it is supplied by preganglionic sympathetic fibres.

Blood supply: Suprarenal is supplied by superior, middle and inferior suprarenal arteries. These form a plexus in its capsule. Cortical capillaries supply cells of the cortex before reaching the sinusoids of medulla. The medullary vessels pass through the cortex to reach the medulla. Thus the sinusoids of medulla receive blood both from cortex and medulla (Fig. 18.5).

CORTEX

The cortex shows three zones, outermost is the *zona glomerulosa*, a thick middle layer is the *zona fasciculata*, and moderately thick inner layer is the *zona reticularis* which is continuous with the medulla. The transition from one zone to the other is gradual and is not well demarcated (Fig. 18.6).

The zona glomerulosa or outer zone consists of closely packed groups and **arches of columnar cells**. The nuclei are spherical and stain deeply. The cytoplasm shows vacuoles. Sinusoids are seen in between the groups of cells. The cells of the zona glomerulosa secrete *mineralocorticoids*.

In the middle zone or zona fasciculata the cells are arranged in vertical columns, with large number of vacuoles in their cytoplasm. These cells are also called **spongiocytes**. The cytoplasm is slightly basophilic and nuclei are central. The sinusoids follow a vertical course in this zone. The cells of the zona fasciculata secrete *glucocorticoids*.

In the inner zone or zona reticularis, the regular parallel arrangement of cords give way to an anastomosing network. The cytoplasm of cells contains fewer lipid droplets and is less vacuolated. Some of the cells contain yellow pigment. The intervening capillaries are irregularly arranged. These cells secrete *sex hormones* (Fig. 18.7).

Another view about the functions of the cortex is that zona glomerulosa is the cell producing zone; zona fasciculata the hormone-producing zone and the zona reticularis the graveyard of the cells.

MEDULLA

Medulla is composed of chromaffin cells or pheochromocytes. These are arranged in irregular rounded groups or short cords isolated by fine septa. These are surrounded by blood capillaries and venules. The cytoplasm of the cells is basophilic. When the tissue is fixed in solution containing potassium bichromate, these cells are seen to be

Endocrine Glands

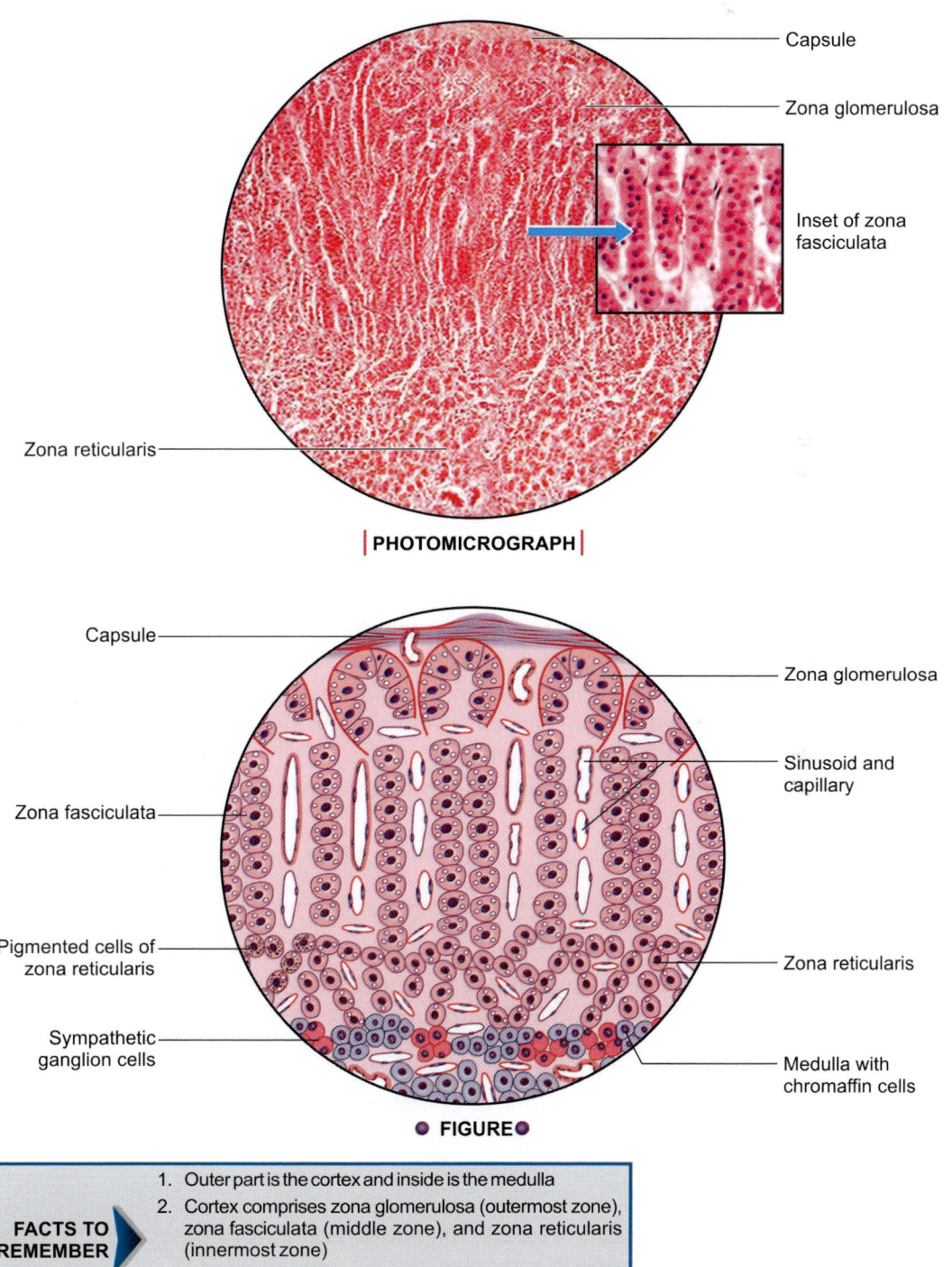

FACTS TO REMEMBER
1. Outer part is the cortex and inside is the medulla
2. Cortex comprises zona glomerulosa (outermost zone), zona fasciculata (middle zone), and zona reticularis (innermost zone)
3. Medulla comprises chromaffin cells and sympathetic ganglion cells

Fig. 18.5: *Suprarenal gland. Stain: Haematoxylin-eosin, 400X*

filled with fine brown granules and this is described as the *chromaffin reaction*. These granules are precursors of the hormone *epinephrine* or *adrenaline* and *norepinephrine* or *noradrenaline*. Norepinephrine producing cells are relatively more densely granulated. Interspersed between these cells are characteristic autonomic ganglion cells which are seen singly or in groups of two to four. The ganglion cells are large with big vesicular nuclei and nucleoli (Fig. 18.7).

Functional Aspect

- The cells of zona glomerulosa secrete mineralo-corticoids, the most active being aldosterone. Aldosterone increases reabsorption of sodium from distal convoluted tubules of kidneys.
- Zona fasciculata secretes glucocorticoids, the important being ones being cortisone and cortisol. These are for combating the stress, by increasing blood glucose levels.
- Zona reticularis secrete minimal levels of sex steroids.
- The adrenal medulla is under the direct control of hypothalamus. During acute stress the medullary cells produce increased amounts of epinephrine and norepinephrine to help fright, flight or fight reactions.

Applied Aspect

- **Cushing's syndrome:** Hyperactivity of suprarenal manifests as Cushing's syndrome.
- **Addison's disease:** Hypofunction of this gland leads to Addison's disease.
- **Adrenal medulla** secretes adrenaline and noradrenaline. Adrenaline stimulates cardiorespiratory system, increases blood sugar and general metabolism. Noradrenaline increase blood pressure.
- During stress, adrenal medulla secretes adrenaline and noradrenaline to combat the emergency.
- Tumour of adrenal medulla is called *pheochromocytoma*.

PINEAL GLAND

The pineal gland is a little cone shaped body about 1 cm in length. It originates from and remains connected to third ventricle and lies dorsal to the midbrain. It contains two types of cells. The neuroectodermal cells give rise to parenchymal cells and are termed *pinealocytes*. The *mesenchymal cells* give rise to connective tissue of capsule of the gland and the incomplete partitions of connective tissue more or less divide the gland into lobules. Pineal gland secretes *serotonin* and *melatonin*.

PANCREAS

Islets of Langerhans of pancreas constitute the **endocrine** part of the gland and have been described with the pancreas gland.

TESTIS AND OVARY

The hormones produced by these glands have been described with the respective reproductive systems.

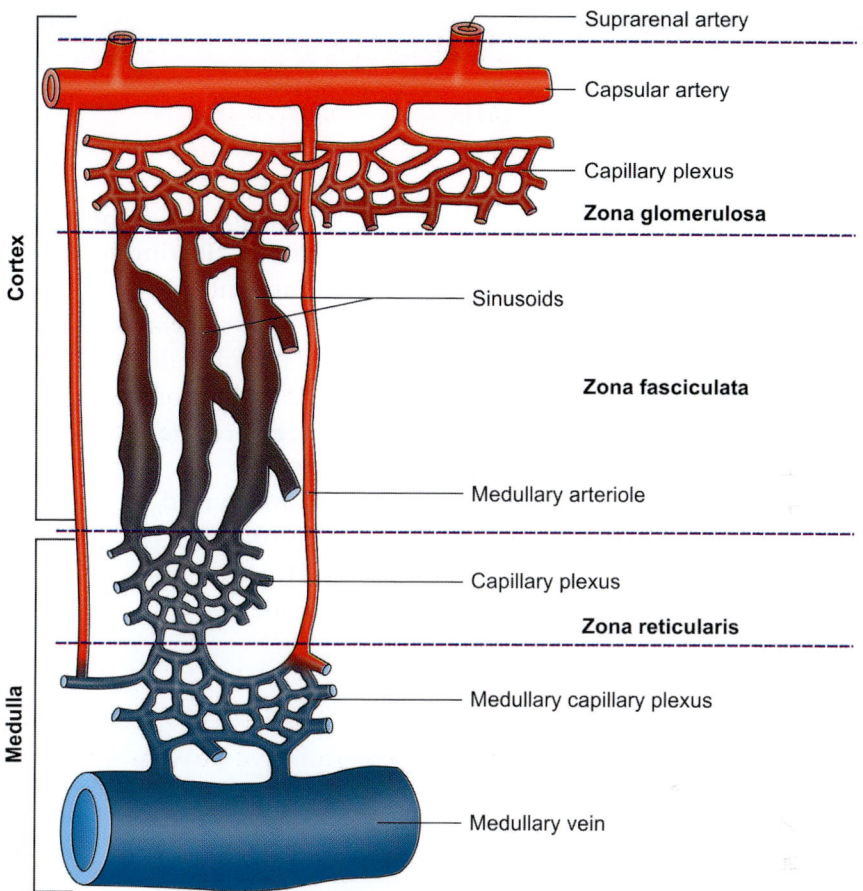

Fig. 18.6: *Suprarenal gland. Stain: Haematoxylin-eosin, 200X*

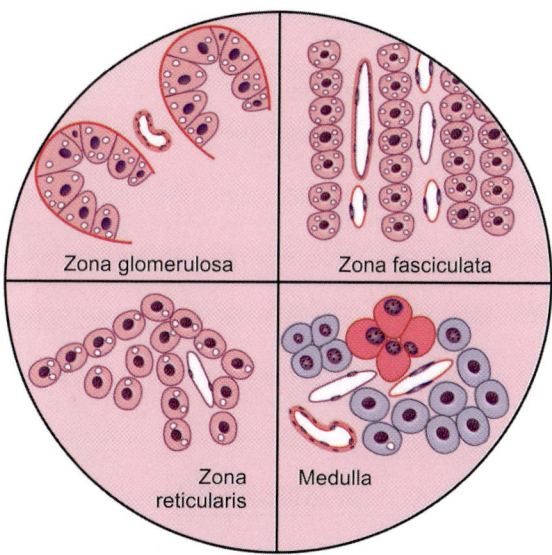

Fig. 18.7: *Suprarenal gland. Stain: Haematoxylin-eosin, 400X*

MULTIPLE CHOICE QUESTIONS

1. **Which gland has secretory cells present in the form of follicles?**
   a. Parathyroid
   b. Thyroid
   c. Suprarenal
   d. Hypophysis cerebri
2. **Adenohypophysis contains all the following types of cells *except*:**
   a. Chromophobes
   b. Acidophils
   c. Basophils
   d. Pituicytes
3. **Acidophils are one of the following types of cells:**
   a. Corticotrophs
   b. Thyrotrophs
   c. Somatotrophs
   d. Gonadotrophs
4. **Which part of hypophysis cerebri contains Herring bodies?**
   a. Pars anterior
   b. Pars posterior
   c. Pars tuberalis
   d. Pars intermedia
5. **Where are the parafollicular cells present:**
   a. Parathyroid
   b. Suprarenal
   c. Thyroid
   d. Pancreas

ANSWERS

1. b   2. d   3. c   4. b
5. c

Organs of Special Senses 19

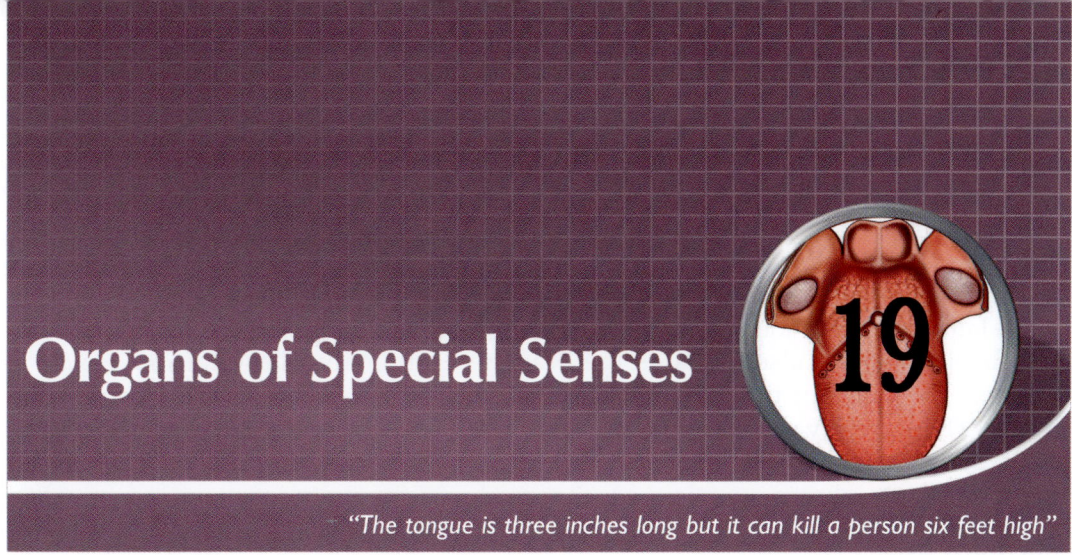

"The tongue is three inches long but it can kill a person six feet high"

Following are the organs of special senses:
1. Olfactory epithelium for sense of smell.
2. Taste buds of tongue for sense of taste (included with tongue).
3. Retina of the eye for sense of sight (included with eyeball).
4. Internal ear for sense of hearing and balance.
5. Skin for sense of touch (*see* Chapter 10).

OLFACTORY EPITHELIUM

The receptors of the sense of smell are located in the olfactory epithelium. The olfactory area extends from the middle of the roof of the nasal cavity, about 8 to 10 mm inferiorly on each side of the septum and on the upper surface of the superior nasal concha.

The epithelium is of tall *pseudostratified columnar* variety. It consists of three types—*basal cells, supporting or sustentacular cells* and *olfactory cells* (Fig. 19.1).

BASAL CELLS

These cells form the deepest layer of the epithelium. They are triangular in shape with dark nuclei and branching processes. They have capability of regeneration.

SUPPORTING OR SUSTENTACULAR CELLS

These are tall cells, narrow at the basal end and wider at the free end. The nucleus is almost in the centre with light staining chromatin and nucleolus. A few gaps are present in between these cells through which olfactory cell processes pass.

OLFACTORY CELLS

These cells are evenly distributed between the supporting cells and are called the *bipolar neurons*. The nuclei of these cells lie towards the basement membrane between the basal cells and sustentacular cells. The apical portion of the bipolar cells is a modified dendron which passes through the gap between the sustentacular cells and reaches the surface of the epithelium. The proximal end tapers into a thin smooth filament, which is the axon, a fibre of the olfactory nerve. It passes into the connective tissue and with similar fibres forms small nerve bundles. Radiating from its apical surface are six to eight olfactory cilia which are non-motile. These cilia are the components of the sense organ and are stimulated by contact with odorous substances.

The **lamina propria** contains a rich plexus of blood capillaries, large veins, lymphatics and elastic fibres. It also contains the branched tubuloalveolar olfactory *glands of Bowman*. The ducts of the glands assume a perpendicular course and open on the surface. The secretory part has mucous acini. The glands secrete a thin mucus secretion which bathes the cilia. The gases first get dissolved in this fluid before they can be smelt.

Functional Aspect

The odorous molecules are dissolved in the watery secretion of the glands. These molecules bind to the receptor proteins on the cilia of olfactory cells or bipolar neurons. The non-myelinated afferent axons from olfactory cells join to form olfactory rootlets in the lamina propria. These rootlets pass through cribriform plate of ethmoid to the **olfactory bulb** of the brain and to end in the *uncus*.

Applied Aspect

Sinusitis: Nasal infection spreads to various air sinuses causing their inflammation. It may be due to allergy.

TASTE BUDS OF TONGUE

TONGUE

The tongue is a muscular organ and its functions are as follows.
  i. To move the bolus of food from side to side.
 ii. To help in articulation of speech.
iii. To perceive the taste of various foodstuffs through the taste buds.

The tongue (Fig. 19.2) consists of interlacing bundles of striated muscles that run in different directions and cross one another. The musculature of the tongue is covered by *stratified squamous non-keratinised epithelium*. The epithelium on the ventral surface is thinner as compared to the epithelium on the dorsal surface which is much thicker.

In the anterior two-thirds on the dorsal surface of tongue, the underlying corium consists of collagen and elastic fibres which project upwards forming *papillae*; whereas in its posterior one-third or pharyngeal part, it presents only irregular bulges due to *lymphoid tissue*. The boundary between the two regions is inverted V-shaped. The principal gustatory region of the tongue is anterior to this line.

PAPILLAE

Three types of papillae are present: The *filiform*, the *fungiform* and the *circumvallate*.
  i. The *filiform papillae* are arranged in more or less distinct rows diverging to the right and left from the middle line.
 ii. The *fungiform papillae* are a few in number. These have short, slightly constricted stalks and flattened hemispherical upper surfaces. The lamina propria core forms

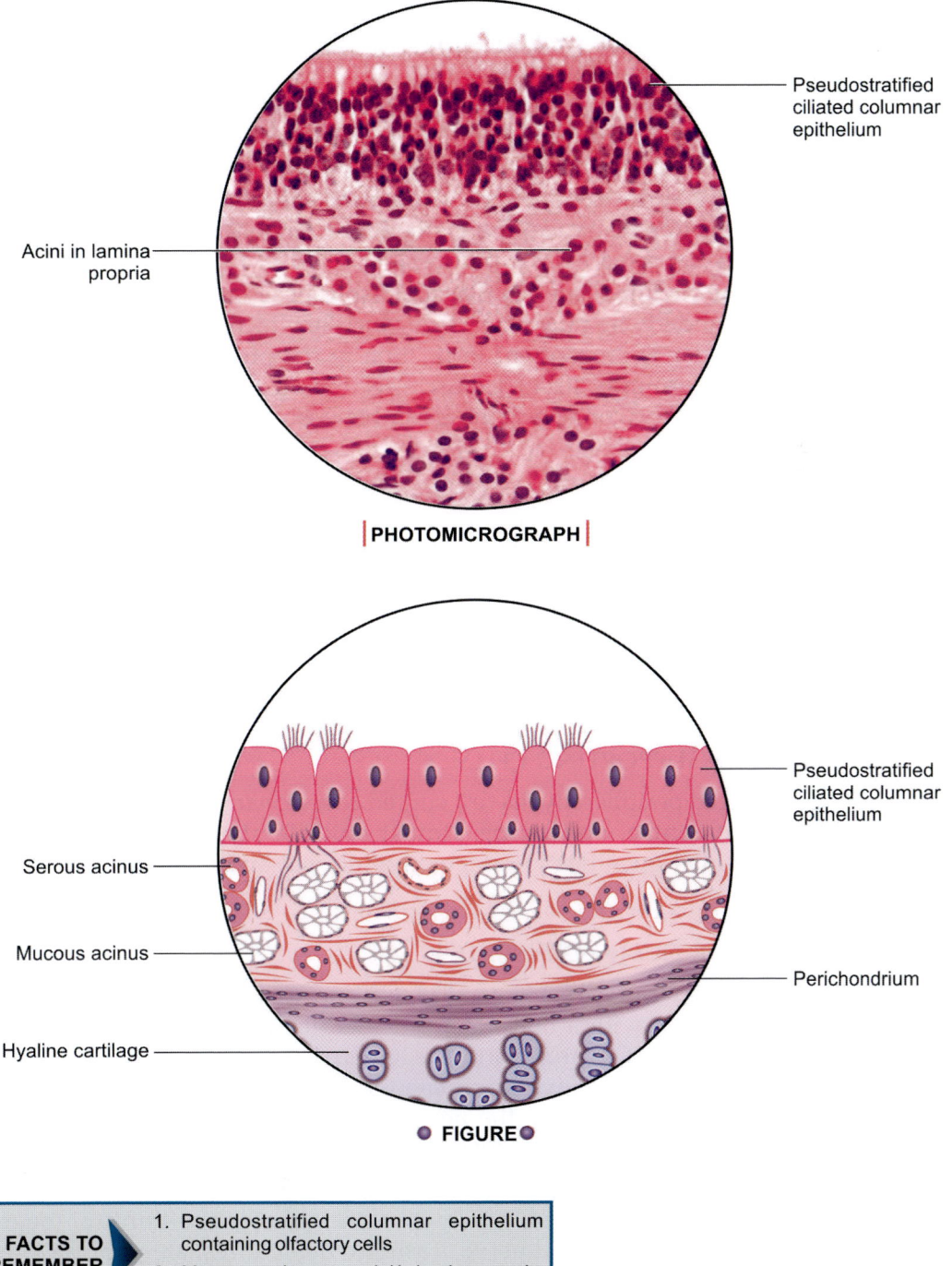

Fig. 19.1: *Olfactory mucous membrane. Stain: Haematoxylin-eosin, 400X*

secondary papillae that project into the recesses on the undersurface of the epithelium. On some of the fungiform papillae the epithelium associated with secondary papillae contains taste buds.

iii. The *circumvallate papillae* (Fig. 19.3) are bigger than the other two types of papillae and lie just anterior to the junction of the anterior two-thirds and the posterior one-third of the tongue. The papillae are surrounded by deep circular furrows and **do not** project above the surface epithelium. The **lamina propria** core forms secondary papillae only on the upper surface. The epithelium is smooth on the lateral surface of papillae, and contains many taste buds.

Connected with the circumvallate papillae are glands of serous type, whose bodies are embedded in the underlying muscular tissue, ducts of which open at the bottom of the furrow. Mucous glands are present in relation to the pharyngeal part, tip and margins. Deep to the corium is striated muscle seen in all planes, i.e. longitudinal, transverse and oblique. The connective tissue in between muscle fasciculi contains blood vessels and nerves.

TASTE BUDS

The taste buds are seen on the lateral sides of the circumvallate papillae; some are also seen on the fungiform papillae. These are also present on the posterior part of the tongue, on the soft palate, on the posterior surface of epiglottis and on the posterior wall of the pharynx. Taste buds are barrel-shaped structures, narrower at the ends and broader in the middle. Two types of cells are distinguished in relation to the taste buds, the *supporting* or *sustentacular cells* and *neuroepithelial* or *gustatory cells.*

SUSTENTACULAR OR SUPPORTING CELLS

These cells are arranged peripherally, have a curved course, narrow at each of its ends and broader in the centre, appearing almost spindle-shaped. At both ends the cells surround small openings known as the internal and external taste pores (Fig. 19.4).

NEUROEPITHELIAL OR GUSTATORY CELLS

These are distributed between the sustentacular cells and are long narrow cells having a slender rod-shaped form with a nucleus in the middle. On the free surface, these cells give rise to short hair which project into the lumen of the pit. The substances to be tasted first get dissolved in the saliva, stimulate the hair of neuroepithelial cells and then the impulse is conducted along the nerves. There are five fundamental taste sensations—sweet, bitter, sour, salty and umami. Last one is pleasant and gets triggered by amino acids, e.g. meat broth or old cheese (Fig. 19.5).

Pathway of taste: The taste is carried from most of the anterior two-thirds of tongue via chorda tympani, branch of facial nerve. Taste from circumvallate papillae lying anterior to sulcus terminalis and posterior one-third of tongue is carried by the glossopharyngeal nerve.

Taste from posterior most part of tongue and epiglottis is carried via vagus nerve. Fibres of all three nerves reach the nucleus of tractus solitarius in medulla oblongata for a relay. The relayed fibres cross mainly to the opposite side for another relay in one

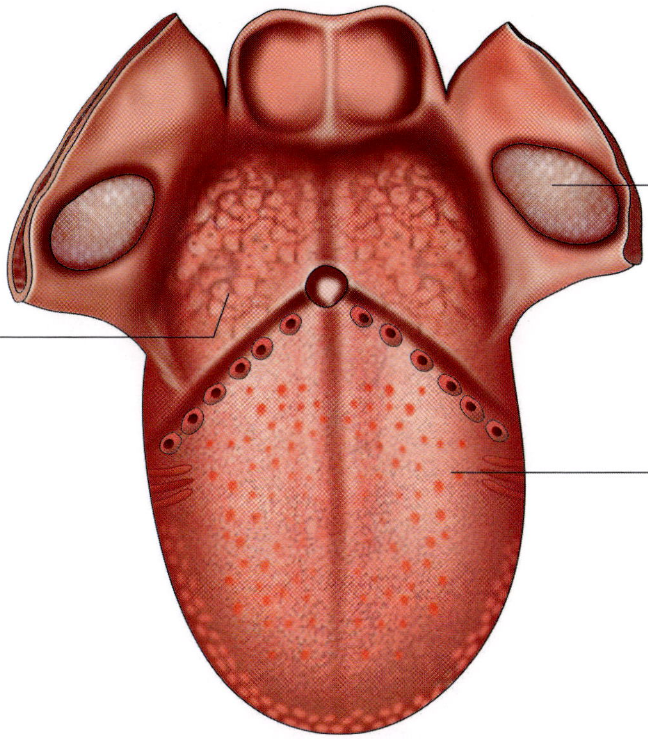

Organs of Special Senses

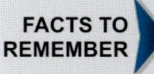

- Palatine tonsil
- Posterior 1/3rd of tongue
- Anterior 2/3rd of tongue

● FIGURE ●

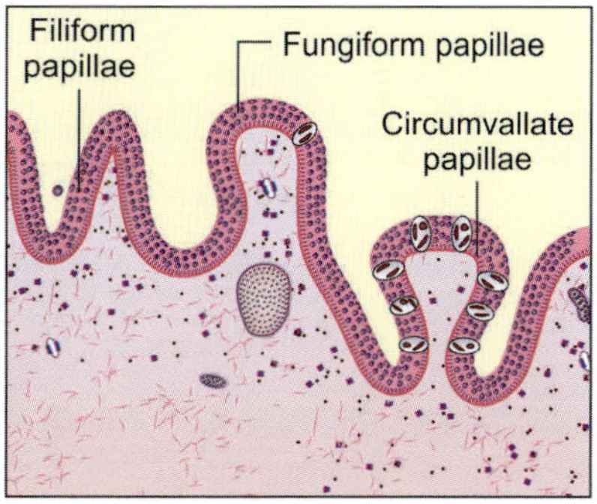

- Filiform papillae
- Fungiform papillae
- Circumvallate papillae

■ INSET ■

FACTS TO REMEMBER
1. Stratified squamous epithelium
2. Filiform, fungiform and circumvallate papillae with taste buds
3. Anterior 2/3rd contains papillae and posterior 1/3rd contains lymphoid follicles

Fig. 19.2: *Tongue with its parts. The inset shows the various types of papillae*

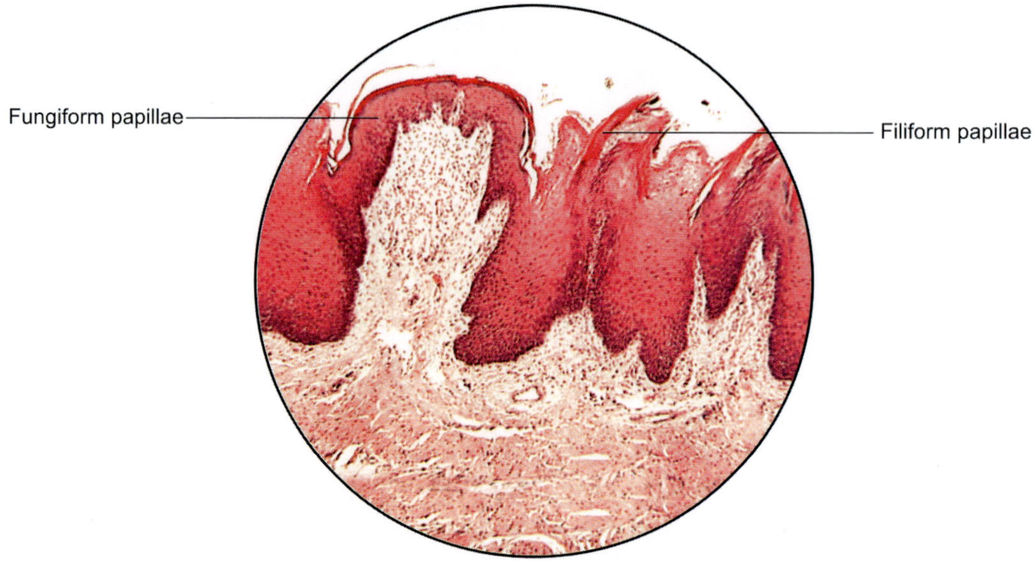

244 | Textbook of Histology

| PHOTOMICROGRAPH |

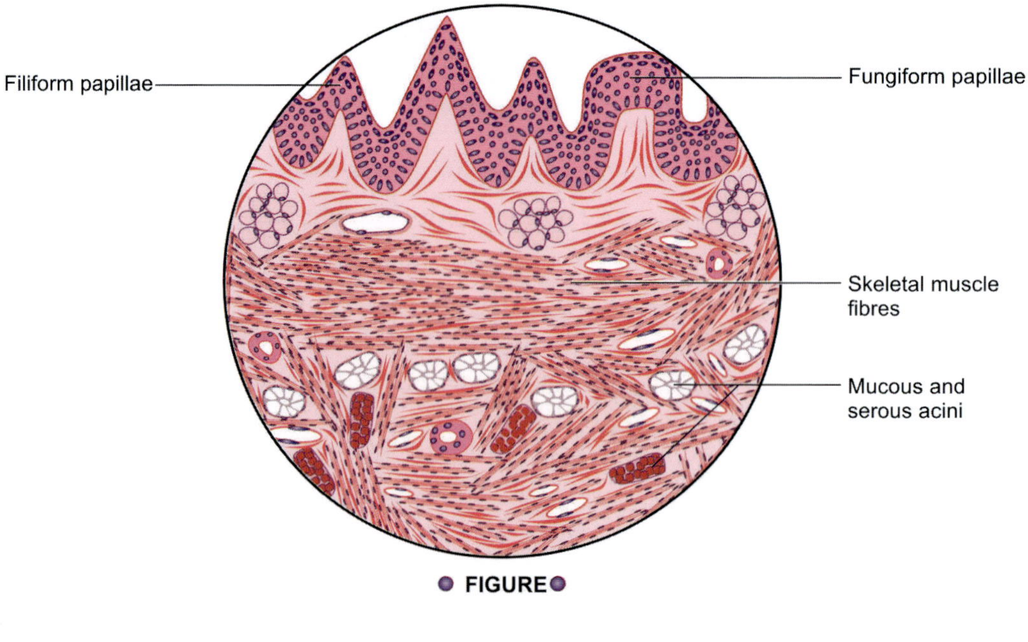

- Fungiform papillae
- Filiform papillae

• FIGURE •

- Filiform papillae
- Fungiform papillae
- Skeletal muscle fibres
- Mucous and serous acini

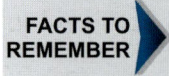
FACTS TO REMEMBER
1. Stratified squamous epithelium
2. Filiform and fungiform papillae seen
3. Striated muscle with mucous and serous acini

Fig. 19.3: *Anterior part of tongue with papillae. Stain: Haematoxylin-eosin, 100X*

Organs of Special Senses

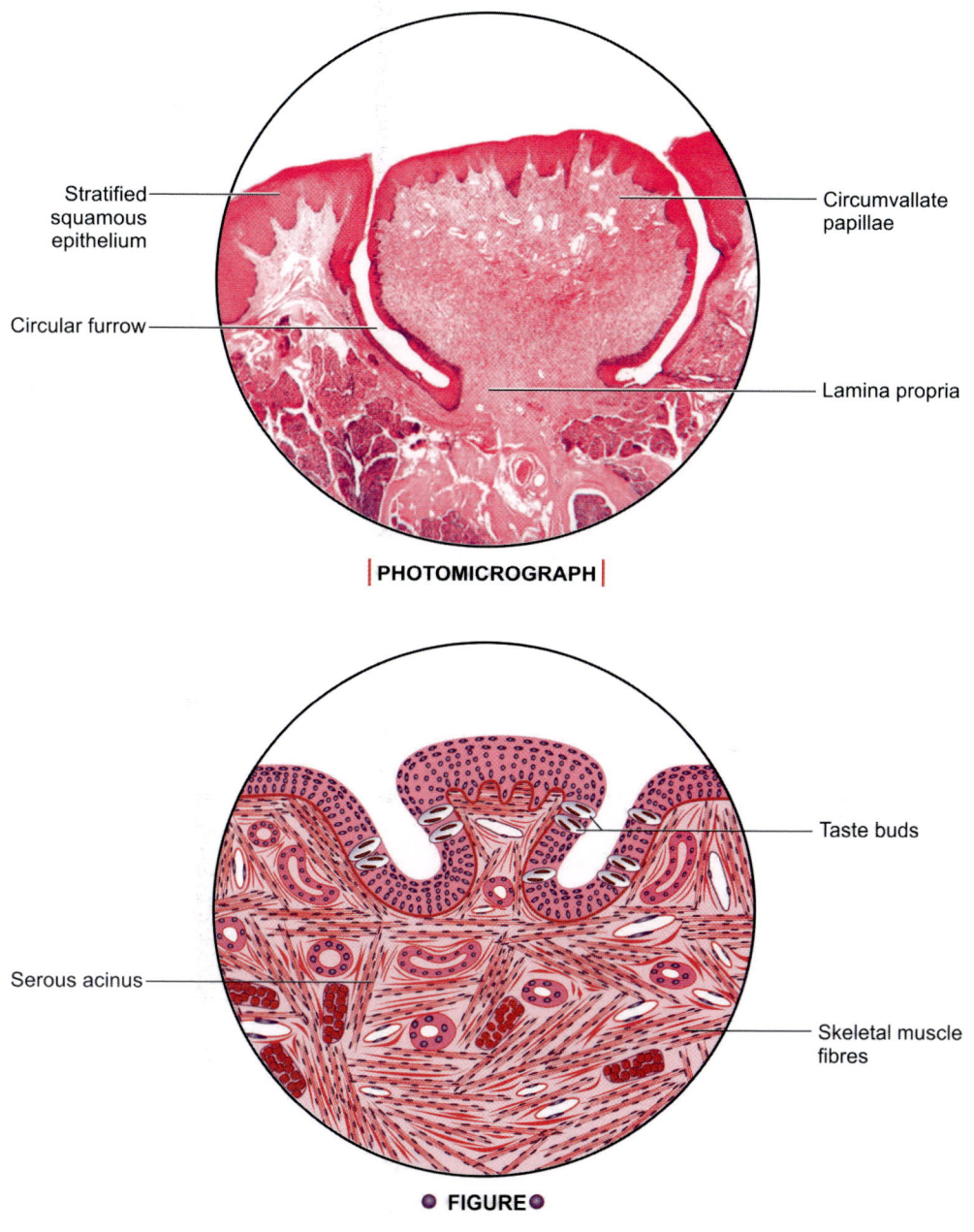

FACTS TO REMEMBER
1. The epithelium is stratified squamous in nature
2. The side walls of the papilla contain numerous taste buds
3. Taste buds comprise sustentacular and gustatory cells

Fig. 19.4: *Circumvallate papilla. Stain: Haematoxylin-eosin, 100X*

of the thalamic nuclei. The final relayed fibres reach the lowest part of the postcentral gyrus.

Applied Aspect

- *Anaemia:* Undersurface of tongue is used to judge anaemia and jaundice.
- *Carcinoma of tongue:* Starts as a nodule on the side of the tongue. It breaks down to form an irregular ulcer with ragged edges. Soon it spreads to deep cervical lymph nodes.

STRUCTURE OF THE EYEBALL

The wall of the eyeball is composed of three concentric layers, the outer protective corneo-scleral coat, the middle vascular coat, and the innermost layer which is the photosensitive retina. The corneo-scleral coat has a large posterior opaque segment, the sclera, and a smaller anterior transparent segment, the cornea.

The eyeball contains three chambers:
1. Anterior chamber lies between cornea, and iris (Fig. 19.6).
2. Posterior chamber lies between iris anteriorly and lens with its suspensory ligament posteriorly. The anterior and posterior chambers communicate through the pupil. Both these contain aqueous humor.
3. Vitreous chamber is large and lies between lens, with suspensory ligament anteriorly and retina posteriorly. Vitreous chamber lodges vitreous humor.

OUTER CORNEO-SCLERAL COAT

Cornea

Cornea consists of five layers:
1. Corneal epithelium which is continuous at its margins with the conjunctiva.
2. The anterior limiting membrane or Bowman's membrane.
3. Substantia propria.
4. The posterior limiting membrane or Descemet's membrane.
5. The posterior epithelium or mesenchymal epithelium of the anterior chamber.

Corneal Epithelium

It covers the front of the cornea and is stratified squamous, having four to five layers of cells. The deepest cells resting on the linear basement membrane are columnar with rod shaped nuclei. In the superficial layers, the cells become progressively squamous. They contain flattened nuclei which do not become keratinised. The epithelium of the cornea is extremely sensitive and contains numerous free nerve endings.

BOWMAN'S MEMBRANE

The corneal epithelium rests on a structureless homogeneous membrane called the Bowman's membrane. It is formed by collagen fibres of substantia propria.

Organs of Special Senses

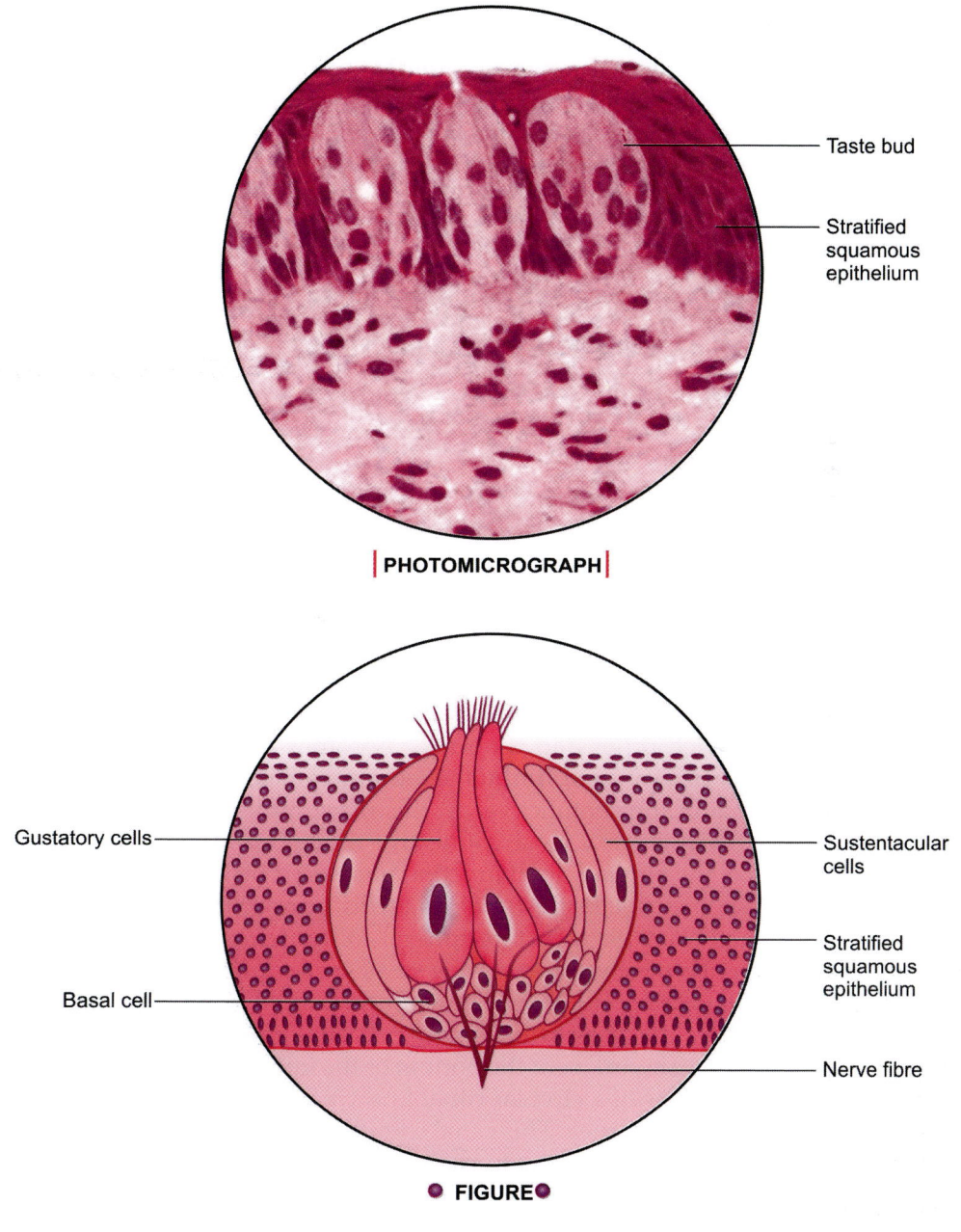

Fig. 19.5: *Taste bud. Stain: Haematoxylin-eosin, 400X*

FACTS TO REMEMBER
1. Central gustatory cells
2. Peripheral sustentacular cells
3. Basal cell at the base

SUBSTANTIA PROPRIA

It is a transparent connective tissue whose bundles form thin lamellae arranged in many layers. Between the lamellae there is a metachromatic protein polysaccharide ground substance, the components of which are *chondroitin sulphate* and *keratosulphate*. The cells of the stroma are long slender fibroblasts lodged in narrow clefts among parallel bundles of collagen fibres.

DESCEMET'S MEMBRANE

It is homogeneous membrane deep to the substantia propria.

POSTERIOR EPITHELIUM OR MESENCHYMAL EPITHELIUM

The inner surface of Descemet's membrane is covered by a layer of low cuboidal cells.

SCLERA

Sclera consists of white fibrous tissue, the fibres of which run in bundles, parallel to the surface, between which are a few elastic and reticular fibres. The cells of the sclera are elongated fibroblasts.

CORNEOSCLERAL JUNCTION

The boundary between the opaque sclera and the transparent cornea is an oblique line. The outer edge of the sclera overlaps slightly the border of the cornea. The collagenous bundles of the sclera continue directly into those of the cornea where they become parallel with each other and the tissue becomes homogeneous as well as transparent. At the marginal zone or **limbus** of the cornea there is a gradual transition of its epithelium to that of the conjunctiva. At this margin the Bowman's membrane ends and the subepithelial layer of loose connective tissue begins.

On its inner surface, the corneoscleral junction is marked by a shallow groove, the internal scleral furrow or sulcus. Its posterior lip forms a projecting ridge to which the ciliary body is fastened (Fig. 19.7). Just peripheral to the termination of Descemet's membrane is the trabecular meshwork enclosing small spaces known as *spaces of Fontana* which are lined by attenuated epithelium. These spaces communicate with the anterior chamber of the eye. There are also several small epithelial lined cavities, anterior and lateral to the trabecular meshwork near the bottom of the internal scleral furrow. These cavities are the cross-sections of a circular canal known as the *canal of Schlemm* which is parallel to the border of the cornea. This canal communicates with the venous system and is usually filled with clear **aqueous humor**.

MIDDLE VASCULAR COAT: CHOROID, CILIARY BODY AND IRIS

From without inwards, choroid consists of the following four layers:
1. *Suprachoroid or epichoroid layer:* It is made up of fine collagenous fibres with elastic fibres and pigment cells called the *chromatophores* (Figs 19.8 and 19.9).
2. *Vascular layer:* Contains large blood vessels. Between the vessels is fine connective tissue containing chromatophores.
3. *Choriocapillary layer:* Contains capillaries in a stroma of fine collagen and elastic fibres. These are the **widest capillaries in the body**. Through these capillaries the retina is constantly being nourished.

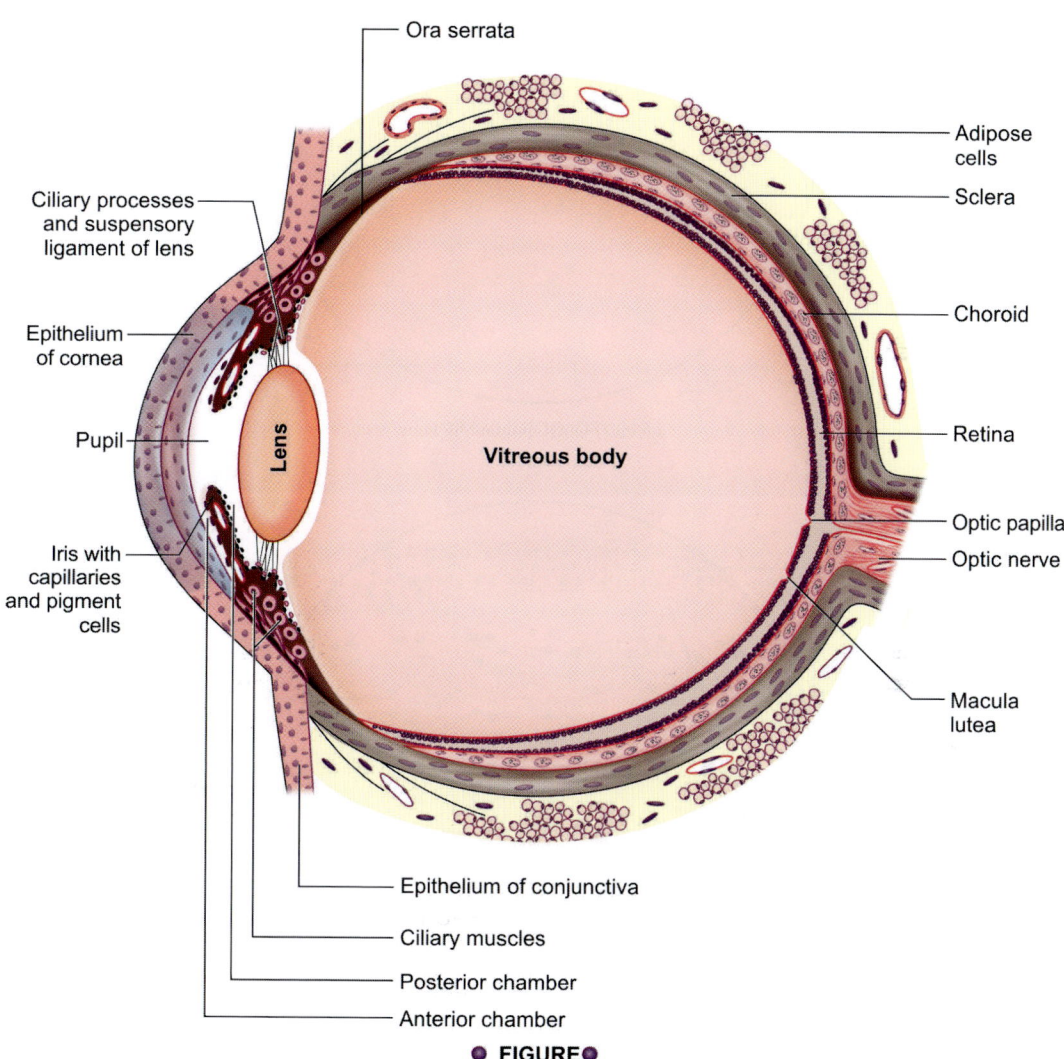

Fig. 19.6: *Structure of the eyeball*

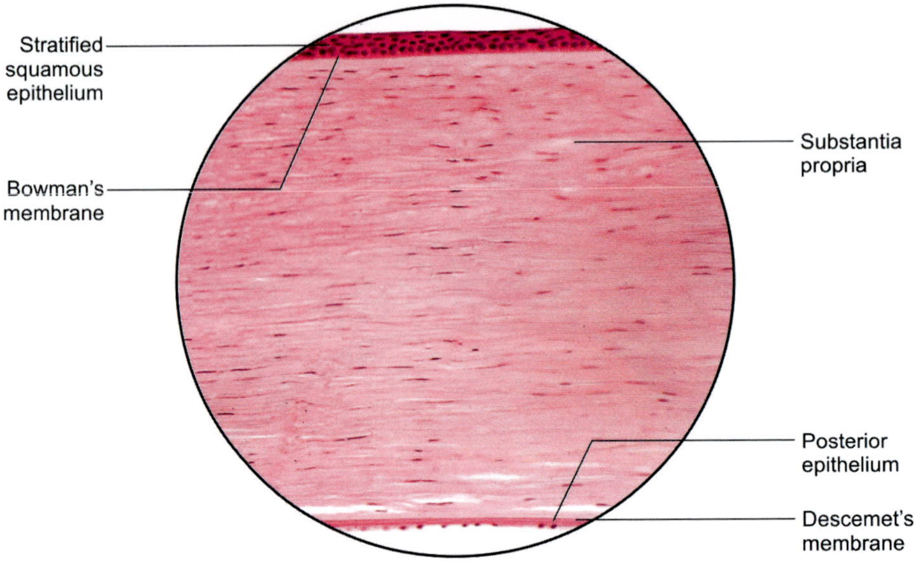

PHOTOMICROGRAPH

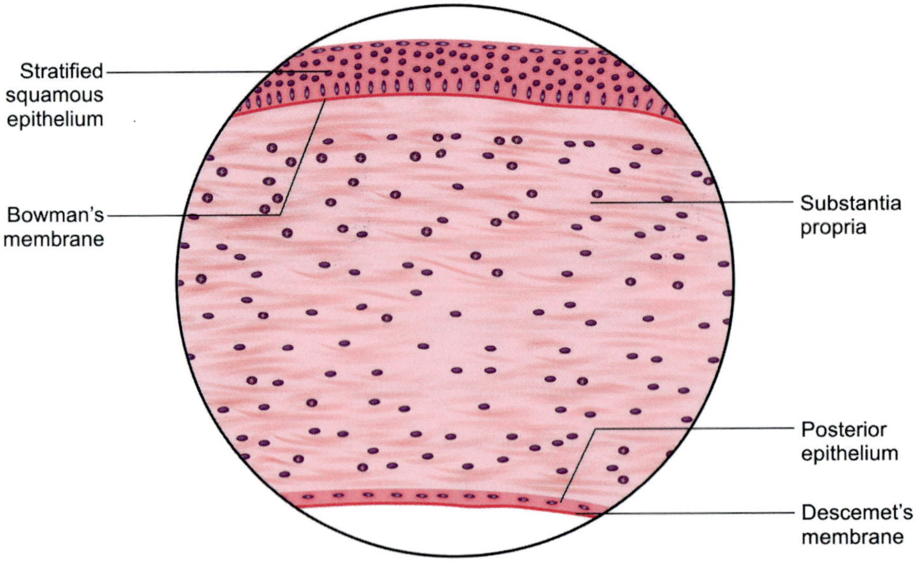

FIGURE

FACTS TO REMEMBER	1. Stratified squamous epithelium 2. Substantia propria is thick 3. Descemet's membrane next to posterior epithelium

Fig. 19.7: *Structure of cornea. Stain: Haematoxylin-eosin, 100X*

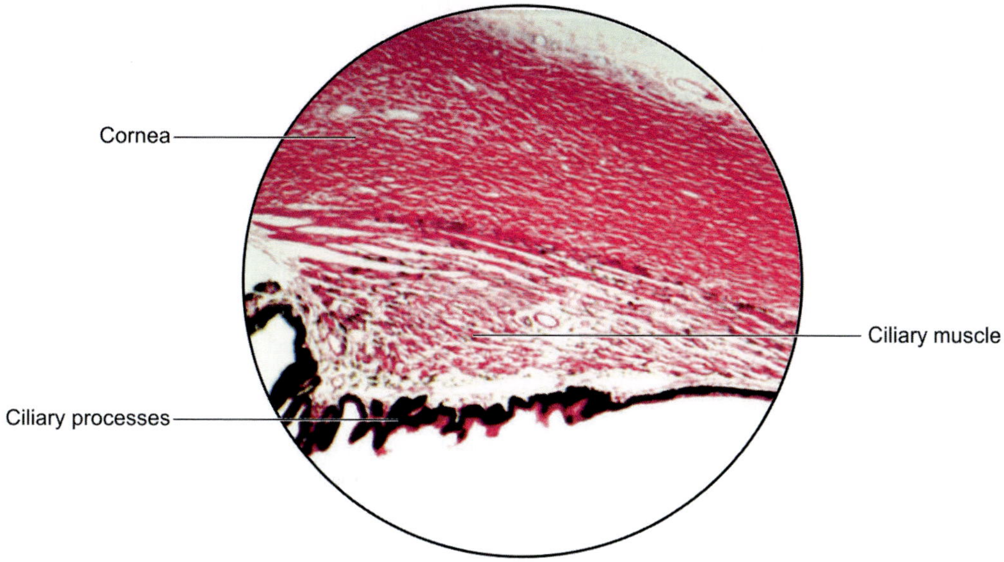

Organs of Special Senses

PHOTOMICROGRAPH

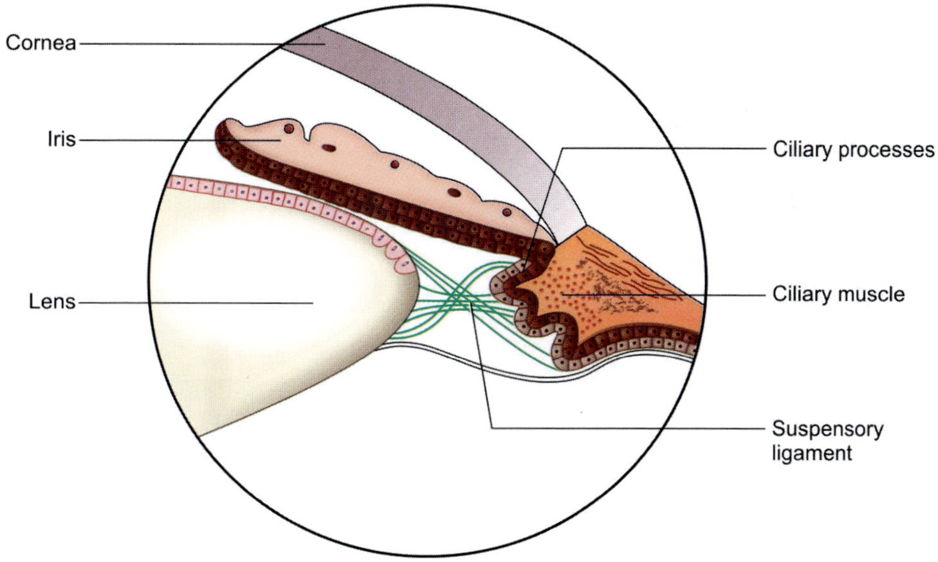

Labels: Cornea, Ciliary muscle, Ciliary processes

FIGURE

Labels: Cornea, Iris, Lens, Ciliary processes, Ciliary muscle, Suspensory ligament

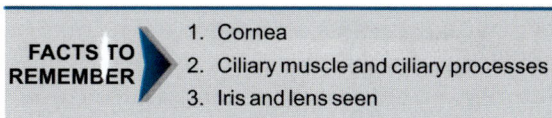

FACTS TO REMEMBER
1. Cornea
2. Ciliary muscle and ciliary processes
3. Iris and lens seen

Fig. 19.8: *Corneoscleral junction. Stain: Haematoxylin-eosin, 100X*

4. *Bruch's membrane:* It a thin glassy layer, which is made up of elastic fibres. It also acts as the basement membrane for the pigment cells of the retina.

CILIARY BODY

It comprises a *ciliary ring*, the *ciliary muscles* which are made up of radial and circular fibres, and vascular *ciliary processes* which secrete the aqueous humor.

Iris

Iris is the anterior continuation of the ciliary body. The iris has an opening in its centre called the *pupil*. Between the iris and the cornea is the *anterior chamber* and between the iris and the lens is the *posterior chamber*. Both chambers are filled with **aqueous humor**.

Anteriorly the iris is lined by the mesothelial layer which is a continuation of the lining of the posterior surface of cornea. Posteriorly the iris is lined by two layers of cells which are the forward continuations of the two original layers of the retina. The stroma of the iris consists of fine connective tissue containing blood vessels, nerves, *sphincter and dilator pupillae muscles* as well as **chromatophores**. The number and distribution of chromatophores gives the appropriate colour to the iris.

INNER COAT—RETINA

Retina is the innermost of the three layers of the eyeball. In the retina ten parallel layers can be distinguished. Starting from the outer layers these are:
1. The pigment epithelium
2. Layer of rods and cones
3. Outer limiting membrane
4. Outer nuclear layer
5. Outer plexiform layer
6. Inner nuclear layer
7. Inner plexiform layer
8. Layer of ganglion cells
9. Layers of optic nerve fibres
10. Inner limiting membrane

1. *Pigment cell layer:* In this layer the cells have round nuclei. The apical cytoplasm is occupied by melanin granules.
2. *Layer of rods and cones:* This layer consists of dendritic cytoplasmic processes of the photoreceptors, i.e. rods and cones. Each rod or cone consists of an external or peripheral process, middle parts containing the nuclei forming the outer nuclear layer.

   The internal or central processes or axons synapse with dendrites of bipolar cells and form outer plexiform layer. The peripheral processes of rods are cylindrical or rod shaped and are responsible for night vision. The peripheral processes of cones are conical in shape and are meant for **aquity, brightness of vision and for colour vision**. The *macula lutea* and *fovea centralis* contain only the **cones**.
3. *Outer limiting membrane:* It is made up of processes of neuroglial cells called *Müller's cells*.

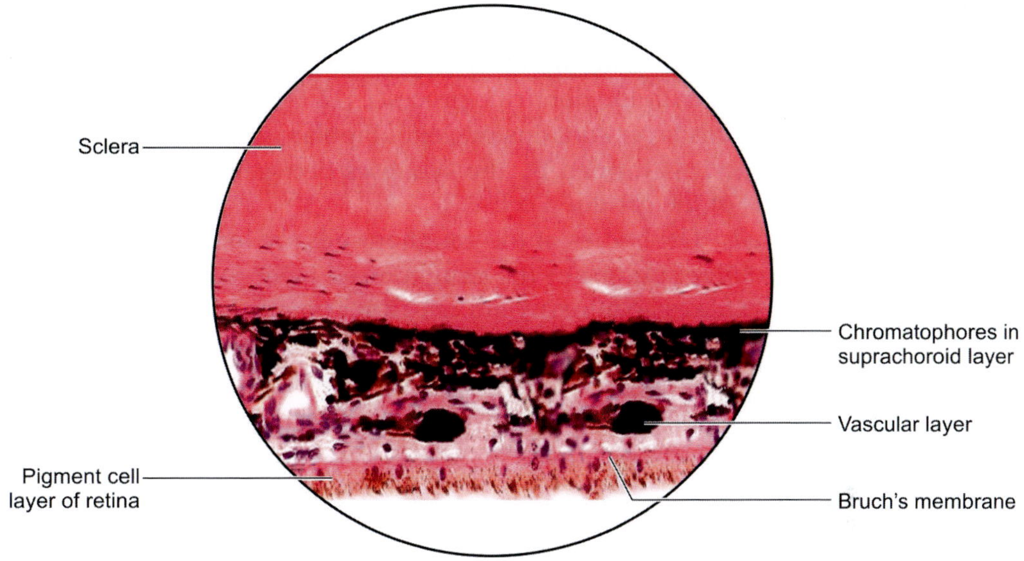

Organs of Special Senses

PHOTOMICROGRAPH

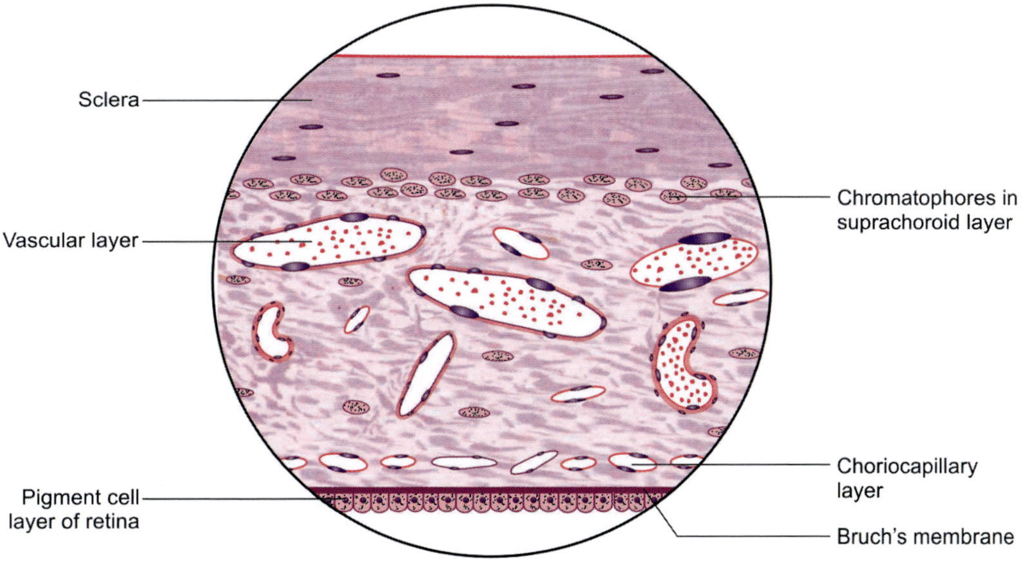

- Sclera
- Chromatophores in suprachoroid layer
- Vascular layer
- Pigment cell layer of retina
- Bruch's membrane

FIGURE

- Sclera
- Chromatophores in suprachoroid layer
- Vascular layer
- Choriocapillary layer
- Pigment cell layer of retina
- Bruch's membrane

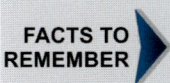

FACTS TO REMEMBER
1. Chromatophores in suprachoroidal layer
2. Blood vessels of choroid
3. Bruch's membrane

Fig. 19.9: *Sclera and choroid. Stain: Haematoxylin-eosin, 100X*

4. *Outer nuclear layer:* The nuclei of rods and cones are present in this layer.
5. *Outer plexiform layer:* It is made up of synapses between the central processes of rods and cones along with the dendritic processes of the bipolar cells.
6. *Inner nuclear layer:* This layer contains nuclei of bipolar cells and Müller's cells.
7. *Inner plexiform layer:* It is formed by the synapses between the axons of bipolar cells and dendrites of the ganglion cells.
8. *Layer of ganglion cells:* The bodies of the ganglion cells are located in this layer.
9. *Layer of optic nerve fibres:* Axons of the ganglion cell layer form the layer of optic nerve fibres. These fibres acquire myelin only after piercing the sclera.
10. *Inner limiting membrane:* It is a thin homogeneous membrane formed by the termination of inner fibres of Müller's cells. It separates the rest of the layers of retina from the vitreous body (Fig. 19.10).

LENS

The lens is biconvex with anterior and posterior poles and an equator. Outermost is the lens capsule. Anteriorly the lens is lined by the *anterior epithelium* which is cuboidal in type. The rest of the lens is made up of *lens fibres* which are transparent (Fig. 19.6).

Functional Aspect

- Eyes are extremely important sense organs. These are very sensitive as well. The cranial nerves involved with eyes are II, III, IV, V_1, V_2, VI and sympathetic fibres. These are protected from all sides. Lacrimal fluid protects, moisten and lubricates. the surface of the eye. Aqueous humor nourishes cornea and lens. Cornea and lens are avascular to maintain transparency.
- Most of the retina is supplied by an "end artery"—the central artery of retina.
- The retina comprises three types of neurons—nuclei of rods and cones, bipolar cells and ganglion cells. The axons of ganglion cells form the optic nerve. The pigmented layer absorbs light rays preventing them from reflecting back through the retina. Cones function under bright light. These are concentrated in the fovea centralis or yellow spot. So this region produces colour differentiation (red, blue or green) and responsible for brightness and visual acuity. Rods function under dim light.

Applied Aspect

- *Corneal ulcer:* Breach in the epithelium of cornea causes *ulcer*. Corneal ulcer, if deep, heals leaving an opacity.
- Sympathetic stimulation causes **dilation** of the pupil.
- *Choroiditis:* Inflammation of choroid or vascular coat.
- *Retinal detachment:* Detachment of the inner nine layers from the outermost layer of retina. It is an inter-retinal detachment.
- *Cataract:* Lens may become opaque due to ageing process or diabetes. It needs to be replaced.

LACRIMAL GLAND

Lacrimal gland is a serous gland situated chiefly in the lacrimal fossa on the anterolateral part of the roof of the bony orbit and partly in the upper eyelid. It secretes lacrimal

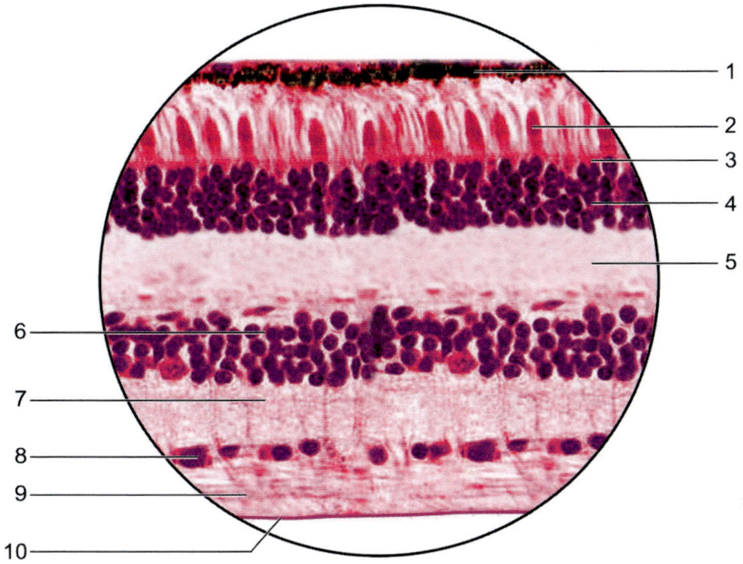

Organs of Special Senses

PHOTOMICROGRAPH

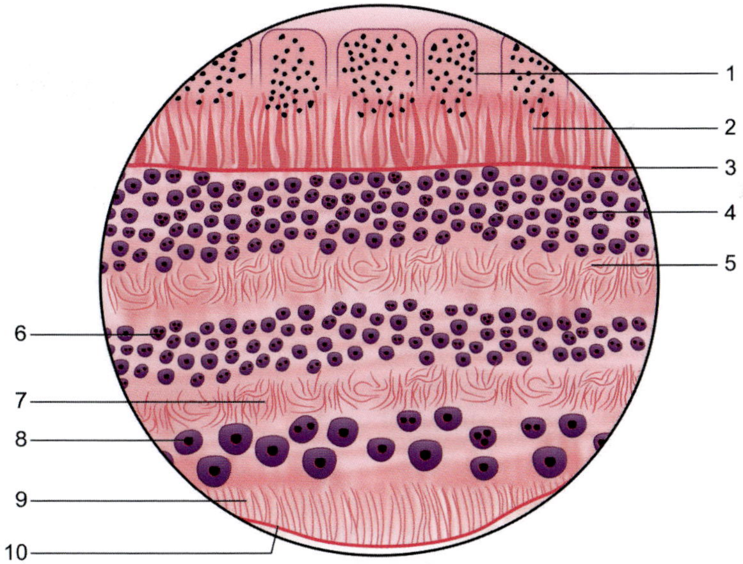

FIGURE

1. Pigment cell layer	6. Inner nuclear layer
2. Layer of rods and cones	7. Inner plexiform layer
3. Outer limiting membrane	8. Ganglion cell layer
4. Outer nuclear layer	9. Optic nerve fibres
5. Outer plexiform layer	10. Inner limiting membrane

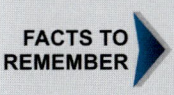

FACTS TO REMEMBER
1. Pigment cell layer
2. Six more layers of retina
3. Optic nerve fibres and two membranes

Fig. 19.10: *Structure of retina. Stain: Haematoxylin-eosin, 400X*

fluid for friction free movements of eyelids. When lacrimal fluid is produced in excess, it is called tears.

STRUCTURE OF EYELID

Each lid is made up of the following layers from without inwards:
1. The *skin* is thin, loose and easily distensible by oedema fluid or blood.
2. The *superficial fascia* is without any fat. It contains the palpebral part of the orbicularis oculi muscle.
3. The *palpebral fascia* of the two lids forms the orbital septum. Its thickenings form tarsal plates or *tarsi* in the lids and the *palpebral ligaments* at the angles. Tarsi are thin plates of condensed fibrous tissue located near the lid margins. They give stiffness to the lids.
4. The *conjunctiva* lines the posterior surface of the tarsus.

Apart from the usual glands of the skin and mucous glands in the conjunctiva, the larger glands found in the lids are:
a. Large sebaceous glands also called *Zeis's glands* at the lid margin associated with cilia.
b. Modified sweat glands or *Moll's glands* at the lid margin closely associated with Zeis's glands and cilia.
c. *Tarsal glands* or meibomian glands are embedded in the posterior surface of the tarsi; their ducts open in a row behind the cilia.

INTERNAL EAR

The internal ear is called labyrinth because of its complex structure. It is composed of a series of fluid-filled sacs and tubules suspended in cavities of corresponding form in the petrous part of the temporal bone.

There are two major cavities in the bony labyrinth—the vestibule which houses the saccule and the utricle of the membranous labyrinth. Anteromedial to it is the spirally coiled cochlea which contains the organ of Corti.

COCHLEA

Cochlea consists of a complex bony canal that makes two and three quarter spiral turns around a central axis formed by a conical pillar of the spongy bone called the *modiolus*. The *spiral ganglion* which receives the nerve fibres from the cochlear division of the statoacoustic (eighth cranial) nerve lies within the modiolus along the inner wall of the cochlear canal. Cell bodies in the spiral ganglion are *bipolar* afferent neurons (Fig. 19.11).

The lumen of the canal of the osseous cochlea is divided along its whole course into upper and lower sections by a *spiral lamina*. The lamina is divided into two zones, the inner zone containing bone (the osseous spiral lamina), and a fibrous outer zone (the membranous spiral lamina); the latter is also called the *basilar membrane*. At the attachment of the basilar membrane to the outer wall of cochlea, the periosteum is

Organs of Special Senses

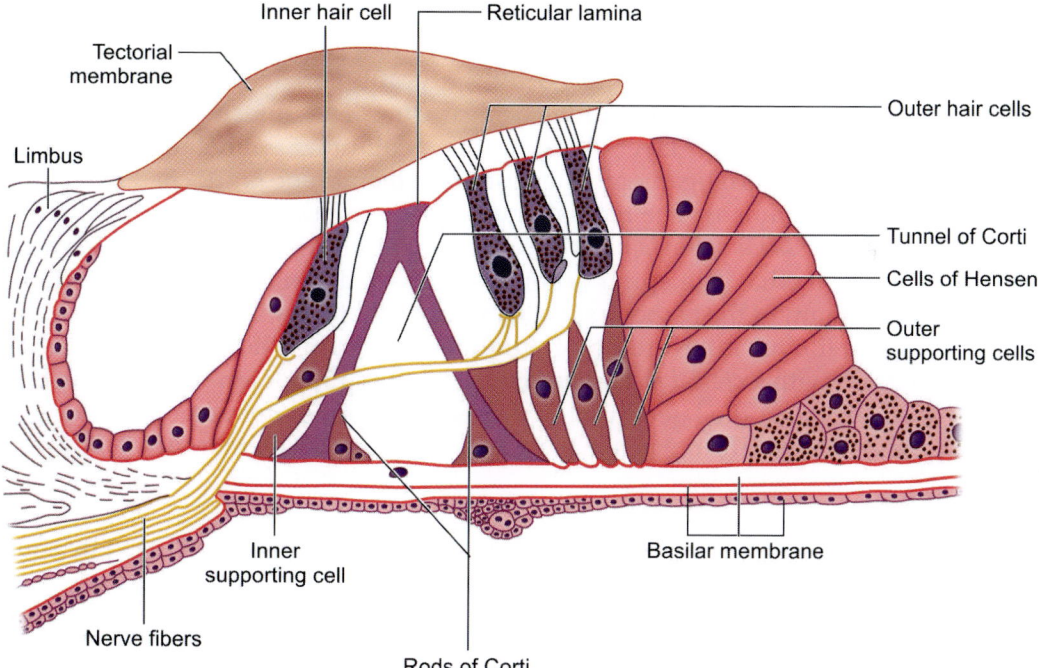

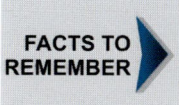

FACTS TO REMEMBER

1. Scala media shown above lies between scala vestibuli above and scala tympani below
2. Organ of Corti rests on the basilar membrane
3. Organ of Corti contains hair cells and supporting cells

Fig. 19.11: *Structure of scala media (diagrammatic). Stain: Haematoxylin-eosin, 400X*

thickened and forms a distinct structure, the *spiral ligament*. The cochlear membrane (*Reissner's membrane*), extends obliquely from spiral lamina to the outer wall of the bony cochlea.

Thus a cross-section of the bony cochlea shows three compartments; an upper cavity the *scala vestibuli*; a lower cavity, the *scala tympani*; and an intermediate cavity the *scala media*. The latter is the cochlear duct, a portion of the endolymphatic system. The scala vestibuli and scala tympani are perilymphatic spaces.

SCALA MEDIA OR COCHLEAR DUCT

The roof of the scala media is formed by the vestibular or Reissner's membrane separating the scala vestibuli from the cochlear duct. The outer wall of the cochlear duct is formed by a vascular layer of the stratified columnar epithelium, under which lies the collagenous spiral ligament. The vestibular membrane is attached to the upper end of this spiral ligament. The medial end of the membrane is continuous with the periosteum of the *osseous spiral lamina*. The osseous spiral lamina bulges into the medial end of the scala media. The spiral limbus is thickened connective tissue continued from the periosteum of the osseous spiral lamina and it forms the floor of the cochlear duct. The spiral limbus is covered by columnar epithelium which is continuous at its lateral extension with *tectorial membrane* overlying the spiral organ of Corti. The *basilar membrane* lies between the lateral end of the osseous spiral lamina and the lower end of the spiral ligament. The *organ of Corti* rests on the basilar membrane.

Organ of Corti

Organ of Corti is composed of hair cells (the receptors of stimuli produced by sound) and various supporting cells. These are tall, slender cells extending from the basilar membrane to the free surface of the organ of Corti. The supporting cells include the **inner and outer pillar cells, inner and outer phalangeal cells** and **Dieter's cells**. The *inner pillar cells* have broad bases that rest on the basilar membrane and conical cell bodies with their apices extending upwards. The cytoplasm contains a nucleus at its inner end. The most distinctive feature of the cells is the darkly staining tonofibril that courses from the cell base through the body to end in the junctional complexes of the other cells at the apex. The *outer pillar cells* are longer than the inner but cell bodies are similar to those of the inner pillar cells. *Inner phalangeal cells* are arranged in a row on the inner surface of the inner pillar cells and completely surround the inner hair cells.

HAIR CELLS

Two types of hair cells are present. The inner hair cells are arranged in a single row along the whole length of the cochlea. The outer hair cells form three rows and are lodged between the outer pillar and outer phalangeal cells. In the second coil of the cochlea, a fourth, and in the upper coil, a fifth row of outer hair cells are present. The peripheral processes of bipolar neurons end in the hair cells of the spiral organ of Corti.

Functional Aspect

- Pinna is almost vestigial in human. It is used for wearing ear rings. It also supports the spectacles. It may be used for pulling as token of punishment and used by acupuncturist also. Hairy pinna—Y chromosome.

- The sound waves traverse the external ear to vibrate the tympanic membrane. These vibrations are then channelised through the ossicles of middle ear to reach the internal ear. These vibrations stimulates the hair cells of organ of Corti. Organ of Corti converts the vibrations into nerve impulses which pass along the dendrites of spiral ganglion cells. Their axons form the cochlear nerve which traverses the medulla, pons, midbrain, medial geniculate body and terminate in part of the temporal lobe.
- The internal ear also controls the equilibrium of the person through *cristae of semicircular canals* and *maculae* of utricle and saccule. These impulses traverse via the vestibular division of VIII nerve to reach the cerebellum.

Applied Aspect

- **Otitis externa:** Inflammation of the pinna or of the external auditory meatus.
- **Otitis media:** Inflammation of the middle ear. Infection may spread and cause meningitis, labyrinthitis, mastoiditis, pharyngitis, etc.

MULTIPLE CHOICE QUESTIONS

1. Taste buds are present in the following *except*:
   a. Epiglottis
   b. Filiform papillae
   c. Fungiform papillae
   d. Circumvallate papillae

2. Which stratified squamous non-keratinised epithelium is devoid of any papillae?
   a. Oesophagus
   b. Oral cavity
   c. Cornea
   d. Vagina

3. Which of the following contain organ of Corti?
   a. Scala vestibuli   b. Scala tympani
   c. Scala media   d. Utricle

4. Axons of which of the following cell layers form the optic nerve:
   a. Bipolar cell layer
   b. Outer nuclear layer
   c. Ganglion cell layer
   d. None of the above

5. Sclera comprises the following:
   a. Reticular   b. Collagen
   c. Elastic   d. All of the above

ANSWERS

1. b   2. c   3. c   4. c
5. d

Histological Techniques
Staining: Haematoxylin-Eosin

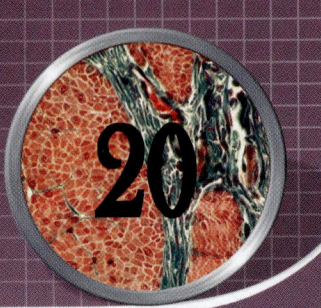

"Repentant tears wash out the stain of guilt"

FIXATION

Preservation of tissues as close as possible to living state in the most important step through the process of histology.

PURPOSE OF FIXATION
- Once the tissue is removed from the body it will go through a process of self destruction called autolysis. Fixation stops autolysis.
- It starts soon after the cell death
- Cells contain digestive enzymes in lysosomes and when cells die these enzymes are released which cause the breakdown of protein and eventual liquefaction of the cell.
- Tissues rich in enzymes, such as liver, brain and kidney are rapidly and severely autolysed
- A bacterial attack will occur when tissues are left without any preservation and this process is called putrefaction.

Fixation is the most essential part in histology to arrest autolysis and putrefaction. The objectives of fixation are:
- To preserve tissue constituents and cells as possible to living condition as possible.
- To stabilise the cellular and tissue constituents so that they withstand subsequent processing of tissues.
- To arrest autolysis and bacterial decomposition.

AN IDEAL FIXATIVE
- Does not swell and shrinks the tissue
- Does not dissolve out any tissue components
- Adequately and properly penetrates
- Kills micro-organisms
- Compatible with subsequent staining methods
- Retains the tissue components in as close a life like state as possible throughout the subsequent stages of tissue processing.

TYPES OF FIXATION

There are main two types of fixation:
1. *Physical method:*
   - Heat—fixing of smears for bacteriology. After the introduction of microwave fixation this method is familiar in the histology laboratories.
   - Desiccation—rarely used in histology.
2. *Chemical method:* Most commonly used in histology and considered as the primary method of fixation.
   - Additive—chemically bind or link to the tissue, e.g. formalin, picric acid.
   - Non-additive act on the tissue without chemically binding or linking with the tissue, e.g. acetone, alcohol.

In addition, chemical reagents may be classified as coagulant and non-coagulant.
- Coagulant—allow the solutions easily to penetrate into the interior of the tissue, e.g. ethanol, methanol, picric acid, acetone, etc.
- Non-coagulant act by forming a gel like barrier that makes solution more difficult to penetrate into the interior of the tissue, e.g. formaldehyde, glutaraldehyde, osmium tetroxide.

Some chemical fixatives
- Aldehydes—formaldehyde, glutaraldehyde
- Oxidising agents—potassium dichromate, osmium tetroxide
- Protein denaturing agents—ethanol, methanol
- Unknown mechanism—mercuric oxide, picric acid

FACTORS AFFECTING THE QUALITY OF FIXATION

- Buffers, pH
- Duration of fixation
- Size of tissue
- Temperature of fixation
- Concentration of fixative
- Osmolality of fixative
- Ionic composition
- Additives
- Additional procedures (decalcification)

COMMONLY USED FIXATIVES

Formaldehyde

Formaldehyde is the most commonly and widely employed universal fixative particularly for routine paraffin embedded section. It is used as 4% buffered formaldehyde or 10% buffered formalin. Aldehydes form cross-links between proteins, creating a gel, thus retaining cellular constituents in their in vivo conditions. Soluble proteins are fixed to structural proteins and rendered insoluble giving some mechanical strength to the entire structure which enables it to withstand subsequent processing.

Reaction with Tissue

- Cross-links with protein molecules
- React slowly and may be reversible for first 24 hours.
- Non-coagulative fixation
- Penetrates rapidly

Advantages

- Preserves tissues for a long time if the solution is buffered to neutrality
- Good general purpose fixative
- Preserves proteins and lipids
- Relatively inexpensive

Disadvantages

- Causes a little shrinkage which is produced when the tissues are subjected to paraffin embedding
- Take much more time
- Unpleasant odor
- Strong eye, skin and mucous membrane irritant
- Moderately flammable.

Glutaraldehyde

Glutaraldehyde has also been used extensively as an agent for protein —protein linkage and hence for fixation. It is, however, the most widely used fixative for standard electron microscopy.

Advantages

- Less distortion, brittleness, shrinkage, more total fixation on concentration/time frame.
- Maintained elasticity during manipulation and sectioning.

Disadvantages

- Comparatively high molecular weight of glutaraldehyde limits its ability to diffuse into thick specimen.
- Four carbon chain of glutaraldehyde may mask amine-containing epitopes, making immunostaining impossible.

Osmium Tetroxide

Mostly used in preservation of lipids, in membranes, organelles and myelin sheaths. It is known to form cross-links with proteins as reflected in the rapid increase in viscosity of a protein solution when they react together. It is now largely employed as a secondary fixative in electron microscopy.

Its main disadvantages are that it is very expensive and has toxic, irritating vapour that can cause corneal opacities.

Chromic Acid

Chromium salts form complexes with water and combine with reactive groups of adjacent protein chains to bring about a cross-linking effect similar to that of formalin. It is a strong oxidiser that is used with other ingredients.

Acetic Acid

It is never used alone but often used in combination with other fixatives that cause shrinkage such as ethanol and methanol. It penetrates the tissue thoroughly and rapidly causes lysis of red blood cell.

Picric Acid

It reacts with base groups of proteins and forms pirates. It causes extreme shrinkage of tissues and has a slow penetration rate. It is toxic and must be stored under water as it is explosive when dry.

Acetone

Acetone is used as a fixative in the acetone-methyl benzoate xylene technique. It has rapid action but causes brittleness in tissue if exposure is prolonged. It has been used as a dehydrating agent in tissue processing and is more volatile than alcohols and other dehydrants.

Alcoholic Fixatives

Mainly methanol and ethanol and rarely used alone except for cytology fixation and for fixing tissues with uric acid or urate deposition (gout). Ethanol can cause excessive hardening and shrinkage of tissues but penetrates rapidly.

DEHYDRATION

Dehydration is the removal of "water from" and is a necessary step to prepare the tissue for subsequent treatment. It is usually achieved by replacing the water in the tissue with dehydrating agent. Tissues after fixation in aqueous fixatives retain high water content which can interfere with the clearing of the tissues. Since water is immiscible with clearing agents and embedding media, it is necessary to dehydrate the tissue completely before proceeding to the next step. A series of solutions of dehydrating agents in water with gradually increasing percentage is used for this purpose.

It is necessary to transfer from one step to another very gradually in the dehydration process, otherwise shrinkage and distortion of the tissue is certain to occur. Ethyl alcohol is the most common reagent used for dehydration.

CLEARING

Clearing is an important intermediary step between dehydration and embedding. It consists of replacing the dehydrating agent with a substance that will be miscible with the embedding medium (paraffin). The term "clearing" represents the fact that the clearing agents often have the same refractive index as proteins. As a result, when the tissue is completely infiltrated with the clearing agent, render it them translucent giving crystalline appearance. This change in appearance is often used as an indication of the completeness of the clearing process.

The most common clearing agent is xylene which is reasonably cost effective. It works well for short-term clearing of small tissue blocks but long-term immersion results in tissue distortions.

Chloroform has been used in some applications but it acts slowly and may lead to sectioning difficulties. It also has a severe health hazard. It causes no undue hardness to the tissues if left in it for 10 hours or longer.

Oils (Cedarwood, clove, terpinol) are good for whole mounts but not suitable for histological purpose. It must not be used to clear the tissues scheduled for embedding in paraffin. Oils are slow in their action but they have the advantage of not hardening the tissues even after prolonged immersion.

TISSUE EMBEDDING

The ultimate stage in tissue preparation is to prepare specimens which allow the cutting of sections thin enough for microscopy. For this purpose, tissue dehydration and clearing is followed by infiltration with suitable matrix. The choice of embedding substance depends mainly on the type of histological study to be performed. Paraffin wax is the usual embedding medium for histopathological study and many other light microscopic purposes.

Tissue embedding is always done with liquid media. In the case of paraffin, tissue blocks are treated with hot liquefied paraffin which becomes solid when cooled down to room temperature. Paraffin with different hardness and melting points are available. Paraffin is the usual embedding medium. For electron microscopy and as well as under certain condition when semithin sections are to be preferred, tissue specimens are embedded in one of the available resins.

SECTIONING

After embedding and block preparation, the tissue must be cut into sections that can be placed on a slide. Microtome is used for this purpose. The microtome is nothing but more than a knife with a mechanism or advancing a paraffin block maintaining a standard distances across it. Microtomes have a mechanism for advancing the block across the knife. Usually this distance can be set, for most paraffin embedded tissues at 6–8 microns.

STAINING

Staining of the tissues is necessary to enhance contrast in the normally colourless tissue sections as most of them become almost transparent or do not retain colour to be visible under minoscope. Apart from that stain also plays an important role in identifying different tissues, their cell types and thus help in pathological diagnosis.

Staining Reactions

The principle of histological staining relies on the treatment of tissue sections with the dyes in solution which will react more or less specifically with defined cell and tissue structures.

Histological Techniques

Dye

A dye is a coloured substance containing two groups, chromophoric and auxochromic. Chromophoric group give the colouring property to the dye and auxochromic group is responsible for attaching dye to tissue structures and their solubility and dissolubility in water. The dye may actually be dissolved in the stained substance.

- A dye may be absorbed on the surface of a structure or may be precipitated within the structure.
- Most staining reactions involve a chemical union between dye and stained substance through salt linkages, hydrogen bonds or others.
- Staining with the dyes results in a predictable colour pattern based in part on the acid–base characteristics of the tissue.

Classification

- Basic stains—a stain in which the colouring agent is in the basic radical. A substance that is stained by the basic dye is considered to be basophilic, it carries acid groups which bind the basic dye through salt linkages, e.g. haematoxylin.
- Acid stain— a stain in which the colouring agent is in the acidic radical. A substance that is stained by an acid dye is referred to as acidophilic, it carries basic groups which bind the acid dye, e.g. eosin.
- Neutral stains—these are compounds of acid dye and basic dye. They are so-called as they contain base and acid—both of which being coloured, e.g. Wright's stain.

Mordant

A mordant is a metallic salt or hydroxide which fixes the dye to a substance by combining with the dye to form an insoluble compound. A lake is formed when the complex of dye and mordant are combined, which is capable of attaching itself to the tissue.

Some of the most frequently used mordant in haematoxylin and carmin dyes are aluminium, ferric and chromium salts and alums.

Accentuators

An accentuators is any chemical which facilities the staining process. Without combining chemically in any way with the dyes or taking part in the formation of lake, it act as catalyst increasing the selectivity or stainability of certain dyes. For example, the use of phenol accentuation in carbol fuscin.

Vital Staining

It is the staining of living tissue without harming or killing the cells. Examples include the use of trypan blue and vital red. Intravital staining involves the injection of a stain into an organism. Some of the living cells take up the dye. Supravital staining involves the removal of living tissue from a multicellular organism and its subsequent staining.

Progressive Staining

Stain applied to the tissue is in strict and specific sequence and for specific times.

The stain is not washed out or decolourised because there is no overstaining of tissue.

Regressive Staining

Tissue is first overstained and then the excess stain is removed by the process of differentiation.

Direct Staining

Application of simple dye to stain the tissues perfectly in varying shades of colours.

Indirect Staining

Many stains including haematoxylin require an additional intermediate substance known as mordant to facilitate a particular staining method. In this type of staining also the accentuator is used to improve either the selectivity or the intensity of stain.

Metachromatic Staining

There are certain basic dyes belonging to aniline group that will differentiate particular tissue element by staining them a different colour to that of the basic colour of the dye. This phenomenon is known a metachromasia. Metachromatic stains help to study the specific tissue components of connective tissue, e.g. toluidine blue and safranin.

Some Commonly Used Stains

Haematoxylin and eosin: Most widely used and general stain is haematoxylin. Haematoxylin stain is a natural dye extracted by boiling the wood of log tree Haematoxylin campechianum and purified through recrystallisation. Dye used for the staining is the oxidised form of haematoxylin called haematin. It is one of the best known nuclear stains. It can also be used to stain myelin sheath, mitotic stages, muscle fibres, etc.

Eosin is an acid aniline dye which stains the more basic proteins within cells (cytoplasm) and in extracellular spaces (collagen) pink to red.

In summary haematoxylin and eosin stain nuclei blue and cytoplasm pink to red.

Masson trichrome stain: It is a good staining procedure involving iron haematoxylin, acid fuscin and light green. It is generally used for distinguishing cellular from extracellular components (Fig. 20.1).

Nuclei stains black or brown where as mucus and ground substances take on varying shades of green. Cytoplasm and collagen fibres stain red and an intense green respectively.

- *Verhoeff's haematoxylin:* It is another variant of the versatile haematoxylin stains. It stains elastic fibres black in addition to nuclei. A good stain for connective tissue, especially elastin.
- *Iron haemotoxylin:* Staining with iron haemotoxylin solution produces selective nuclei staining that is stable and requires no additional differentiation. This type of stain contains iron salts which are used both as mordant and as oxidising agent.

Commonly used iron haematoxylins are:
- Weigert's haematoxylin
- Heidenhain's haematoxylin

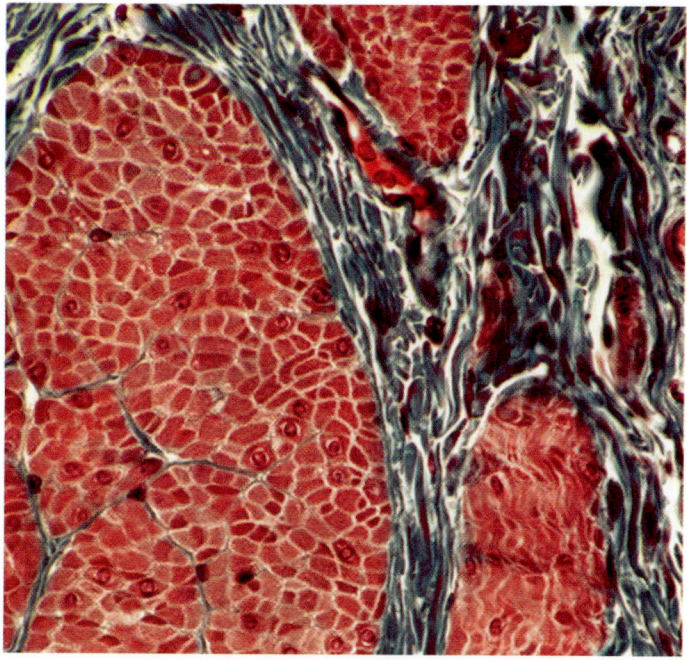

Fig. 20.1: *Tissue stained by Masson trichrome stain*

- Loyez haematoxylin
- Verhoeff's haematoxylin.

Wright's Stain

It is a neutral stain produced by the interaction of an acidic dye and a basic dye, producing a large salt molecule with a coloured dye in both of its parts. General stains for blood and bone marrow smears.

According to the number of acid and basic groups present, cell components take up the dyes from the mixture in various proportions. Romanovsky type mixtures including Wright's and Giemsa stains are the best known of these neutral stains. They are formed by the interaction of methylene blue and eosin.

Periodic acid Schiff (PAS): This is versatile stain and has been used to stain many structures including glycogen, mucin, mucoprotein, glycoprotein. Adjacent hydroxyl groups (1, 2 glycols) or amino and hydroxyl groups are oxidised to aldehyde groups with periodic acid. The aldehydes are then detected by the Schiff reagent, which stains them reddish purple (Fig. 20.2). Other tissue components stain according to counter stain used.

Sudan stains: These are used to stain lipids. The Sudan dyes, e.g. Sudan IV, dissolve in droplet containing triglycerides and colour them intensely. For staining with sudan dyes, care must be taken during tissue preparation to retain the lipid which is often washed out by standard tissue preparation procedures.

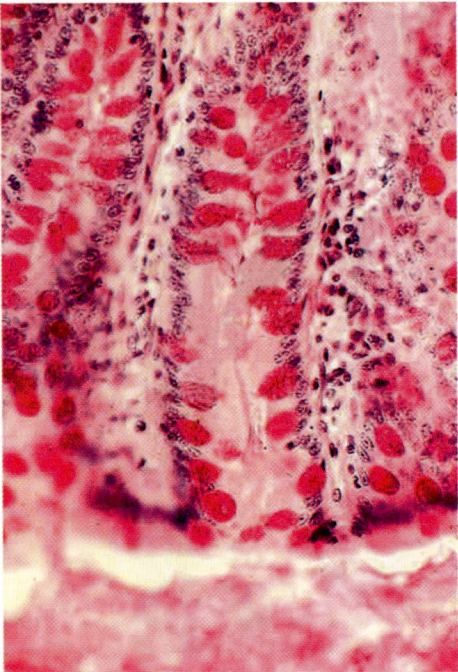

Fig. 20.2: *Tissue stained by PAS stain*

STAINING: HAEMATOXYLIN-EOSIN

REQUIREMENTS FOR STAINING

Ehrlich's haematoxylin stain tested for five to seven minutes; water soluble eosin stain tested for half to one minute, Coplin jars containing xylol, absolute alcohol, 90 per cent alcohol, 70 per cent alcohol, 1 per cent acid alcohol, Canada balsam, slide rack, burner, coverslip, tap water, and blotting paper.

Procedure

Before proceeding with staining, the side of the tissue on the slide should be determined. The steps are as follows.

1. *Removal of Paraffin*
  i. Warm the slide on the reverse side of the tissue on a burner in order to melt the paraffin completely. The time varies according to the weather. Care should be taken not to burn the tissue.
  ii. Dip the slide in xylol for 2–3 minutes to remove the paraffin.

2. *Hydration of Tissue*

Dip the slide in descending series of alcohol, i.e. absolute alcohol, 90 per cent alcohol, 70 per cent alcohol and water for one minute each respectively. This procedure hydrates the tissue so that it is ready for staining with haematoxylin and eosin which are water soluble stains.

3. Staining of the Slide

  i. **_Haematoxylin stain:_** Place the slide on the slide-rack and cover the tissue with drops of haematoxylin stain for five to seven minutes. It stains the nucleus as well as the cytoplasm of the tissue.

  Bluing: The haematoxylin stained slide is placed in a beaker of running tap water (alkaline pH) for ten to fifteen minutes. During this time the nucleus retains the stain whereas the stain is washed off from the cytoplasm. The differentiation of the cells is checked under low power of the microscope. If the tissue is seen to be overstained with haematoxylin, the slide is dipped in 1 per cent acid alcohol and then in water to remove the excess of stain.

  ii. **_Eosin stain:_** Stain the tissue with a few drops of water soluble eosin solution for half to one minute and wash the slide with water. If the tissue gets overstained, the slide should be washed with running water till excess of stain is removed.

4. Dehydration of Tissue

The slide is passed through the ascending grades of alcohol, i.e. 70 per cent, 90 per cent and absolute alcohol for one minute each. Finally it is dipped in xylol (clearing agent) to get rid of the alcohol. The section is blotted for mounting.

5. Mounting the Slide

One drop of Canada balsam is put on the slide. A clean cover slip is gradually lowered on it so that air bubbles do not enter between the tissue and the coverslip.

Precautions

1. The slide should never be allowed to get dry.
2. If the tissue is overstained with haematoxylin, it should be treated with 1 per cent acid alcohol and then water.
3. In case of overstaining of tissue with eosin, the slide should be washed with water to remove excess of stain.
4. Cover slip should be gradually lowered on the slide in order to prevent entry of air bubbles.
5. During the process of staining care should be taken to avoid the tissue being washed off from the slide.
6. The slide should be examined under the microscope for proper differentiation.

Index

Acid hydrolases 4
Adipose cells 25
Adipose tissue 32
Alveoli 128
Anal canal 164
Appendages of skin 114
Areolar tissue 32
Arrector pili muscle 116
Arteries 82
Arterioles 84
Astrocytes 66
Atria, alveolar ducts and alveolar sacs 128

Barr body 4
Basement membrane 8
Blood vessels 82
Bone 44
    cells of 44
    functions 44
Bronchial tubes 126

Capillaries 86
Cardiac muscle 58
Cartilage 39
    cells 39
    fibres 40
    ground substance 40
Cell 1, 6
Cell membrane 1
Cells of connective tissue
    fixed cells 25
    wandering cells 26
Centrioles 4
Cerebellum 78
Cerebrum 74
Cervix 212
Chromatin 5
Chromosomes 5
Cilia 4
Classification of cartilage 40
Clearing 263

Collagen fibres 28
Colon 160
Columnar epithelium 9
Compound epithelium 8, 16
Connective tissue 25
Corneoscleral junction 246, 248
Cuboidal epithelium 9
Cytoplasm 1
    cytoplasmic inclusions 4
    cytoplasmic organelles 1
Cytoskeleton 4

Dehydration 263
Dense connective tissue 36
Dermis 114
Desmosome 8
Digestive system 135
Ductus deferens 191
Duodenum 154

Elastic arteries 82
Elastic cartilage 40
Elastic fibres 30
Endocrine glands 225
Endoplasmic reticulum 1
    rough surface 1
    smooth surface 2
Ependymal cells 68
Epidermis 113
Epididymis 191
Epithelial tissue 6
Epithelium 6, 9
    characters 8
    classification 8
    functions 6
    special features 6
Eyeball 246

Fallopian tube 204
Female reproductive system 201
Female urethra 184
Fibres 28

Fibrocartilage 42
Fibroblasts 25
Fixation 260
    commonly used 261
    purpose of 260
    types of 261
Flagellum 4
Fundus and body of stomach 142

Gall bladder 170
Ganglia 74
Gap junction 8
Gastro-oesophageal junction 142
General plan of gastrointestinal tract 137
Glands 105
Golgi apparatus 2
Ground substance 30

Haematoxylin-eosin 268
Hair follicles 114
Histiocytes 26
Histological techniques 260
Histology 6
Hyaline cartilage 40
Hypophysis cerebri 225
    blood supply of 226

Ileum 156
Inner coat-retina 252
Integumentary system 113
Internal ear 256
    cochlea 256
    organ of Corti 258
Intrapulmonary bronchus 126

Jejunum 156
Junctional complexes 6

Kidney 177
    circulation of blood 177
    structure of 178

Lacrimal gland 256
Large intestine 158
    parts of 160
Larynx 124
Lens 254
Liver 167
    circulation of blood 170
Loose connective tissue 32

Lymph node 92
Lymphatic system 92
Lysosomes 4

Macrophages/histiocytes 26
Male reproductive system 187
Male urethra 198
Mammary glands 214
    lactating phase 214
    resting phase 214
Mast cells 28
Mesenchymal cells 26
Microfilaments 4
Microglia 68
Microscopic structure 47
    compact bone 47
    spongy bone 47
Microtubules 4
Middle vascular coat: choroid, ciliary body and iris 248
Mitochondria 2
Mucous gland 108
Muscular arteries 84
Muscular tissue 53
Myxomatous tissue 32

Nasopharynx 124
Nerve fibres 69
Nerve trunk 69
Nervous tissue 62
Neuroglia 64
Neuron 62
    cell processes 64
    classification 64
Nose 123
Nuclear membrane 4
Nuclear sap 5
Nucleolus 5
Nucleus 4

Oesophagus 140
Olfactory epithelium 239
Oligodendrocytes 66
Organs of special senses 239
Ossification of bones 47
    intracartilaginous 50
    intramembranous 47
Ovary 201, 236
    corpus luteum 202

Index

Palatine tonsil 101
Pancreas 172, 236
Parathyroid gland 232
Parotid gland 106
Pars distalis 225
Pars intermedia 226
Pars nervosa 226
Parts of the nervous system 72
Parts of the small intestine 154
Penis 196
Pigment cells 26
Pineal gland 236
Placenta 219
Plasma cells 28
Polyribosomes 4
Prostate gland 194
Pseudostratified epithelium 8, 16
Pyloric part 144

Rectum 164
Respiratory bronchiole 128
Respiratory part 128
Respiratory system 123
Reticular fibres 30
Reticular tissue 32
Ribosomes 4

Salivary glands 106
Satellite or capsular cells 68
Schwann cells 68
Sebaceous gland 116
Sectioning 264
Seminal vesicle 196
Simple epithelium 8, 9
Sinusoids 88
Skeletal muscle 53
   structure of 53
Small intestine 150
   general plan 150
Smooth muscle 56
Some commonly used stains 266
Spinal cord 72
Spleen 94
   splenic circulation 96

Squamous epithelium 9
Staining 264
Stomach 142
Stratified columnar epithelium 18
Stratified squamous keratinised epithelium 18
Stratified squamous non-keratinised epithelium 18
Structure of eyelid 256
Sublingual gland 108
Submandibular gland 106
Suprarenal gland 234

Taste buds 240, 242
Teeth 136
Terminal bronchiole 126
Testis 187, 236
Thymus 98
Thyroid gland 230
Tissue embedding 264
Tongue 240
   papillae 240
Trachea 124
Transitional epithelium 18
Types of 118
   thick skin 118
   thin skin 118

Umbilical cord 220
Unit membrane 1
Ureter 182
Urinary bladder 184
Urinary system 177
Uterus 206
   menstrual phase 208
   myometrium 208
   progestational phase 208
   proliferative phase 206

Vagina 212
Veins 88
Vermiform appendix 160

White blood cells 28

Zonula adherens 8
Zonula occludens 6, 8

Reader's Notes

Reader's Notes

Reader's Notes